REFERENCE EDITION

ENDOCRINE BOARD REVIEW

Serge A. Jabbour, MD, Program Chair
Professor of Medicine
Director, Division of Endocrinology,
Diabetes & Metabolic Diseases
Sidney Kimmel Medical College
Thomas Jefferson University

Andrea D. Coviello, MD
Associate Professor of Medicine
Division of Endocrinology,
Metabolism, and Nutrition
Duke University School of Medicine

Natalie Cusano, MD, MS
Associate Professor of Medicine
Zucker School of Medicine
at Hofstra/Northwell
Director of the Bone
Metabolism Program
Division of Endocrinology
at Lenox Hill Hospital

Tobias Else, MD
Associate Professor
Division of Metabolism,
Endocrinology, and Diabetes
University of Michigan

Frances J. Hayes, MB BCh, BAO
Clinical Director
Endocrine Division
Massachusetts General Hospital

Jacqueline Jonklaas, MD, PhD, MPH
Professor
Division of Endocrinology
Georgetown University Medical Center

Laurence Katznelson, MD
Professor of Neurosurgery
and Medicine
Division of Endocrinology
Stanford University

Michelle F. Magee, MD
Director
MedStar Diabetes, Research
and Innovation Institutes
Professor of Medicine
Georgetown University
School of Medicine

Kathryn A. Martin, MD
Assistant Professor of Medicine
Harvard Medical School
Practicing Clinician
Massachusetts General Hospital
Senior Physician Editor,
Endocrinology and Diabetes
UpToDate

Abbie L. Young, MS, CGC, ELS(D)
Medical Editor

Endocrine Society
2055 L Street NW, Suite 600, Washington, DC 20036
1-888-ENDOCRINE • www.endocrine.org

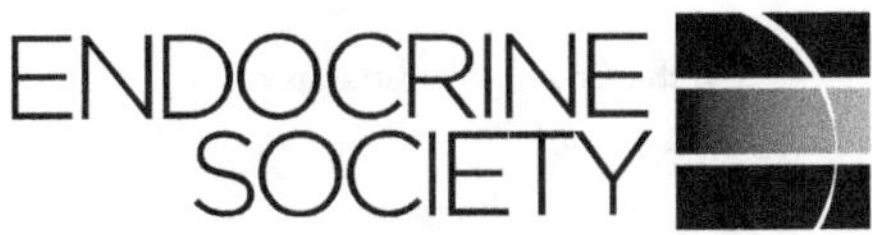

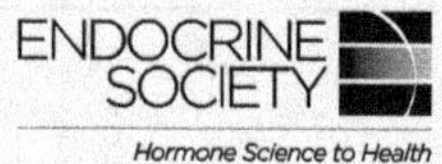

The Endocrine Society is the world's largest, oldest, and most active organization working to advance the clinical practice of endocrinology and hormone research. Founded in 1916, the Society now has more than 18,000 global members across a range of disciplines. The Society has earned an international reputation for excellence in the quality of its peer-reviewed journals, educational resources, meetings, and programs that improve public health through the practice and science of endocrinology.

Visit us at:
education.endocrine.org
endocrine.org

Other Publications:
endocrine.org/publications

The statements and opinions expressed in this publication are those of the individual authors and do not necessarily reflect the views of the Endocrine Society. The Endocrine Society is not responsible or liable in any way for the currency of the information, for any errors, omissions, or inaccuracies, or for any consequences arising therefrom. With respect to any drugs mentioned, the reader is advised to refer to the appropriate medical literature and the product information currently provided by the manufacturer to verify appropriate dosage, method and duration of administration, and other relevant information. In all instances, it is the responsibility of the treating physician or other health care professional, relying on independent experience and expertise, as well as knowledge of the patient, to determine the best treatment for the patient.

PERMISSIONS: For permission to reuse material, please visit the Copyright Clearance Center (CCC) at www.copyright.com or call 978-750-8400. CCC is a non-for-profit organization that provides licenses and registration for a variety of uses.

Copyright © 2020 by the Endocrine Society, 2055 L Street NW, Suite 600, Washington, DC 20036. All rights reserved. No part of this publication may be reproduced, stored in a retrieval system, posted on the Internet, or transmitted in any form, by any means, electronic, mechanical, photocopying, recording, or otherwise, without written permission of the publisher.

TRANSLATIONS AND LICENSING: Rights to translate and reproduce Endocrine Society publications internationally are extended through a licensing agreement on full or partial editions. To request rights for a local edition, please visit: https://www.endocrine.org/publications/ or licensing@endocrine.org.

ISBN: 978-1-879225-69-5
Library of Congress Control Number: 2020945022

On the Cover: © Shutterstock. High Quality Digital Media Asset. (By tsyhun).

OVERVIEW

Endocrine Board Review (EBR) 12th Edition (2020) is a board examination preparation book designed for endocrine fellows who have completed or are nearing completion of their fellowship and are preparing to sit for the board certification exam, and for practicing endocrinologists in search of a comprehensive self-assessment of endocrinology, either to prepare for recertification or to update their practice. EBR consists of approximately 240 case-based, American Board of Internal Medicine (ABIM) style, multiple-choice questions. Each section follows the ABIM Endocrinology, Diabetes, and Metabolism Certification Examination blueprint, covering the breadth and depth of the certification and recertification examinations. Each case is discussed in detail with detailed answer explanations and references provided.

The EBR 12th Edition (2020) reference book is intended primarily for consultation and self-assessment of knowledge relating to endocrinology. As a reference book, educational credits are not available upon completion of the multiple-choice questions included. For information on educational products that include educational credit, please visit endocrine.org/store.

LEARNING OBJECTIVES

Upon completion of this educational activity, learners will be able to demonstrate enhanced medical knowledge and clinical skills across all major areas of endocrinology; apply knowledge and skills in diagnosing, managing, and treating a wide spectrum of endocrine disorders; and successfully complete the board examination for certification or recertification in the subspecialty of endocrinology, diabetes, and metabolism.

TARGET AUDIENCE

This activity should be of substantial interest to endocrinologists, internists, and endocrine fellows preparing for the board examination or recertification; or endocrinologists and other health care practitioners seeking a review in endocrinology.

STATEMENT OF INDEPENDENCE

The Endocrine Society has a policy of ensuring that the content and quality of this educational activity are balanced, independent, objective, and scientifically rigorous. The scientific content of this activity was developed under the supervision of the Endocrine Society's EBR faculty. There are no commercial supporters of this activity and no commercial entities have had an influence over the planning of this activity.

DISCLOSURE POLICY

The faculty, committee members, and staff who are in position to control the content of this activity are required to disclose to the Endocrine Society and to learners and relevant financial relationship(s) of the individual or spouse/partner that have occurred within the last 12 months with any commercial interest(s) whose products or services are related to the content. Financial relationships are defined by remuneration in any amount from the commercial interest(s) in the form of grants; research support; consulting fees; salary; ownership interest (eg, stocks, stock options, or ownership interest excluding diversified mutual funds); honoraria or other payments for participation in speakers' bureaus, advisory boards, or boards of directors; or other financial benefits. The intent of this disclosure is not to prevent planners with relevant financial relationships from planning or delivery of content, but rather to provide learners with information that allows them to make their own judgments of whether these financial relationships may have influenced the educational activity with regard to exposition or conclusion.

The Endocrine Society has reviewed all disclosures and resolved or managed all identified conflicts of interest, as applicable.

The faculty reported the following relevant financial relationship(s) during the content development process for this activity:

Natalie Cusano, MD, MS, has served as a consultant to Shire/Takeda and Radius Pharmaceuticals and has served as a speaker for Shire/Takeda and Alexion.

Tobias Else, MD, has served as an advisory board member to Corcept Therapeutics and HRA Pharma, and his institution has received research support from Corcept Therapeutics, Merck and Strongbridge Biopharma.

Serge A. Jabbour, MD, has served as a consultant to AstraZeneca and Janssen, and his institution has received research support from the National Institutes of Health.

Laurence Katznelson, MD, has served as a consultant and principal investigator to Chiasma and Camarus, and he has served as an advisory board member to Novo Nordisk.

Michelle F. Magee, MD, receives research support from the NIH Diabetes Prevention Program Observational Study and the NIH Grade Study as an investigator on behalf of MedStar Health Research Institute. She serves as a speaker for the American Diabetes Association, the American College of Cardiology, and the Endocrine Society.

Kathryn A. Martin, MD, has served as a physician editor for UpToDate.

The following faculty reported no relevant financial relationships: Andrea D. Coviello, MD; Frances J. Hayes, MB BCh, BAO; and Jacqueline Jonklaas, MD, PhD, MPH

The medical editor for this activity reported no relevant financial relationships: Abbie L. Young, MS, CGC, ELS(D)

Endocrine Society staff associated with the development of content for this activity reported no relevant financial relationships.

DISCLAIMERS

The information presented in this activity represents the opinion of the faculty and is not necessarily the official position of the Endocrine Society.

Use of professional judgment:

The educational content in this activity relates to basic principles of diagnosis and therapy and does not substitute for individual patient assessment based on the health care provider's examination of the patient and consideration of laboratory data and other factors unique to the patient. Standards in medicine change as new data become available.

Drugs and dosages:

When prescribing medications, the physician is advised to check the product information sheet accompanying each drug to verify conditions of use and to identify any changes in drug dosage schedule or contraindications.

POLICY ON UNLABELED/OFF-LABEL USE

The Endocrine Society has determined that disclosure of unlabeled/off-label or investigational use of commercial product(s) is informative for audiences and therefore requires this information to be disclosed to the learners at the beginning of the presentation. Uses of specific therapeutic agents, devices, and other products discussed in this educational activity may not be the same as those indicated in product labeling approved by the Food and Drug Administration (FDA). The Endocrine Society requires that any discussions of such "off-label" use be based on scientific research that conforms to generally accepted standards of experimental design, data collection, and data analysis. Before recommending or prescribing any therapeutic agent or device, learners should review the complete prescribing information, including indications, contraindications, warnings, precautions, and adverse events.

ACKNOWLEDGMENT OF COMMERCIAL SUPPORT

The activity is not supported by educational grant(s) or other funds from any commercial supporters.

Publication Date: August 2020

Contents

LABORATORY REFERENCE RANGES

Reference ranges vary among laboratories. Conventional units are listed first with SI units in parentheses.

Lipid Values

High-density lipoprotein (HDL) cholesterol

- Optimal ---- >60 mg/dL (>1.55 mmol/L)
- Normal ---- 40-60 mg/dL (1.04-1.55 mmol/L)
- Low ---- <40 mg/dL (<1.04 mmol/L)

Low-density lipoprotein (LDL) cholesterol

- Optimal ---- <100 mg/dL (<2.59 mmol/L)
- Low ---- 100-129 mg/dL (2.59-3.34 mmol/L)
- Borderline-high ---- 130-159 mg/dL (3.37-4.12 mmol/L)
- High ---- 160-189 mg/dL (4.14-4.90 mmol/L)
- Very high ---- ≥190 mg/dL (≥4.92 mmol/L)

Non-HDL cholesterol

- Optimal ---- <130 mg/dL (<3.37 mmol/L)
- Borderline-high ---- 130-159 mg/dL (3.37-4.12 mmol/L)
- High ---- ≥240 mg/dL (≥6.22 mmol/L)

Total cholesterol

- Optimal ---- <200 mg/dL (<5.18 mmol/L)
- Borderline-high ---- 200-239 mg/dL (5.18-6.19 mmol/L)
- High ---- ≥240 mg/dL (≥6.22 mmol/L)

Triglycerides

- Optimal ---- <150 mg/dL (<1.70 mmol/L)
- Borderline-high ---- 150-199 mg/dL (1.70-2.25 mmol/L)
- High ---- 200-499 mg/dL (2.26-5.64 mmol/L)
- Very high ---- ≥500 mg/dL (≥5.65 mmol/L)

Lipoprotein (a) ---- ≤30 mg/dL (≤1.07 μmol/L)

Apolipoprotein B ---- 50-110 mg/dL (0.5-1.1 g/L)

Hematologic Values

Erythrocyte sedimentation rate ---- 0-20 mm/h

Haptoglobin ---- 30-200 mg/dL (300-2000 mg/L)

Hematocrit ---- 41%-50% (0.41-0.51) (male); 35%-45% (0.35-0.45) (female)

Hemoglobin A_{1c} ---- 4.0%-5.6% (20-38 mmol/mol)

Hemoglobin ---- 13.8-17.2 g/dL (138-172 g/L) (male); 12.1-15.1 g/dL (121-151 g/L) (female)

International normalized ratio ---- 0.8-1.2

Mean corpuscular volume (MCV) ---- 80-100 μm^3 (80-100 fL)

Platelet count ---- 150-450 × 10^3/μL (150-450 × 10^9/L)

Protein (total) ---- 6.3-7.9 g/dL (63-79 g/L)

Reticulocyte count ---- 0.5%-1.5% of red blood cells (0.005-0.015)

White blood cell count ---- 4500-11,000/μL (4.5-11.0 × 10^9/L)

Thyroid Values

Thyroglobulin ---- 3-42 ng/mL (3-42 μg/L) (after surgery and radioactive iodine treatment: <1.0 ng/mL [<1.0 μg/L])

Thyroglobulin antibodies ---- ≤4.0 IU/mL (≤4.0 kIU/L)

Thyrotropin (TSH) ---- 0.5-5.0 mIU/L

Thyrotropin-receptor antibodies (TRAb) ---- ≤1.75 IU/L

Thyroid-stimulating immunoglobulin ---- ≤120% of basal activity

Thyroperoxidase (TPO) antibodies ---- <2.0 IU/mL (<2.0 kIU/L)

Thyroxine (T_4) (free) ---- 0.8-1.8 ng/dL (10.30-23.17 pmol/L)

Thyroxine (T_4) (total) ---- 5.5-12.5 μg/dL (94.02-213.68 nmol/L)

Free thyroxine (T_4) index ---- 4-12

Triiodothyronine (T_3) (free) ---- 2.3-4.2 pg/mL (3.53-6.45 pmol/L)

Triiodothyronine (T_3) (total) ---- 70-200 ng/dL (1.08-3.08 nmol/L)

Triiodothyronine (T_3), reverse ---- 10-24 ng/dL (0.15-0.37 nmol/L)

Triiodothyronine uptake, resin ---- 25%-38%

Radioactive iodine uptake ---- 3%-16% (6 hours); 15%-30% (24 hours)

Endocrine Values

Serum

Aldosterone ---- 4-21 ng/dL (111.0-582.5 pmol/L)

Alkaline phosphatase ---- 50-120 U/L (0.84-2.00 μkat/L)

Alkaline phosphatase (bone-specific) ---- ≤20 μg/L (adult male); ≤14 μg/L (premenopausal female); ≤22 μg/L (postmenopausal female)

Androstenedione ---- 65-210 ng/dL (2.27-7.33 nmol/L) (adult male); 30-200 ng/dL (1.05-6.98 nmol/L) (adult female)

Antimullerian hormone ---- 0.7-19.0 ng/mL (5.0-135.7 pmol/L) (male, >12 years); 0.9-9.5 ng/mL (6.4-67.9 pmol/L) (female, 13-45 years); <1.0 ng/mL (<7.1 pmol/L) (female, >45 years)

Calcitonin ---- <16 pg/mL (<4.67 pmol/L) (basal, male); <8 pg/mL (<2.34 pmol/L) (basal, female); ≤130 pg/mL (≤37.96 pmol/L) (peak calcium infusion, male); ≤90 pg/mL (≤26.28 pmol/L) (peak calcium infusion, female)

Carcinoembryonic antigen ---- <2.5 ng/mL (<2.5 μg/L)

Chromogranin A ---- <93 ng/mL (<93 μg/L)

Corticosterone ---- 53-1560 ng/dL (1.53-45.08 nmol/L) (>18 years)

Corticotropin (ACTH) ---- 10-60 pg/mL (2.2-13.2 pmol/L)

Cortisol (8 AM) ---- 5-25 μg/dL (137.9-689.7 nmol/L)

Cortisol (4 PM) -------------------- 2-14 μg/dL (55.2-386.2 nmol/L)

C-peptide ----------------------- 0.9-4.3 ng/mL (0.30-1.42 nmol/L)

C-reactive protein -------------- 0.8-3.1 mg/L (7.62-29.52 nmol/L)

Cross-linked N-telopeptide of type 1 collagen -------------------------

5.4-24.2 nmol BCE/mmol creat (male);

6.2-19.0 nmol BCE/mmol creat (female)

Dehydroepiandrosterone sulfate (DHEA-S)

Patient Age	Female	Male
18-29 years	44-332 μg/dL (1.19-9.00 μmol/L)	89-457 μg/dL (2.41-12.38 μmol/L)
30-39 years	31-228 μg/dL (0.84-6.78 μmol/L)	65-334 μg/dL (1.76-9.05 μmol/L)
40-49 years	18-244 μg/dL (0.49-6.61 μmol/L)	48-244 μg/dL (1.30-6.61 μmol/L)
50-59 years	15-200 μg/dL (0.41-5.42 μmol/L)	35-179 μg/dL (0.95-4.85 μmol/L)
≥60 years	15-157 μg/dL (0.41-4.25 μmol/L)	25-131 μg/dL (0.68-3.55 μmol/L)

Deoxycorticosterone -------<10 ng/dL (<0.30 nmol/L) (>18 years)

1,25-Dihydroxyvitamin D_3 ------ 16-65 pg/mL (41.6-169.0 pmol/L)

Estradiol ---------------- 10-40 pg/mL (36.7-146.8 pmol/L) (male);

10-180 pg/mL (36.7-660.8 pmol/L) (follicular, female);

100-300 pg/mL (367.1-1101.3 pmol/L) (midcycle, female);

40-200 pg/mL (146.8-734.2 pmol/L) (luteal, female);

<20 pg/mL (<73.4 pmol/L) (postmenopausal, female)

Estrone ----------------- 10-60 pg/mL (37.0-221.9 pmol/L) (male);

17-200 pg/mL (62.9-739.6 pmol/L) (premenopausal female);

7-40 pg/mL (25.9-147.9 pmol/L) (postmenopausal female)

α-Fetoprotein ---------------------------------- <6 ng/mL (<6 μg/L)

Follicle-stimulating hormone (FSH) ------------------------------

1.0-13.0 mIU/mL (1.0-13.0 IU/L) (male);

<3.0 mIU/mL (<3.0 IU/L) (prepuberty, female);

2.0-12.0 mIU/mL (2.0-12.0 IU/L) (follicular, female);

4.0-36.0 mIU/mL (4.0-36.0 IU/L) (midcycle, female);

1.0-9.0 mIU/mL (1.0-9.0 IU/L) (luteal, female);

>30.0 mIU/mL (>30.0 IU/L) (postmenopausal, female)

Free fatty acids ----------------- 10.6-18.0 mg/dL (0.4-0.7 nmol/L)

Gastrin ------------------------------------<100 pg/mL (<100 ng/L)

Growth hormone (GH) -- 0.01-0.97 ng/mL (0.01-0.97 μg/L) (male);

0.01-3.61 ng/mL (0.01-3.61 μg/L) (female)

Homocysteine -------------------------- ≤1.76 mg/L (≤13 μmol/L)

β-Human chorionic gonadotropin (β-hCG) -----------------------

<3.0 mIU/mL (<3.0 IU/L) (nonpregnant female);

>25 mIU/mL (>25 IU/L) indicates a positive pregnancy test

β-Hydroxybutyrate ------------------- <3.0 mg/dL (<288.2 μmol/L)

17-Hydroxypregnenolone ------ 29-189 ng/dL (0.87-5.69 nmol/L)

17α-Hydroxyprogesterone ---------------------------------------

<220 ng/dL (<6.67 nmol/L) (adult male);

<80 ng/dL (<2.42 nmol/L) (follicular, female);

<285 ng/dL (<8.64 nmol/L) (luteal, female);

<51 ng/dL (1.55 nmol/L) (postmenopausal, female)

25-Hydroxyvitamin D ---

<20 ng/mL (<49.9 nmol/L) (deficiency);

21-29 ng/mL (52.4-72.4 nmol/L) (insufficiency);

30-80 ng/mL (74.9-199.7 nmol/L) (optimal levels);

>80 ng/mL (>199.7 nmol/L) (toxicity possible)

Inhibin B ---------------------------- 15-300 pg/mL (15-300 ng/L)

Insulinlike growth factor 1 (IGF-1)

Patient Age	Female	Male
18 years	162-541 ng/mL (21.2-70.9 nmol/L)	170-640 ng/mL (22.3-83.8 nmol/L)
19 years	138-442 ng/mL (18.1-57.9 nmol/L)	147-527 ng/mL (19.3-69.0 nmol/L)
20 years	122-384 ng/mL (16.0-50.3 nmol/L)	132-457 ng/mL (17.3-59.9 nmol/L)
21-25 years	116-341 ng/mL (15.2-44.7 nmol/L)	116-341 ng/mL (15.2-44.7 nmol/L)
26-30 years	117-321 ng/mL (15.3-42.1 nmol/L)	117-321 ng/mL (15.3-42.1 nmol/L)
31-35 years	113-297 ng/mL (14.8-38.9 nmol/L)	113-297 ng/mL (14.8-38.9 nmol/L)
36-40 years	106-277 ng/mL (13.9-36.3 nmol/L)	106-277 ng/mL (13.9-36.3 nmol/L)
41-45 years	98-261 ng/mL (12.8-34.2 nmol/L)	98-261 ng/mL (12.8-34.2 nmol/L)
46-50 years	91-246 ng/mL (11.9-32.2 nmol/L)	91-246 ng/mL (11.9-32.2 nmol/L)
51-55 years	84-233 ng/mL (11.0-30.5 nmol/L)	84-233 ng/mL (11.0-30.5 nmol/L)
56-60 years	78-220 ng/mL (10.2-28.8 nmol/L)	78-220 ng/mL (10.2-28.8 nmol/L)
61-65 years	72-207 ng/mL (9.4-27.1 nmol/L)	72-207 ng/mL (9.4-27.1 nmol/L)
66-70 years	67-195 ng/mL (8.8-25.5 nmol/L)	67-195 ng/mL (8.8-25.5 nmol/L)
71-75 years	62-184 ng/mL (8.1-24.1 nmol/L)	62-184 ng/mL (8.1-24.1 nmol/L)
76-80 years	57-172 ng/mL (7.5-22.5 nmol/L)	57-172 ng/mL (7.5-22.5 nmol/L)
≥80 years	53-162 ng/mL (6.9-21.2 nmol/L)	53-162 ng/mL (6.9-21.2 nmol/L)

Insulinlike growth factor binding protein 3 ----------- 2.5-4.8 mg/L

Insulin-------------------------- 1.4-14.0 µIU/mL (9.7-97.2 pmol/L)

Islet-cell antibody assay--
0 Juvenile Diabetes Foundation units

Luteinizing hormone (LH)---
1.0-9.0 mIU/mL (1.0-9.0 IU/L) (male);
<1.0 mIU/mL (<1.0 IU/L) (prepuberty, female);
1.0-18.0 mIU/mL (1.0-18.0 IU/L) (follicular, female);
20.0-80.0 mIU/mL (20.0-80.0 IU/L) (midcycle, female);
0.5-18.0 mIU/mL (0.5-18.0 IU/L) (luteal, female);
>30.0 mIU/mL (>30.0 IU/L) (postmenopausal, female)

Metanephrines (plasma fractionated)
Metanephrine------------------------ <99 pg/mL (<0.50 nmol/L)
Normetanephrine------------------<165 pg/mL (<0.90 nmol/L)

75-g oral glucose tolerance test blood glucose values --------------
60-100 mg/dL (3.3-5.6 mmol/L) (fasting);
<200 mg/dL (<11.1 mmol/L) (1 hour);
<140 mg/dL (<7.8 mmol/L) (2 hour);
between 140-200 mg/dL (7.8-11.1 mmol/L) is considered impaired glucose tolerance or prediabetes. Greater than 200 mg/dL (11.1 mmol/L) is a sign of diabetes mellitus.

50-g oral glucose tolerance test for gestational diabetes -----------
<140 mg/dL (<7.8 mmol/L) (1 hour)

100-g oral glucose tolerance test for gestational diabetes -----------
<95 mg/dL (<5.3 mmol/L) (fasting);
<180 mg/dL (<10.0 mmol/L) (1 hour);
<155 mg/dL (<8.6 mmol/L) (2 hour);
<140 mg/dL (<7.8 mmol/L) (3 hour)

Osteocalcin ------------------------9.0-42.0 ng/mL (9.0-42.0 µg/L)

Parathyroid hormone, intact (PTH)-----10-65 pg/mL (10-65 ng/L)

Parathyroid hormone–related protein (PTHrP)--------<2.0 pmol/L

Progesterone --------------------≤1.2 ng/mL (≤3.8 nmol/L) (male);
≤1.0 ng/mL (≤3.2 nmol/L) (follicular, female);
2.0-20.0 ng/mL (6.4-63.6 nmol/L) (luteal, female);
≤1.1 ng/mL (≤3.5 nmol/L) (postmenopausal, female);
>10.0 ng/mL (>31.8 nmol/L) (evidence of ovulatory adequacy)

Proinsulin -------------------- 26.5-176.4 pg/mL (3.0-20.0 pmol/L)

Prolactin -------------------4-23 ng/mL (0.17-1.00 nmol/L) (male);
4-30 ng/mL (0.17-1.30 nmol/L) (nonlactating female);
10-200 ng/mL (0.43-8.70 nmol/L) (lactating female)

Prostate-specific antigen (PSA) -----------------------------------
<2.0 ng/mL (<2.0 µg/L) (≤40 years);
<2.8 ng/mL (<2.8 µg/L) (≤50 years);
<3.8 ng/mL (<3.8 µg/L) (≤60 years);
<5.3 ng/mL (<5.3 µg/L) (≤70 years);
<7.0 ng/mL (<7.0 µg/L) (≤79 years);
<7.2 ng/mL (<7.2 µg/L) (≥80 years)

Renin activity, plasma, sodium replete, ambulatory --------------
0.6-4.3 ng/mL per h

Renin, direct concentration ---------- 4-44 pg/mL (0.1-1.0 pmol/L)

Sex hormone–binding globulin (SHBG) ---------------------------
1.1-6.7 µg/mL (10-60 nmol/L) (male);
2.2-14.6 µg/mL (20-130 nmol/L) (female)

α-Subunit of pituitary glycoprotein hormones ------------------------
<1.2 ng/mL (<1.2 µg/L)

Testosterone (bioavailable)---------------------------------------
0.8-4.0 ng/dL (0.03-0.14 nmol/L)
(20-50 years, female on oral estrogen);
0.8-10.0 ng/dL (0.03-0.35 nmol/L)
(20-50 years, female not on oral estrogen);
83.0-257.0 ng/dL (2.88-8.92 nmol/L) (male 20-29 years);
72.0-235.0 ng/dL (2.50-8.15 nmol/L) (male 30-39 years);
61.0-213.0 ng/dL (2.12-7.39 nmol/L) (male 40-49 years);
50.0-190.0 ng/dL (1.74-6.59 nmol/L) (male 50-59 years);
40.0-168.0 ng/dL (1.39-5.83 nmol/L) (male 60-69 years)

Testosterone (free)------9.0-30.0 ng/dL (0.31-1.04 nmol/L) (male);
0.3-1.9 ng/dL (0.01-0.07 nmol/L) (female)

Testosterone (total)---- 300-900 ng/dL (10.4-31.2 nmol/L) (male);
8-60 ng/dL (0.3-2.1 nmol/L) (female)

Vitamin B_{12} -------------------- 180-914 pg/mL (133-674 pmol/L)

Chemistry Values

Alanine aminotransferase-----------10-40 U/L (0.17-0.67 µkat/L)

Albumin----------------------------------- 3.5-5.0 g/dL (35-50 g/L)

Amylase --------------------------- 26-102 U/L (0.43-1.70 µkat/L)

Aspartate aminotransferase --------20-48 U/L (0.33-0.80 µkat/L)

Bicarbonate ------------------------ 21-28 mEq/L (21-28 mmol/L)

Bilirubin (total)--------------------0.3-1.2 mg/dL (5.1-20.5 µmol/L)

Blood gases
Po_2, arterial blood ------------80-100 mm Hg (10.6-13.3 kPa)
Pco_2, arterial blood --------------- 35-45 mm Hg (4.7-6.0 kPa)

Blood pH-- 7.35-7.45

Calcium -------------------------8.2-10.2 mg/dL (2.1-2.6 mmol/L)

Calcium (ionized) -------------- 4.60-5.08 mg/dL (1.2-1.3 mmol/L)

Carbon dioxide --------------------- 22-28 mEq/L (22-28 mmol/L)

CD_4 cell count-----------------------500-1400/µL (0.5-1.4 × 10^9/L)

Chloride------------------------- 96-106 mEq/L (96-106 mmol/L)

Creatine kinase -------------------- 50-200 U/L (0.84-3.34 µkat/L)

Creatinine-------------- 0.7-1.3 mg/dL (61.9-114.9 µmol/L) (male);
0.6-1.1 mg/dL (53.0-97.2 µmol/L) (female)

Ferritin ----------------------- 15-200 ng/mL (33.7-449.4 pmol/L)

Folate -------------------------------------- ≥4.0 ng/mL (≥4.0 µg/L)

Glucose ---------------------------- 70-99 mg/dL (3.9-5.5 mmol/L)

γ-Glutamyltransferase --------------- 2-30 U/L (0.03-0.50 µkat/L)

Iron --

50-150 μg/dL (9.0-26.8 μmol/L) (male);

35-145 μg/dL (6.3-26.0 μmol/L) (female)

Lactate dehydrogenase -------------100-200 U/L (1.7-3.3 μkat/L)

Lactic acid ----------------------5.4-20.7 mg/dL (0.6-2.3 mmol/L)

Lipase ------------------------------10-73 U/L (0.17-1.22 μkat/L)

Magnesium ---------------------- 1.5-2.3 mg/dL (0.6-0.9 mmol/L)

Osmolality ---------------275-295 mOsm/kg (275-295 mmol/kg)

Phosphate ----------------------- 2.3-4.7 mg/dL (0.7-1.5 mmol/L)

Potassium ----------------------- 3.5-5.0 mEq/L (3.5-5.0 mmol/L)

Prothrombin time --------------------------------------8.3-10.8 s

Serum urea nitrogen----------------8-23 mg/dL (2.9-8.2 mmol/L)

Sodium -----------------------136-142 mEq/L (136-142 mmol/L)

Transferrin saturation -------------------------------- 14%-50%

Troponin I -------------------------------- <0.6 ng/mL (<0.6 μg/L)

Tryptase -------------------------------<11.5 ng/mL (<11.5 μg/L)

Uric acid -------------------- 3.5-7.0 mg/dL (208.2-416.4 μmol/L)

Urine

Albumin-------------30-300 μg/mg creat (3.4-33.9 μg/mol creat)

Albumin-to-creatinine ratio ---------------------- <30 mg/g creat

Aldosterone---------------------- 3-20 μg/24 h (8.3-55.4 nmol/d)

(should be <12 μg/24 h [<33.2 nmol/d] with oral sodium loading—confirmed with 24-hour urinary sodium >200 mEq)

Calcium --------------------- 100-300 mg/24 h (2.5-7.5 mmol/d)

Catecholamine fractionation

Normotensive normal ranges:

Dopamine --------------------- <400 μg/24 h (<2610 nmol/d)

Epinephrine----------------------- <21 μg/24 h (<115 nmol/d)

Norepinephrine ------------------- <80 μg/24 h (<473 nmol/d)

Citrate ------------------- 320-1240 mg/24 h (16.7-64.5 mmol/d)

Cortisol ----------------------------4-50 μg/24 h (11-138 nmol/d)

Cortisol following dexamethasone suppression test

(low-dose: 2 day, 2 mg daily)------- 10 μg/24 h (<27.6 nmol/d)

Creatinine-----------------------1.0-2.0 g/24 h (8.8-17.7 mmol/d)

Glomerular filtration rate (estimated) ---->60 mL/min per 1.73 m^2

5-Hydroxyindole acetic acid------ 2-9 mg/24 h (10.5-47.1 μmol/d)

Iodine (random)-->100 μg/L

17-Ketosteroids -----6.0-21.0 mg/24 h (20.8-72.9 μmol/d) (male);

4.0-17.0 mg/24 h (13.9-59.0 μmol/d) (female)

Metanephrine fractionation

Normotensive normal ranges:

Metanephrine---------- <261 μg/24 h (<1323 nmol/d) (male);

<180 μg/24 h (<913 nmol/d) (female)

Normetanephrine-------------------- age and sex dependent

Total metanephrine------------------ age and sex dependent

Osmolality ------------ 150-1150 mOsm/kg (150-1150 mmol/kg)

Oxalate ------------------------------<40 mg/24 h (<456 mmol/d)

Phosphate -------------------- 0.9-1.3 g/24 h (29.1-42.0 mmol/d)

Potassium ----------------------17-77 mEq/24 h (17-77 mmol/d)

Sodium ---------------------- 40-217 mEq/24 h (40-217 mmol/d)

Uric acid ---------------------------- <800 mg/24 h (<4.7 mmol/d)

Saliva

Cortisol (salivary), midnight ----------- <0.13 μg/dL (<3.6 nmol/L)

Semen

Semen analysis------------ >20 million sperm/mL; >50% motility

COMMON ABBREVIATIONS USED IN ENDOCRINE BOARD REVIEW

ACTH = corticotropin
ACE inhibitor = angiotensin-converting enzyme inhibitor
ALT = alanine aminotransferase
AST = aspartate aminotransferase
BMI = body mass index
CNS = central nervous system
CT = computed tomography
DHEA = dehydroepiandrosterone
DHEA-S = dehydroepiandrosterone sulfate
DNA = deoxyribonucleic acid
DPP-4 inhibitor = dipeptidyl-peptidase 4 inhibitor
DXA = dual-energy x-ray absorptiometry
FDA = Food and Drug Administration
FGF-23 = fibroblast growth factor 23
FNA = fine-needle aspiration
FSH = follicle-stimulating hormone
GH = growth hormone
GHRH = growth hormone–releasing hormone
GLP-1 receptor agonist = glucagonlike peptide 1 receptor agonist
GnRH = gonadotropin-releasing hormone
hCG = human chorionic gonadotropin
HDL = high-density lipoprotein
HIV = human immunodeficiency virus
HMG-CoA reductase inhibitor = 3-hydroxy-3-methylglutaryl coenzyme A reductase inhibitor
IGF-1 = insulinlike growth factor 1
LDL = low-density lipoprotein
LH = luteinizing hormone
MCV = mean corpuscular volume
MIBG = *meta*-iodobenzylguanidine
MRI = magnetic resonance imaging
NPH insulin = neutral protamine Hagedorn insulin
PCSK9 inhibitor = proprotein convertase subtilisin/kexin 9 inhibitor
PET = positron emission tomography
PSA = prostate-specific antigen
PTH = parathyroid hormone
PTHrP = parathyroid hormone–related protein
SGLT-2 inhibitor = sodium-glucose cotransporter 2 inhibitor
SHBG = sex hormone–binding globulin
T_3 = triiodothyronine
T_4 = thyroxine
TPO antibodies = thyroperoxidase antibodies
TRH = thyrotropin-releasing hormone
TRAb = thyrotropin-receptor antibodies
TSH = thyrotropin
VLDL = very low-density lipoprotein

ENDOCRINE BOARD REVIEW

QUESTIONS

Adrenal Board Review

Tobias Else, MD

1 An endocrine surgery colleague requests a consult to evaluate a 38-year-old woman who was referred to him for surgery to remove a possible pheochromocytoma. She has episodic hypertension with blood pressure values ranging up to 210/110 mm Hg accompanied by headaches, nausea, lightheadedness, and diaphoresis. These episodes started in her early 20s, occur several times per week, and last from hours to days.

She has a PhD degree in engineering and works as an executive for a local company. She brings a detailed log listing up to 20 blood pressure measurements per day. Her family history is negative for paraganglioma, pheochromocytoma, or cancers. At today's visit, her blood pressure is 132/81 mm Hg and pulse rate is 78 beats/min.

The laboratory workup and imaging that her primary care physician ordered are available for review. The CT shows a thickened left adrenal gland with a probable central 1-cm nodule (*see images, arrows*).

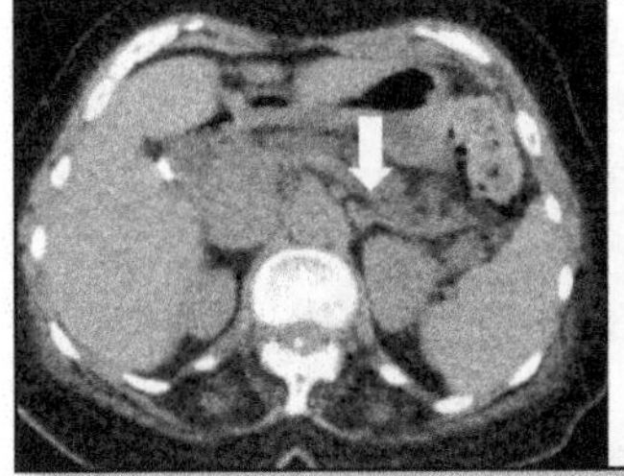

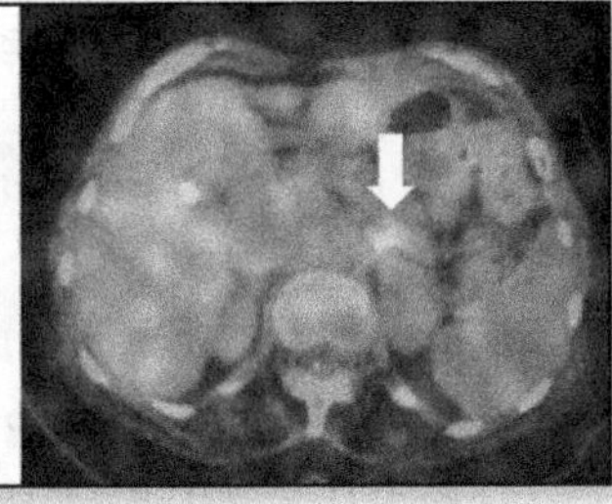

The ^{123}I-MIBG-SPECT/CT shows avidity of the left adrenal gland, presence of a cardiac silhouette, and no other MIBG-avid lesion (*see image*).

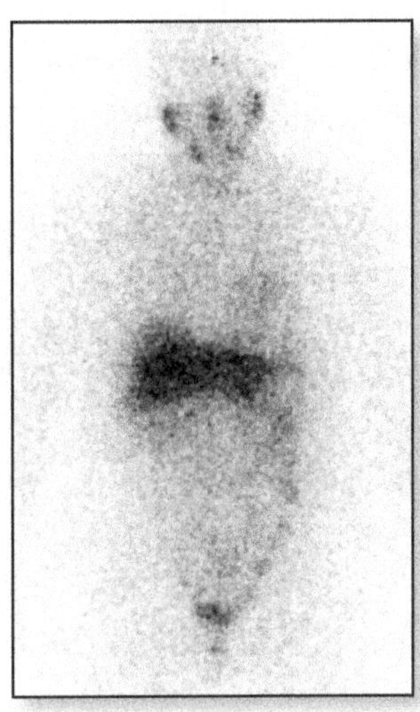

Laboratory test results:

- Plasma normetanephrine = 205.1 pg/mL (<164.8 pg/mL) (SI: 1.12 nmol/L [<0.90 nmol/L])
- Plasma metanephrine = 39.4 pg/mL (<98.6 pg/mL) (SI: 0.20 nmol/L [<0.50 nmol/L])
- Sodium = 140 mEq/L (136-142 mEq/L) (SI: 140 mmol/L [136-142 mmol/L])
- Potassium = 4.2 mEq/L (3.5-5.0 mEq/L) (SI: 4.2 mmol/L [3.5-5.0 mmol/L])
- Serum aldosterone = 6 ng/dL (4-21 ng/dL) (SI: 166.4 pmol/L [111.0-582.5 pmol/L])
- Plasma renin activity = <0.6 ng/mL per h (0.6-4.3 ng/mL per h)

Which of the following is the best next step in this patient's care?

A. Obtain a 24-hour urine collection for metanephrine and normetanephrine
B. Perform a ^{68}Ga-DOTATATE PET-CT
C. Discuss the diagnosis of pseudopheochromocytoma
D. Proceed with left adrenalectomy
E. Perform MRI with in-phase/out-of-phase imaging

2 A 55-year-old man is referred for endocrine consultation after a recent emergency department visit for hypertensive urgency. He has a 20-year history of hypertension controlled with hydrochlorothiazide. However, he has recently been experiencing headaches and has measured his blood pressure more often. These measurements document values ranging between 160 and 190 mm Hg systolic and between 95 and 110 mm Hg diastolic. His primary care physician intensified his antihypertensive regimen to include amlodipine, losartan, and doxazosin.

He describes worsening headaches, loss of libido, tiredness, and fatigue over the last few months. He has gained more than 40 lb (>18.1 kg) over the last 5 years, and his current BMI is 37 kg/m^2.

On physical examination, he is a well-developed, obese patient with typical fat distribution and no striae, bruising, or skin atrophy. His blood pressure is 142/92 mm Hg.

Laboratory test results after the emergency department visit:

Urinary metanephrine = 66 μg/24 h (<261 μg/24 h)
Urinary normetanephrine = 920 μg/24 h (<484 μg/24 h)
Plasma metanephrine = 39.4 pg/mL (<98.6 pg/mL) (SI: 0.2 nmol/L [<0.50 nmol/L])
Plasma normetanephrine = 183.2 pg/mL (<164.8 pg/mL) (SI: 1.0 nmol/L [<0.90 nmol/L])
Sodium = 140 mEq/L (136-142 mEq/L) (SI: 140 mmol/L [136-142 mmol/L])
Potassium = 3.5 mEq/L (3.5-5.0 mEq/L) (SI: 3.5 mmol/L [3.5-5.0 mmol/L])
Serum aldosterone = 18 ng/dL (4-21 ng/dL) (SI: 499.3 pmol/L [111.0-582.5 pmol/L])
Plasma renin activity = 1.0 ng/mL per h (0.6-4.3 ng/mL per h)
Serum testosterone = 240 ng/dL (300-900 ng/dL) (SI: 8.3 nmol/L [10.4-31.2 nmol/L])

Which of the following is the best next step in this patient's evaluation?

A. 24-Hour urine collection for cortisol measurement
B. Sleep study
C. ^{68}Ga-DOTATATE PET-CT
D. ^{123}I-MIBG SPECT-CT
E. Repeated measurement of plasma metanephrine levels after holding doxazosin

3 A general surgeon requests a consult to evaluate a 68-year-old woman for adrenal insufficiency. The patient had a left hemicolectomy for colon cancer with construction of a transient colostomy the night before. Overnight she had episodes of hypotension with blood pressure as low as 90/50 mm Hg (baseline blood pressure is 130/80 mm Hg), mild fever, tachycardia of 110 beats/min, and increased output through her colostomy. She was treated with intravenous fluids and 50 mg of tramadol. She developed mild hyponatremia, and a morning cortisol concentration was documented to be 0.9 μg/dL (24.8 nmol/L).

She does not smoke cigarettes and was healthy before her surgery. She has a diagnosis of mild hypertension and diet-controlled diabetes (most recent hemoglobin A_{1c} = 6.8% [51 mmol/mol]).

She is resting comfortably and does not have any nausea. She would like to eat. On physical examination, she is obese (BMI = 32 kg/m^2) and does not appear ill. Her blood pressure is 124/85 mm Hg, and pulse rate is 90 beats/min.

Her most recent basic metabolic profile shows the following results:

Sodium = 133 mEq/L (136-142 mEq/L) (SI: 133 mmol/L [136-142 mmol/L])
Potassium = 3.8 mEq/L (3.5-5.0 mEq/L) (SI: 3.8 mmol/L [3.5-5.0 mmol/L])
Glucose = 168 mg/dL (70-99 mg/dL) (SI: 9.3 mmol/L [3.9-5.5 mmol/L])
Serum creatinine = 0.7 mg/dL (0.6-1.1 mg/dL) (SI: 61.9 μmol/L [53.0-97.2 μmol/L])

Which of the following is the most likely cause for the low cortisol level?

A. Medication given as a prophylaxis for postoperative nausea
B. Overnight use of tramadol
C. Primary autoimmune adrenal insufficiency
D. Metastasis from the colon cancer
E. Delayed effect of inhaled anesthetics

4 A 48-year old man has recently been diagnosed with adrenocortical carcinoma. He reports no history of malignancy, but states that his brother had colon cancer at age 38 years and that his mother died of uterine cancer at age 51 years. His mother had 5 siblings: a brother with colon cancer in his late 50s, a sister with stomach cancer in her 40s, and 3 brothers who are alive and well in their 60s without any cancer diagnosis. The patient's maternal grandfather had prostate cancer in his 60s and his maternal grandmother had colon cancer at age 47 years. There are no family members with adrenal tumors.

The patient's family is wondering whether they could have a familial cancer syndrome.

Which hereditary syndrome is most likely in this patient's family?

A. Li-Fraumeni syndrome
B. Lynch syndrome (hereditary nonpolyposis colon cancer)
C. Familial adenomatous polyposis
D. Carney complex
E. Multiple endocrine neoplasia type 1

5 A 52-year-old man is referred for evaluation of bilateral adrenal masses. Over the last 6 months, he has lost 30 lb (13.6 kg) and developed night sweats. He has been increasingly fatigued and has had dizziness and nausea. He lives in a northern state and has not traveled outside the United States. He is a lifelong nonsmoker. He has had no sick contacts and works in an office setting.

On physical examination, the patient appears chronically ill and thin. His blood pressure is 98/50 mm Hg (sitting) and 75/45 mm Hg (standing). He can move all extremities but has generalized weakness. Lungs are clear, and no skin lesions are appreciated.

As part of the initial workup, he had an abdominal CT (*see image*), which documented bilateral adrenal masses, and a chest CT, which showed no abnormalities. The following laboratory test results were documented:

Sodium = 129 mEq/L (136-142 mEq/L)
(SI: 129 mmol/L [136-142 mmol/L])
Potassium = 5.4 mEq/L (3.5-5.0 mEq/L)
(SI: 5.4 mmol/L [3.5-5.0 mmol/L])
Serum aldosterone = <2 ng/dL (4-21 ng/dL)
(SI: 55.5 pmol/L [111.0-582.5 pmol/L])
Plasma renin activity = 64 ng/mL per h
(0.6-4.3 ng/mL per h)
Plasma ACTH = 252 pg/mL (10-60 pg/mL)
(SI: 55.4 pmol/L [2.2-13.2 pmol/L])
Serum cortisol (8 AM) = 1.2 μg/dL (5-25 μg/dL)
(SI: 106.1 nmol/L [137.9-689.7 nmol/L])
Serum DHEA-S = 23 μg/dL (35-179 μg/dL)
(SI: 0.62 μmol/L [0.95-4.85 μmol/L])

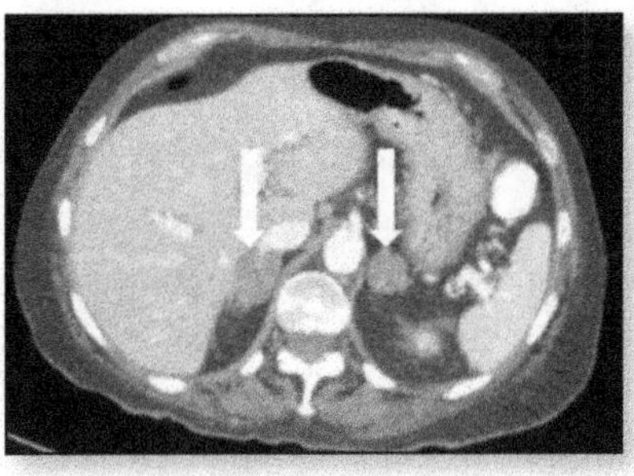

Which of the following is the most likely diagnosis underlying this patient's presentation?

A. Congenital adrenal hyperplasia
B. Autoimmune adrenalitis
C. Melanoma metastatic to the adrenal gland
D. Adrenal lymphoma
E. Histoplasmosis

6 A 37-year-old woman with primary adrenal insufficiency presents for routine follow-up. She describes worsening anorexia and nausea. She has been on steady dosages of hydrocortisone, 15 mg in the morning upon awakening and 5 mg in the afternoon, and fludrocortisone, 0.1 mg daily. Adrenal insufficiency was initially diagnosed at age 24 years. She follows "sick day rules" and has injectable hydrocortisone at home. She has always been slightly hyperpigmented since diagnosis, but she has noticed worsening hyperpigmentation over the last 6 months.

Over the last year, she started the following medications: combined oral contraceptives; biotin supplement (for subjective hair loss); omeprazole, 40 mg daily; and cholestyramine, 8 g daily (for postcholecytectomy diarrhea). Diarrhea improved slightly, but still persists. Over the course of the last 6 weeks, she has lost 13.2 lb (6 kg). Her current weight is 127.9 lb (58 kg).

On physical examination, she appears less healthy than you remember from prior visits. She is generally pale and has hyperpigmentation. Her blood pressure is 110/78 mm Hg, and pulse rate is 89 beats/min.

Laboratory test results:

Sodium = 130 mEq/L (136-142 mEq/L)
(SI: 130 mmol/L [136-142 mmol/L])
Potassium = 5.4 mEq/L (3.5-5.0 mEq/L)
(SI: 5.4 mmol/L [3.5-5.0 mmol/L])
Plasma renin activity = 60 ng/mL per h
(0.6-4.3 ng/mL per h)
Plasma ACTH = 644 pg/mL (10-60 pg/mL)
(SI: pmol/L [2.2-13.2 pmol/L])
TSH = 5.2 mIU/L (0.5-5.0 mIU/L)
Free T_4 = 1.0 ng/dL (0.8-1.8 ng/dL)
(SI: 12.9 pmol/L [10.30-23.17 pmol/L])

Which of the following is the most likely cause of this patient's concerns?

A. Cholestyramine
B. Omeprazole
C. Hashimoto disease
D. Combined oral contraceptive
E. Atrophic gastritis

7 A 32-year-old woman is referred for evaluation of an incidental adrenal mass that was identified on CT performed as part of the workup for an episode of painless hematuria 4 weeks ago. In taking a history, you elicit a 14-lb (6.5-kg) weight gain over the past year associated with the onset of irregular menses, hirsutism, and poor sleep. She takes no medications.

On physical examination, her blood pressure is 140/88 mm Hg. She has mild to moderate facial fullness and plethora and supraclavicular fat accumulation.

CT demonstrates a 1.4-cm left adrenal mass (*see image; right and left adrenal glands are identified by arrows*).

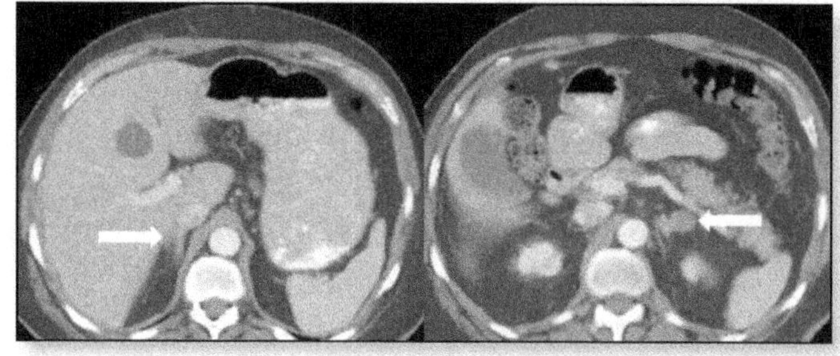

Laboratory test results:

Sodium = 138 mEq/L (136-142 mEq/L)
(SI: 138 mmol/L [136-142 mmol/L])
Potassium = 3.7 mEq/L (3.5-5.0 mEq/L)
(SI: 3.7 mmol/L [3.5-5.0 mmol/L])
Late-night salivary cortisol (2 measurements) = 0.43 μg/dL (SI: 11.9 nmol/L)
Serum cortisol after overnight 1-mg dexamethasone = 8.2 μg/dL (SI: 226.2 nmol/L)
Serum aldosterone = 4 ng/dL (4-21 ng/dL)
(SI: 111.0 pmol/L [111.0-582.5 pmol/L])
Pregnancy test, negative

Which of the following studies should be ordered next?

A. Plasma renin activity
B. Adrenal MRI
C. Dexamethasone corticotropin-releasing hormone test
D. Biopsy of the adrenal tumor
E. Plasma ACTH measurement

8 A primary care physician refers a 32-year-old man because of an elevated plasma ACTH concentration. He has a 10-year history of primary adrenal insufficiency due to autoimmune adrenalitis. He also has primary hypothyroidism due to Hashimoto thyroiditis. The patient feels well and has no concerns. His medications include hydrocortisone, 12.5 mg every morning and 5 mg every afternoon; fludrocortisone, 50 mcg daily; and levothyroxine, 125 mcg daily.

On physical examination, he is a healthy appearing man with a blood pressure of 122/76 mm Hg, a regular pulse rate of 70 beats/min, and a BMI of 24 kg/m^2. His skin is well pigmented in sun-exposed areas. Examination findings are otherwise normal.

Laboratory test results:

Electrolytes, normal
Plasma renin activity = 2.1 ng/mL per h (0.6-4.3 ng/mL per h)
Serum TSH = 2.8 mIU/L (0.5-5.0 mIU/L)
Plasma ACTH = 312 pg/mL (10-60 pg/mL) (SI: 68.6 pmol/L [2.2-13.2 pmol/L])

In addition to reviewing sick-day corticosteroid management, which of the following should you recommend?

A. Discontinue hydrocortisone and substitute prednisone, 5 mg in the morning and 2.5 mg in the afternoon
B. Add dexamethasone, 0.75 mg orally at bedtime
C. Increase the hydrocortisone dosage to 20 mg in the morning and 10 mg in the afternoon
D. Increase the fludrocortisone dosage to 100 mcg daily
E. Make no changes in his corticosteroid dosages

9 A 59-year-old woman is referred for a second opinion regarding primary aldosteronism. She developed resistant hypertension in her early 50s and was found to be hypokalemic 6 months ago on routine blood testing.

Screening laboratory test results:

Sodium = 142 mEq/L (136-142 mEq/L) (SI: 142 mmol/L [136-142 mmol/L])
Potassium = 3.2 mEq/L (3.5-5.0 mEq/L) (SI: 3.2 mmol/L [3.5-5.0 mmol/L])
Serum aldosterone = 22 ng/dL (4-21 ng/dL) (SI: 610.3 pmol/L [111.0-582.5 pmol/L])
Plasma renin activity = <0.6 ng/mL per h (0.6-4.3 ng/mL per h)

On the third day of a high-salt diet, the 24-hour urine collection documents a sodium excretion of 240 mEq/24 h (240 mmol/d) and an aldosterone excretion of 24 µg/24 h (66.6 nmol/d). CT with fine cuts of the adrenals shows normal glands. She undergoes adrenal venous sampling with continuous infusion of cosyntropin at 50 mcg per h. The results are shown (*see table*).

She is told that the source is the left adrenal gland on the basis of the high left adrenal vein aldosterone concentration and the aldosterone-to-cortisol ratio.

How should the results of the adrenal venous sampling study be interpreted?

A. Unable to localize
B. Left adrenal gland is the source (left adenoma)
C. Both adrenal glands are sources (bilateral, idiopathic hyperaldosteronism)
D. Insufficient information to interpret whether the study was successful
E. Right adrenal gland is the source (right adenoma)

Measurement	Right Adrenal Vein	Left Adrenal Vein	Inferior Vena Cava
Aldosterone	36 ng/dL (SI: 998.6 pmol/L)	6400 ng/dL (SI: 177,536 pmol/L)	34 ng/dL (SI: 943.2 pmol/L)
Cortisol	21 µg/dL SI: 579.4 nmol/L)	2000 µg/dL (SI: 55,176 nmol/L)	19 µg/dL (SI: 524.2 nmol/L)
Aldosterone-to-Cortisol Ratio	1.7	3.2	1.8

10 A 25-year-old woman with congenital adrenal hyperplasia due to 21-hydroxylase deficiency diagnosed at birth is transitioning to adult care from her pediatric endocrinologist. Her current treatment consists of hydrocortisone, 10 mg 3 times daily with meals, and fludrocortisone acetate, 0.2 mg every evening. She has regular menses, is not sexually active, and is not attempting to become pregnant.

On physical examination, she has no acne or unwanted facial hair, purple striae, or skin thinning. Her BMI is 25 kg/m^2. Her blood pressure is 117/74 mm Hg. She feels well and has no concerns.

She took her hydrocortisone today at 6 AM and 12 PM, and her blood is drawn at 5:30 PM.

Laboratory test results (5:30 PM blood draw):

Sodium = 138 mEq/L (136-142 mEq/L) (SI: 138 mmol/L [136-142 mmol/L])
Potassium = 4.2 mEq/L (3.5-5.0 mEq/L) (SI: 4.2 mmol/L [3.5-5.0 mmol/L])
Serum DHEA-S = <15 µg/dL (44-332 µg/dL) (SI: <0.4 µmol/L [1.19-9.00 µmol/L])
Serum testosterone = 40 ng/dL (8-60 ng/dL) (SI: 1.4 nmol/L [0.3-2.1 nmol/L])
Plasma renin activity = 2.4 ng/mL per h (0.6-4.3 ng/mL per h)
Serum androstenedione = 90 ng/dL (80-240 ng/dL) (SI: 3.0 nmol/L [2.79-8.38 nmol/L])
Serum 17-hydroxyprogesterone = 4500 ng/dL (<80 ng/dL) (SI: 136.4 nmol/L [2.42 nmol/L])

Which of the following changes to her management should be recommended?

A. No changes
B. Increase the second dose of hydrocortisone to 15 mg
C. Switch hydrocortisone to dexamethasone, 1 mg at bedtime
D. Divide hydrocortisone as 7.5 mg 4 times daily
E. Stop fludrocortisone acetate

11 A 56-year-old man is referred for evaluation of an incidentally discovered adrenal mass. He had not seen a physician in 10 years, and he sought medical attention for postprandial abdominal pain. Abdominal CT without contrast was obtained (*see image*). The official interpretation is "1.2-cm left adrenal mass, MRI can further characterize." His abdominal pain has since resolved with a 6-week course of omeprazole. His medical history is unremarkable.

On physical examination, he has no cushingoid stigmata. Blood pressure measurements obtained in the clinic since he first presented have ranged as follows: systolic 144-162 mm Hg and diastolic 92-98 mm Hg (even after resolution of his abdominal pain).

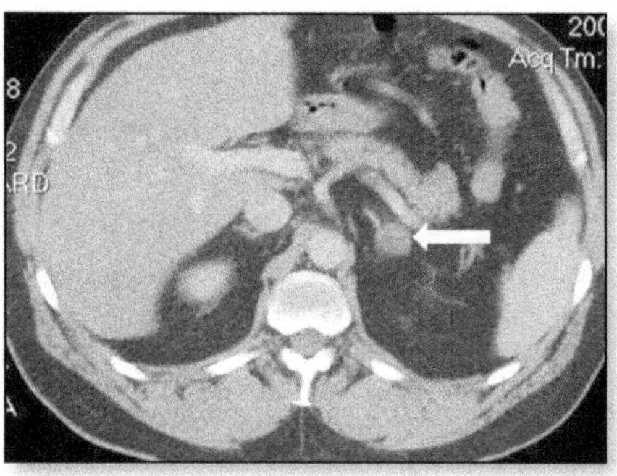

Laboratory test results:

Potassium = 3.8 mEq/L (3.5-5.0 mEq/L) (SI: 3.8 mmol/L [3.5-5.0 mmol/L])
Plasma normetanephrine = 150 pg/mL (<165 pg/mL) (SI: 0.82 nmol/L [<0.90 nmol/L])
Plasma metanephrine = 40 pg/mL (<99 pg/mL) (SI: 0.20 nmol/L [<0.50 nmol/L])
Serum cortisol (8 AM) after overnight 1-mg dexamethasone-suppression test = 0.4 µg/dL (SI: 11.0 nmol/L)
Fasting glucose = 80 mg/dL (70-99 mg/dL) (SI: 4.4 mmol/L [3.9-5.5 mmol/L])

Which of the following is the best next step in this patient's management?

A. Obtain 24-hour urine collection to measure metanephrines
B. Perform adrenal MRI
C. Measure serum DHEA-S and plasma ACTH
D. Repeat adrenal CT in 1 year
E. Measure serum aldosterone and plasma renin activity

12 You are asked to evaluate for Cushing syndrome in a 49-year-old man in the intensive care unit. Over the preceding 8 weeks, he experienced rapid onset of hyperglycemia, hypertension, muscle weakness, and psychosis. He was taken to the emergency department by ambulance, where he was confused and hypoxic. Chest CT shows a 3-cm upper right lung mass and hilar lymphadenopathy. Both adrenal glands are uniformly enlarged to double normal size.

Laboratory test results:

Plasma ACTH = 420 pg/mL (10-60 pg/mL) (SI: 92.4 pmol/L [2.2-13.2 pmol/L])
Serum cortisol = 180 μg/dL (5-25 μg/dL) (SI: 4966 nmol/L [137.9-689.7 nmol/L])
Serum potassium = 2.4 mEq/L (3.5-5.0 mEq/L) (SI: 2.4 mmol/L [3.5-5.0 mmol/L])
ALT = 150 U/L (10-40 U/L) (SI: 2.5 μkat/L [0.17-0.67 μkat/L])

In the emergency department, he was intubated and ventilated before transfer to the intensive care unit. You suspect ectopic ACTH syndrome, but the patient is too ill for further evaluation.

Which of the following medications should be recommended immediately to treat his hypercortisolemia?

A. Mitotane
B. Pasireotide
C. Etomidate
D. Ketoconazole
E. Mifepristone

13 A 43-year-old woman is seen for follow-up of Cushing disease. She initially presented with hypertension, hypokalemia, muscle weakness, hirsutism, oligomenorrhea, and weight gain over the last 2 years.

Preoperative laboratory test results:

Late-night salivary cortisol = 0.82 μg/dL (<0.13 μg/dL) (SI: 22.6 nmol/L [<3.6 nmol/L])
Urinary free cortisol = 850 μg/24 h (4-50 μg/24 h) (SI: 2346 nmol/d [11-138 nmol/d])
Basal plasma ACTH = 102 pg/mL (10-60 pg/mL) (SI: 22.4 pmol/L [2.2-13.2 pmol/L])

Inferior petrosal sinus sampling and MRI confirmed a pituitary tumor, and she underwent transsphenoidal surgery 6 weeks ago. Postoperatively, serial morning cortisol values were less than 0.5 μg/dL (<13.8 nmol/L), and she was discharged on the third postoperative day and instructed to take hydrocortisone, 25 mg on arising and 10 mg in the early afternoon (without her antihypertensive medications).

Her blood pressure has normalized, and she has lost 8 lb (3.6 kg). She describes diffuse muscle aches, fatigue, and anorexia. She states, "I am sleeping all day and feel worse than when I had Cushing's."

On physical examination, her blood pressure is 120/80 mm Hg and pulse rate is 70 beats/min without orthostatic changes. Her cushingoid features are beginning to resolve.

Laboratory test results:

Serum sodium = 136 mEq/L (136-142 mEq/L) (SI: 136 mmol/L [136-142 mmol/L])
Serum potassium = 4.4 mEq/L (3.5-5.0 mEq/L) (SI: 4.4 mmol/L [3.5-5.0 mmol/L])
Fasting glucose = 80 mg/dL (70-99 mg/dL) (SI: 4.4 mmol/L [3.9-5.5 mmol/L])
Serum cortisol (8 AM) before first dose of hydrocortisone = <0.5 μg/dL (5-25 μg/dL) (SI: <13.8 nmol/L [137.9-689.7 nmol/L])
DHEA-S = <15 μg/dL (18-244 μg/dL) (SI: <0.41 μmol/L [0.49-6.61 μmol/L])
Basal plasma ACTH = <4 pg/mL (10-60 pg/mL) (SI: <0.9 pmol/L [2.2-13.2 pmol/L])

Which of the following should be done next to address her symptoms?

A. Perform another pituitary MRI
B. Add fludrocortisone, 0.1 mg daily
C. Measure late-night salivary cortisol
D. Increase the hydrocortisone dosage to 40 mg on arising and 20 mg in the early afternoon
E. Add DHEA, 25 mg daily

14 A 42-year-old woman with recurrent Cushing disease is commencing mifepristone therapy, 300 mg daily. Her comorbidities from Cushing disease include hypertension and diabetes mellitus for which she takes amlodipine, 5 mg daily, and metformin, 1500 mg daily. Her blood pressure is 135/85 mm Hg. Her menses have been irregular.

Laboratory test results:

Fasting glucose = 185 mg/dL (70-99 mg/dL) (SI: 10.3 mmol/L [3.9-5.5 mmol/L])
Potassium = 3.7 mEq/L (3.5-5.0 mEq/L) (SI: 3.7 mmol/L [3.5-5.0 mmol/L])
Serum cortisol = 22 µg/dL (5-25 µg/dL) (SI: 606.9 nmol/L [137.9-689.7 nmol/L])
Hemoglobin A_{1c} = 8.5% (4.0%-5.6%) (69 mmol/mol [20-38 mmol/mol])
Plasma ACTH = 65 pg/mL (10-60 pg/mL) (SI: 14.3 pmol/L [2.2-13.2 pmol/L])
Urinary free cortisol = 360 µg/24 h (4-50 µg/24 h) (SI: 993.6 nmol/d [11-138 nmol/d])

Which of the following parameters should be used to titrate the mifepristone dosage in this patient?

A. Urinary free cortisol excretion
B. Return of regular monthly menses
C. Plasma ACTH level
D. Blood pressure
E. Fasting serum glucose level

15 An endocrine consult is requested for a 72-year-old man who is in the medical intensive care unit for hypovolemic shock from sepsis. Before hospital admission, his only medications were metformin, 1000 mg daily; lisinopril, 20 mg daily; and atorvastatin, 5 mg daily. He remains intubated and has been treated with pressors and saline boluses for 3 days. His systolic blood pressure is 85 mm Hg, and pulse rate is 118 beats/min. The team has performed a cosyntropin-stimulation test and asks for assistance with interpretation of the results.

Results of cosyntropin-stimulation testing:

Basal serum cortisol = 15 µg/dL (5-25 µg/dL) (SI: 413.8 nmol/L [137.9-689.7 nmol/L])
Stimulated serum cortisol = 16 µg/dL (SI: 441.4 nmol/L)
Serum glucose = 134 mg/dL (70-99 mg/dL) (SI: 7.4 mmol/L [3.9-5.5 mmol/L])
Serum albumin = 2.3 g/dL (3.5-5.0 g/dL) (SI: 23 g/L [35-50 g/L])

Which of the following do you recommend as the best next step in this patient's evaluation and management?

A. Insulin tolerance test
B. Serum DHEA-S measurement
C. Plasma ACTH measurement
D. Low-dose cosyntropin-stimulation test
E. No further testing

16 A 33-year-old woman presents for evaluation of weight gain, depression, hirsutism, irregular menses, and hypertension. Her symptoms began 2 years ago and have been gradually progressive. Her medications are an oral contraceptive (ethinylestradiol and drospirenone); sertraline, 100 mg daily; and omeprazole, 20 mg daily.

On physical examination, she has facial plethora, disproportionate supraclavicular fat pads, 1- to 2-cm nonblanching purple striae on the abdomen and upper arms, central obesity, and proximal muscle weakness.

Laboratory test results:

Serum cortisol after 1 mg dexamethasone = 25 µg/dL (SI: 690 nmol/L)
Plasma ACTH = 188 pg/mL (10-60 pg/mL) (SI: 41.4 pmol/L [2.2-13.2 pmol/L])
Late-night salivary cortisol = 0.42 µg/dL (<0.13 µg/dL) (SI: 11.6 nmol/L [<3.6 nmol/L])

Repeat late-night salivary cortisol = 0.48 μg/dL (<0.13 μg/dL) (SI: 13.2 nmol/L [<3.6 nmol/L])
Serum glucose = 125 mg/dL (70-99 mg/dL) (SI: 6.9 mmol/L [3.9-5.5 mmol/L])

MRI of the sella without and with contrast shows an irregular 2-mm area of delayed contrast enhancement on the right side of the pituitary gland found only on the dynamic scans, which the radiology report describes as "consistent with pituitary adenoma."

Which of the following is the best next step in this patient's management?

A. Stop the contraceptive for 6 weeks and repeat the dexamethasone-suppression test
B. Refer for pituitary surgery
C. Measure 24-hour urinary free cortisol excretion
D. Start mifepristone, 600 mg daily
E. Refer for inferior petrosal sinus sampling

17 A 34-year-old woman presents with rapidly progressive hirsutism, secondary amenorrhea, balding, voice deepening, and hypertension over the last 6 months. Her primary care physician has obtained some initial laboratory test results:

Sodium = 143 mEq/L (136-142 mEq/L) (SI: 143 mmol/L [136-142 mmol/L])
Potassium = 3.1 mEq/L (3.5-5.0 mEq/L) (SI: 3.1 mmol/L [3.5-5.0 mmol/L])
Serum aldosterone = <4 ng/dL (4-21 ng/dL) (SI: <111.0 pmol/L [111.0-582.5 pmol/L])
Plasma renin activity = <0.6 ng/mL per h (0.6-4.3 ng/mL per h)
Plasma ACTH = 11 pg/mL (10-60 pg/mL) (SI: 2.4 pmol/L [2.2-13.2 pmol/L])
Serum cortisol (8 AM) = 14 μg/dL (5-25 μg/dL) (SI: 386.2 nmol/L [137.9-689.7 nmol/L])
Serum DHEA-S = 2833 μg/dL (44-352 μg/dL) (SI: 76.8 μmol/L [1.2-9.5 μmol/L])
Serum 11-deoxycortisol = 282 ng/dL (10-79 ng/dL) (SI: 8.5 nmol/L [0.30-2.39 nmol/L])
Serum total testosterone = 310 ng/dL (8-60 ng/dL) (SI: 10.8 nmol/L [0.3-2.1 nmol/L])
SHBG = 1.0 μg/mL (2.2-14.6 μg/mL) (SI: 8.9 nmol/L [20-130 nmol/L])

Which of the following is the most likely diagnosis?

A. Macronodular adrenocortical hyperplasia
B. Nonclassic 11β-hydroxylase deficiency
C. Adrenocortical carcinoma
D. Ovarian hyperthecosis
E. Anabolic steroid abuse

18 A 22-year-old woman is referred for evaluation of severe hypertension and adrenal masses. She has new-onset hypertension and mild hyperglycemia. Her mother and a maternal uncle also developed severe hypertension before age 40 years. The uncle died of a myocardial infarction, and the patient's mother underwent adrenalectomy for bilateral pheochromocytoma and ultimately died of metastatic renal cell cancer.

Laboratory test results:

Sodium = 138 mEq/L (136-142 mEq/L) (SI: 138 mmol/L [136-142 mmol/L])
Potassium = 3.8 mEq/L (3.5-5.0 mEq/L) (SI: 3.8 mmol/L [3.5-5.0 mmol/L])
Plasma normetanephrine = 1502 pg/mL (<165 pg/mL) (SI: 8.2 nmol/L [<0.90 nmol/L])
Plasma metanephrine = 60 pg/mL (<99 pg/mL) (SI: 0.30 nmol/L [<0.50 nmol/L])
Serum aldosterone = 5 ng/dL (4-21 ng/dL) (SI: 138.7 pmol/L [111.0-582.5 pmol/L])
Plasma renin activity = 2.4 ng/mL per h (0.6-4.3 ng/mL per h)

CT scan after intravenous contrast is shown (*see image*).

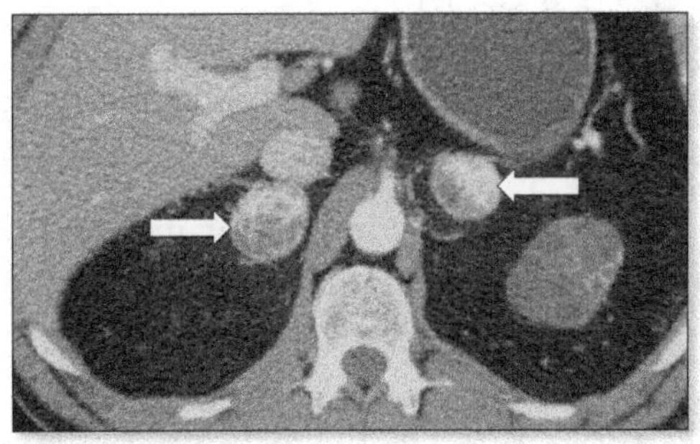

A pathogenic variant in which of the following genes is most likely responsible for pheochromocytoma in this kindred?

A. *RET*
B. *MEN1*
C. *VHL*
D. *SDHD*
E. *TMEM127*

19 A 55-year-old woman is referred for evaluation of an incidentally discovered right adrenal mass. The mass measures 3.4 cm in diameter, the precontrast attenuation value is –5 Hounsfield units, and there is more than 60% contrast medium 15 minutes after contrast administration. The left adrenal gland has no nodularity. Her only medication is alendronate for osteoporosis.

On physical examination, she has borderline hypertension (144/92 mm Hg). Her weight is 169 lb (76.8 kg) (BMI = 29 kg/m^2). She has no facial plethora, dermal atrophy, bruising, or supraclavicular fat pads.

Initial laboratory test results:
- Plasma ACTH (8 AM) = 7 pg/mL (10-60 pg/mL) (SI: 1.5 pmol/L [2.2-13.2 pmol/L])
- Repeated plasma ACTH = 8 pg/mL (SI: 1.8 pmol/L)
- Serum DHEA-S = 58 µg/dL (15-200 µg/dL) (SI: 1.57 µmol/L [0.41-5.42 µmol/L])
- Serum cortisol after 1 mg dexamethasone = 4.2 µg/dL (SI: 115.9 nmol/L)
- Repeated serum cortisol = 4.2 µg/dL (SI: 115.9 nmol/L)
- Urinary free cortisol = 22 µg/24 h (4-50 µg/24 h) (SI: 60.7 nmol/d [11-138 nmol/d])

Two years later, the patient has gained 32 lb (14.5 kg) (BMI = 34 kg/m^2). She has no facial plethora, dermal atrophy, bruising, or supraclavicular fat pads. Hypertension is controlled on amlodipine and losartan (132/80 mm Hg). She is still taking alendronate and has started metformin to treat diabetes (hemoglobin A_{1c} = 6.9% [52 mmol/mol]).

Repeated laboratory test results:
- Plasma ACTH (8 AM) = 8 pg/mL (SI: 1.8 pmol/L)
- Repeated plasma ACTH = 6 pg/mL (SI: 1.3 pmol/L)
- Serum DHEA-S = <15 µg/dL (SI: <0.41 µmol/L)
- Serum cortisol after 1 mg dexamethasone = 4.1 µg/dL (SI: 113.1 nmol/L)
- Urinary free cortisol = 28 µg/24 h (SI: 77.3 nmol/d)

Which of the following is the best recommendation for this patient's care?

A. Delay medical or surgical therapy until urinary free cortisol is clearly elevated
B. Refer for petrosal sinus sampling
C. Start medical treatment with mifepristone, 300 mg daily
D. Refer for laparoscopic right adrenalectomy
E. Perform fluorodeoxyglucose-PET scan to evaluate for malignant transformation

20 A 55-year-old woman presents for follow-up of adrenocortical cancer. She initially presented with ACTH-independent hypercortisolism and androgen excess, and a 9-cm adrenocortical cancer was excised by open resection 12 weeks ago. She developed adrenal insufficiency postoperatively. Due to aggressive histologic features, she was treated with mitotane 3 months ago and advanced to a dosage of 1 g 6 times daily. Her last serum mitotane measurement was therapeutic at 16 mg/L. During the mitotane titration, she experienced fatigue and anorexia, and based on information she learned in an Internet chat group, she experimented with raising her hydrocortisone dosage to 60 mg on arising and 20 mg with lunch and supper. At today's appointment, she reports feeling much better taking the higher dosage of hydrocortisone. A serum cortisol value 3 hours after the morning hydrocortisone dose is 12 µg/dL (331.1 nmol/L).

Her serum cortisol level is not higher after a 60-mg hydrocortisone dose because mitotane:

A. Decreases corticosteroid-binding globulin
B. Induces hepatic CYP3A4 activity
C. Impairs cortisol absorption
D. Increases urinary cortisol excretion
E. Increases 5α-reductase activity

21 A 24-year-old man is referred for evaluation of hypertension and hypokalemia. He has recently moved from the Middle East, where he was treated with potassium supplements and calcium-channel blockers with only fair response. On physical examination, he is short (59 in [149.9 cm]) and muscular with a full beard. His blood pressure is 152/106 mm Hg, and heart examination reveals a 2/6 holosystolic, nonradiating murmur and an S_4. He has no edema or flank bruits, and his skin is well tanned.

Laboratory test results:

Sodium = 144 mEq/L (136-142 mEq/L) (SI: 144 mmol/L [136-142 mmol/L])
Potassium = 3.2 mEq/L (3.5-5.0 mEq/L) (SI: 3.2 mmol/L [3.5-5.0 mmol/L])
Plasma ACTH = 210 pg/mL (10-60 pg/mL) (SI: 46.2 pmol/L [2.2-13.2 pmol/L])
Serum testosterone = 480 ng/dL (300-900 ng/dL) (SI: 16.7 nmol/L [10.4-31.2 nmol/L])
Serum 17-hydroxyprogesterone = 1960 ng/dL (<220 ng/dL) (SI: 59.4 nmol/L [<6.67 nmol/L])
Serum aldosterone = <4 ng/dL (4-21 ng/dL) (SI: <111.0 pmol/L [111.0-582.5 pmol/L])
Plasma renin activity = <0.6 ng/mL per h (0.6-4.3 ng/mL per h)
Serum cortisol = <1 µg/dL (5-25 µg/dL) (SI: <27.6 nmol/L [137.9-689.7 nmol/L])

Which of the following additional laboratory tests will reveal this patient's diagnosis?

A. Serum 17-hydroxypregnenolone measurement
B. Determination of the urinary cortisol-to-cortisone ratio
C. Genotyping the *CYP21A2* gene
D. Serum 18-hydroxycortisol measurement
E. Serum 11-deoxycortisol measurement

22 A 60-year-old woman is referred for evaluation of a left adrenal mass that was incidentally discovered during an evaluation performed for a transient episode of flank pain. She is normotensive and has no signs or symptoms of adrenal gland dysfunction. Her only medication is a bisphosphonate to treat osteoporosis. The mass measures 3.2 cm in diameter, the precontrast attenuation value is –5 Hounsfield units, and there is more than 50% contrast medium washout 10 minutes after contrast administration. The right adrenal gland is normal, and plasma metanephrines are normal.

Which of the following is the best test to screen for cortisol excess in this case?

A. Overnight dexamethasone-suppression test (1 mg)
B. 24-Hour urinary free cortisol measurement
C. Morning and evening serum cortisol measurement
D. Serum DHEA measurement
E. Plasma ACTH measurement

Calcium & Bone Board Review

Natalie Cusano, MD, MS

1 A 72-year-old woman with a history of myocardial infarction status post drug-eluting stent 8 months ago presents to discuss osteoporosis therapy. She had a fall at home resulting in fractures of T12 through L2. She is taking aspirin, clopidogrel, metoprolol, atorvastatin, and a calcium supplement with vitamin D. She has no history of radiation therapy. Recent DXA demonstrated T-scores of –3.7 at the lumbar spine, –3.2 at the femoral neck, and –2.9 at the total hip. Recent laboratory test results in the hospital were normal, including serum calcium, PTH, vitamin D, alkaline phosphatase, and renal function.

Which of the following osteoporosis therapies is contraindicated in this patient?

A. Alendronate
B. Zoledronic acid
C. Denosumab
D. Abaloparatide
E. Romosozumab

2 A 21-year-old woman is referred for a second opinion regarding hypercalcemia. She was noted to have a serum calcium concentration of 12.5 mg/dL (3.1 mmol/L) in the emergency department after presenting with nausea and vomiting due to gastrointestinal illness. Hypercalcemia has persisted in the subsequent months after recovery with calcium concentrations ranging from 11.9 to 12.3 mg/dL (3.0-3.1 mmol/L). She is otherwise healthy and has no history of kidney stones or fractures. She brings the following laboratory test results to her appointment:

Serum calcium = 12.3 mg/dL (8.2-10.2 mg/dL) (SI: 3.1 mmol/L [2.1-2.6 mmol/L])
PTH = 60 pg/mL (10-65 pg/mL) (SI: 60 ng/L [10-65 ng/L])
25-Hydroxyvitamin D = 31 ng/mL (30-80 ng/mL [optimal]) (SI: 77.4 nmol/L [74.9-199.7 nmol/L])
Magnesium = 2.3 mg/dL (1.5-2.3 mg/dL) (SI: 0.95 mmol/L [0.6-0.9 mmol/L])
Phosphate = 2.3 mg/dL (2.3-4.7 mg/dL) (SI: 0.7 mmol/L [0.7-1.5 mmol/L])
24-hour urinary calcium clearance-to-creatinine clearance ratio = 0.006
Calcium-sensing receptor (*CASR*) gene testing, negative for pathogenic variants

Her mother is normocalcemic. Her father is deceased, and she has no siblings or children. Neck ultrasonography and parathyroid sestamibi scan are negative for parathyroid abnormalities.

Which of the following is the best next step?

A. 4D CT of the neck and mediastinum
B. MRI of the neck and mediastinum
C. Referral to a surgeon for 4-gland parathyroid exploration
D. Genetic testing for *GNA11* and *AP2S1* pathogenic variants
E. Genetic testing for *PHEX* pathogenic variants

3 A 72-year-old woman with a history of breast cancer diagnosed at age 45 years status post lumpectomy, chemotherapy, and external beam radiation therapy with incidental radiation to the ribs presents for follow-up of osteoporosis. Osteoporosis was diagnosed at age 62 years after she presented with back pain due to nontraumatic fractures of T10 through T12. She has received

therapy with denosumab, 60 mg subcutaneously every 6 months for the past 10 years, and her last injection was 6 months ago. Her most recent bone density measurement demonstrates T-scores of −1.6 at the lumbar spine (+20.8% from baseline), −1.9 at the femoral neck (+9.1% from baseline), −1.1 at the total hip (+8.9% from baseline), and −1.8 at the one-third radius (+2.8% from baseline).

Which of the following should be recommended for this patient now?

A. "Drug holiday" from antiresorptive therapy
B. Alendronate, 70 mg weekly for 1 year
C. Ibandronate, 150 mg monthly indefinitely
D. Teriparatide, 20 mcg daily for 24 months
E. Romosozumab, 120 mg subcutaneously monthly for 12 months

4 A 45-year-old woman with a history of postoperative hypoparathyroidism following total thyroidectomy for benign goiter presents to the emergency department for perioral numbness and tingling. Her treatment regimen for hypoparathyroidism has remained stable over many years and includes calcium carbonate, 600 mg 3 times daily; calcitriol, 0.5 mcg twice daily; and vitamin D, 1000 IU daily. She states that she has had good treatment adherence. Her medical history is otherwise remarkable only for gastroesophageal reflux disease, and 3 days ago her treatment was changed from ranitidine to omeprazole, 20 mg twice daily.

Laboratory test results:

Serum calcium = 6.8 mg/dL (8.2-10.2 mg/dL) (SI: 1.7 mmol/L [2.1-2.6 mmol/L])
Albumin = 3.8 g/dL (3.5-5.0 g/dL) (SI: 38 g/L [35-50 g/L])
Intact PTH = <3 pg/mL (10-65 pg/mL) (SI: <3 ng/L [10-65 ng/L])
25-Hydroxyvitamin D = 32 ng/mL (30-80 ng/mL [optimal]) (SI: 79.9 nmol/L [62.4-199.7 nmol/L])
Phosphate = 5.3 mg/dL (2.3-4.7 mg/dL) (SI: 1.7 mmol/L [0.7-1.5 mmol/L])
Magnesium = 1.5 mEq/L (1.5-2.2 mEq/L) (SI: 0.6 mmol/L [0.6-0.9 mmol/L])

In addition to intravenous calcium gluconate infusion and calcitriol, 0.5 mg twice daily, which of the following therapies should she receive?

A. Calcium carbonate, 600 mg 4 times daily
B. Calcium citrate, 600 mg 4 times daily
C. rhPTH (1-84), 100 mcg subcutaneously daily, and calcium carbonate, 600 mg 4 times daily
D. PTH (1-34), 20 mcg subcutaneously twice daily, and calcium carbonate, 600 mg 4 times daily
E. Calcium carbonate, 600 mg 4 times daily, and hydrochlorothiazide, 25 mg daily

5 An 18-year-old woman presents for evaluation of a suspected calcium disorder and nephrolithiasis. She had a recent kidney stone that prompted laboratory testing, which revealed hypocalcemia, low PTH, and hypercalciuria. She has perioral numbness/tingling with exercise but has no other symptoms. Medical and surgical history is otherwise unremarkable.

Physical examination demonstrates negative Chvostek sign, no mucocutaneous candidiasis, no vitiligo, no neck scar, and normal nail beds.

Laboratory test results:

Serum calcium = 7.7 mg/dL (8.2-10.2 mg/dL) (SI: 1.9 mmol/L [2.1-2.6 mmol/L])
PTH = 9 pg/mL (10-65 pg/mL) (SI: 9 ng/L [10-65 ng/L])
25-Hydroxyvitamin D = 29 ng/mL (30-80 ng/mL [optimal]) (SI: 72.4 nmol/L [74.9-199.7 nmol/L])
Serum urea nitrogen = 13 mg/dL (8-23 mg/dL) (SI: 4.6 mmol/L [2.9-8.2 mmol/L])
Creatinine = 0.5 mg/dL (0.6-1.1 mg/dL) (SI: 44.2 μmol/L [53.0-97.2 μmol/L])
Estimated glomerular filtration rate = 167 mL/min per 1.73 m^2 (>60 mL/min per 1.73 m^2)
Phosphate = 4.8 mg/dL (2.3-4.7 mg/dL) (SI: 1.6 mmol/L [0.7-1.5 mmol/L])
Magnesium = 1.6 mg/dL (1.5-2.3 mg/dL) (SI: 0.7 mmol/L [0.6-0.9 mmol/L])
Urinary calcium = 380 mg/24 h (100-300 mg/24 h) (SI: 9.5 mmol/d [2.5-7.5 mmol/d])

Genetic evaluation documents an activating pathogenic variant in the *CASR* gene.

Which of the following is the best therapy for this patient?

A. Calcium carbonate, 500 mg 3 times daily, and calcitriol, 0.5 mcg daily
B. Calcium carbonate, 500 mg 3 times daily; calcitriol, 0.5 mcg daily; and hydrochlorothiazide, 25 mg daily
C. Calcium citrate, 500 mg 3 times daily, and calcitriol, 0.5 mcg daily
D. Hydrochlorothiazide, 25 mg daily, and calcium carbonate, 500 mg only with exercise
E. Calcium carbonate, 500 mg 3 times daily, and rhPTH (1-84), 25 mcg daily

6 A 69-year-old woman presents for follow-up of osteoporosis. Evaluation for secondary causes of bone loss at her initial visit last year was unremarkable, including a normal serum calcium and concurrent PTH concentration. She has had 2 injections of denosumab, 60 mg subcutaneously 6 months apart, with the last injection 1 month before her current visit. She is taking calcium, 500 mg twice daily, and vitamin D, 2000 IU daily. She has no other medical problems and is not taking any other medications.

Laboratory test results:

Calcium = 9.4 mg/dL (8.2-10.2 mg/dL) (SI: 2.4 mmol/L [2.1-2.6 mmol/L])
PTH = 121 pg/mL (10-65 pg/mL) (SI: 121 ng/L [10-65 ng/L])
25-Hydroxyvitamin D = 44 ng/mL (30-80 ng/mL [optimal]) (SI: 110 nmol/L [74.9-199.7 nmol/L])
Serum urea nitrogen = 13 mg/dL (8-23 mg/dL) (SI: 4.6 mmol/L [2.9-8.2 mmol/L])
Creatinine = 0.5 mg/dL (0.6-1.1 mg/dL) (SI: 44.2 μmol/L [53.0-97.2 μmol/L])
Estimated glomerular filtration rate = 167 mL/min per 1.73 m^2 (>60 mL/min per 1.73 m^2)

Which of the following is the best next step?

A. Order a parathyroid sestamibi scan
B. Refer to a parathyroid surgeon
C. Stop denosumab therapy
D. Increase vitamin D supplementation to 4000 IU daily
E. Measure PTH again in 5 months (before her next denosumab injection)

7 A 20-year-old woman is referred from orthopedics after a recent tibial stress fracture. Her fracture has successfully healed, and she has resumed regular activities. She runs 25 miles per week, with no increase in physical activity before her fracture. She follows a healthy diet rich in protein and fiber, although she avoids fats. She has amenorrhea.

Physical examination is notable for a BMI of 19.1 kg/m^2 and is otherwise normal, including findings on pelvic examination. Bone density is significant for Z-scores of −2.6 at the lumbar spine, −1.6 at the femoral neck, and −1.5 at the total hip. Laboratory evaluation is notable for low levels of estradiol and FSH but is otherwise negative for secondary causes of oligomenorrhea and bone loss.

Which of the following is the best treatment for this patient's bone health?

A. Combined oral contraceptive pill
B. Alendronate, 70 mg weekly
C. Denosumab, 60 mg subcutaneously every 6 months
D. Teriparatide, 20 mcg daily
E. Working with a dietician to resolve energy deficiency

8 A 72-year-old man is referred for evaluation of hypercalcemia incidentally noted on routine laboratory testing. He feels well and has no concerns. He was treated for tuberculosis 40 years ago, and a basal cell skin cancer was excised 20 years ago. There is no personal or family history of hypercalcemia. Physical examination findings are unremarkable.

Laboratory test results:

Serum calcium = 11.1 mg/dL (8.2-10.2 mg/dL) (SI: 2.8 mmol/L [2.1-2.6 mmol/L])
PTH = 40 pg/mL (10-65 pg/mL) (SI: 40 ng/L [10-65 ng/L])
25-Hydroxyvitamin D = 18 ng/mL (30-80 ng/mL [optimal]) (SI: 44.9 nmol/L [74.9-199.7 nmol/L])
1,25-Dihydroxyvitamin D = 75 pg/mL (16-65 pg/mL) (SI: 195 pmol/L [41.6-169.0 pmol/L])
Creatinine = 1.2 mg/dL (0.7-1.3 mg/dL) (SI: 106.1 μmol/L [61.9-114.9 μmol/L])

Urinary calcium = 90 mg/24 h (100-300 mg/24 h) (SI: 2.3 mmol/d [2.5-7.5 mmol/d])

24-Hour urine calcium clearance-to-creatinine clearance ratio = 0.011

Which of the following is the most likely diagnosis for this patient's hypercalcemia?

A. A. Familial hypocalciuric hypercalcemia
B. Primary hyperparathyroidism
C. Granulomatous disease
D. Calcitriol toxicity
E. Hypercalcemia of malignancy

9 A 65-year-old postmenopausal woman with stage 1 breast cancer and no evidence of metastatic disease has completed surgery and radiation therapy to the breast. She has no history of fractures. Her oncologist would now like to treat her with anastrozole (an aromatase inhibitor) for at least 5 years. The oncologist orders DXA, which demonstrates T-scores of −2.2 at the lumbar spine, −1.7 at the femoral neck, and −1.5 at the total hip. Vertebral fracture assessment is negative for fracture. The FRAX results do not meet treatment thresholds for either major osteoporotic fractures or hip fractures. The oncologist refers the patient for advice regarding bone health.

In addition to optimizing calcium and vitamin D, which of the following interventions should be recommended?

A. Zoledronic acid
B. Calcitonin
C. Teriparatide
D. Raloxifene
E. No intervention needed

10 A 62-year-old woman with osteoporosis has been taking risedronate, 35 mg weekly, for the past 2 years. She has been adherent to this regimen, other than 2 missed doses. She has not had any adverse effects. Repeated bone density testing is performed at the same center as her initial study. The report indicates a significant loss of bone mineral density in the spine and increases in bone mineral density in the femoral neck and total hip. The DXA images and numeric results are shown (*see images and table*).

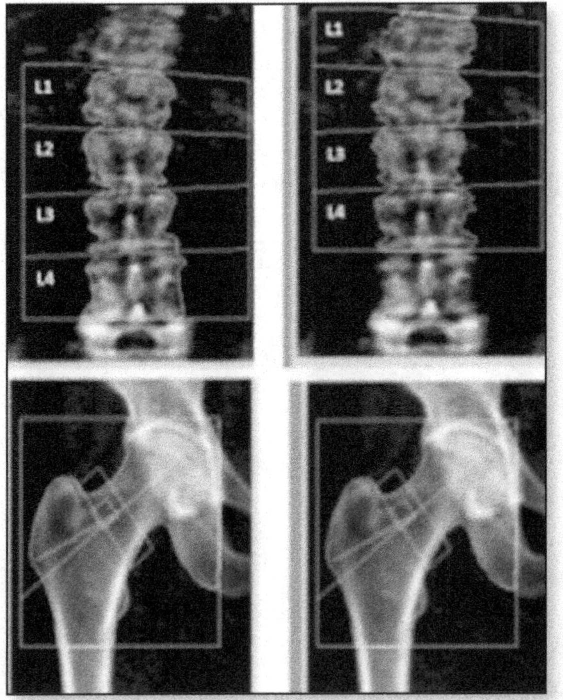

Site	Baseline bone mineral density	Follow-up bone mineral density
L1	0.451	0.423
L2	0.548	0.449
L3	0.593	0.549
L4	0.617	0.591
Total L1-L4	0.557	0.507
Femoral neck	0.480	0.532
Total hip	0.590	0.595

Which of the following is the best explanation for these findings?

A. She is not taking risedronate correctly
B. She is not responding to risedronate
C. She has an underlying cause of secondary osteoporosis
D. Her hip bone mineral density was measured incorrectly
E. Her spine bone mineral density was measured incorrectly

11 A 45-year-old woman presents with bilateral hip pain and the radiographic findings shown (*see image*). She underwent Roux-en-Y gastric bypass surgery for obesity 3 years ago and has lost more than 100 lb (45.5 kg).

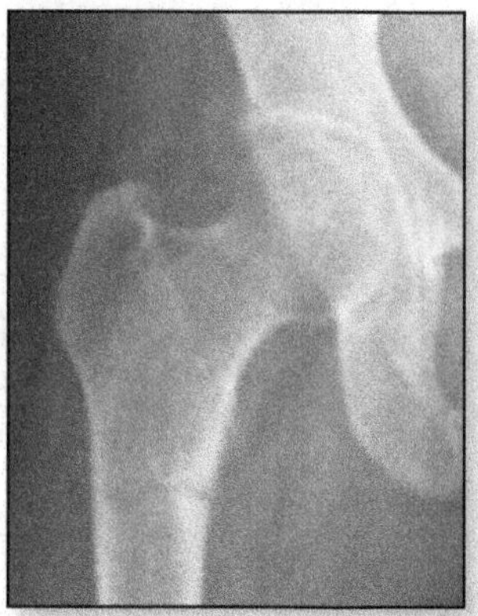

Laboratory test results:

- Serum calcium = 8.2 mg/dL (8.2-10.2 mg/dL) (SI: 2.1 mmol/L [2.1-2.6 mmol/L])
- Phosphate = 2.2 mg/dL (2.3-4.7 mg/dL) (SI: 0.7 mmol/L [0.7-1.5 mmol/L])
- Creatinine = 0.9 mg/dL (0.7-1.3 mg/dL) (SI: 79.6 µmol/L [61.9-114.9 µmol/L])
- Serum alkaline phosphatase = 346 U/L (50-120 U/L) (SI: 5.78 µkat/L [0.84-2.00 µkat/L])

Measurement of which of the following is most likely to provide this patient's diagnosis?

A. 25-Hydroxyvitamin D
B. 1,25-Dihydroxyvitamin D
C. FGF-23
D. Intact PTH
E. C-telopeptide

12 A 72-year-old man presents for evaluation after diagnosis of an L1 fracture that occurred when lifting a heavy package. He underwent pelvic irradiation for bladder cancer 5 years ago. He is otherwise in good health. He has regular follow-up with his oncologist.

On physical examination, he has tenderness over his lower spine. Four years ago, DXA revealed T-scores of −2.0 at the lumbar spine and −1.5 at the femoral neck with FRAX scores that did not meet treatment thresholds.

Current laboratory test results, including complete blood cell count, routine chemistries, alkaline phosphatase, PSA, 25-hydroxyvitamin D, serum/urine protein electrophoresis, and PTH, are all normal. Serum testosterone on a morning specimen is 270 ng/dL (300-900 ng/dL) (SI: 9.4 nmol/L [10.4-31.2 nmol/L]). SHBG is within the reference range.

Which of the following is the best next step in this patient's care?

A. Begin alendronate
B. Begin testosterone
C. Begin teriparatide
D. Refer for bone biopsy and possible kyphoplasty at L1
E. Obtain another DXA

13 A 64-year-old man with end-stage renal disease due to hypertension has been receiving hemodialysis for 10 years. He is referred for evaluation because of multiple vertebral fractures and a femoral neck T-score of −3.8 on DXA. Long-term medications include calcitriol, 0.5 mcg twice daily, and cinacalcet, 90 mg twice daily.

Laboratory test results:

- Serum calcium = 8.1 mg/dL (8.2-10.2 mg/dL) (SI: 2.0 mmol/L [2.1-2.6 mmol/L])
- Phosphate = 5.2 mg/dL (2.3-4.7 mg/dL) (SI: 1.7 mmol/L [0.7-1.5 mmol/L])
- 25-Hydroxyvitamin D = 24 ng/mL (25-80 ng/mL [optimal]) (SI: 59.9 nmol/L [62.4-199.7 nmol/L])
- PTH = 78 pg/mL (10-65 pg/mL) (SI: 78 ng/L [10-65 ng/L])
- Total alkaline phosphatase = 48 U/L (50-120 U/L) (SI: 0.80 µkat/L [0.84-2.00 µkat/L])

An iliac crest biopsy is done after double-tetracycline labeling.

While awaiting bone biopsy results, which of the following changes in management should be made immediately?

A. Increase the calcitriol dosage
B. Decrease the calcitriol dosage
C. Begin teriparatide
D. Begin denosumab
E. Decrease the cinacalcet dosage

14 A 55-year-old man with rheumatoid arthritis has been on a stable dosage of methotrexate and prednisone, 5 mg daily, for the past 3 years. DXA performed last month shows his lowest T-score to be −2.0 at the femoral neck. According to the FRAX calculator, his risk for major osteoporosis-related fracture is 12% and his risk for hip fracture is 1.1%. His only other health issue is Barrett esophagus for which he takes long-term proton-pump inhibitor therapy.

In addition to optimizing calcium and vitamin D, which of the following is the best therapeutic intervention?

A. Ibandronate
B. Zoledronic acid
C. Teriparatide
D. Denosumab
E. No intervention needed now

15 A 74-year-old man with osteoporosis has been on oral alendronate, 70 mg weekly, for 5 years. He has no known history of fracture. Current DXA shows T-scores of −2.0 at the lumbar spine, −2.2 at the femoral neck, and −1.6 at the total hip.

On physical examination, his height is 67 in (170 cm) (a decrease of 2.5 in [6.4 cm] over the past 4 years). He has moderate kyphosis without tenderness; gait and balance are normal. Laboratory testing documents normal levels of serum calcium, phosphate, creatinine, and 25-hydroxyvitamin D. Testosterone is at the lower end of normal. He expresses concerns about long-term adverse effects from bisphosphonates.

Which of the following should be the next step in this patient's management?

A. Continue oral alendronate
B. Discontinue alendronate but reassess in 1 to 2 years
C. Measure fasting serum C-telopeptide
D. Obtain lateral spine radiographs
E. Obtain radiographs of both proximal femurs

16 A 71-year-old man is referred after DXA documented a femoral neck T-score of −2.9. His only other medical issue is mild benign prostatic hypertrophy. He thinks he has a healthy sex drive and has no problems achieving or maintaining erections for intercourse. His overall strength and energy are good, and he is still working full time. His current height is 1.5 in (3.8 cm) less than his peak height. On physical examination, his BMI is 24 kg/m^2. He has no kyphosis and there is room for 2 fingers in the space between the ribs and iliac crests in the midaxillary line.

Laboratory test results:

Complete blood cell count, normal
Chemistry panel, normal
25-Hydroxyvitamin D = 35 ng/mL (30-80 ng/mL [optimal]) (SI: 87.4 nmol/L [62.4-199.7 nmol/L])
Urinary calcium excretion = 285 mg/24 h (100-300 mg/24 h) (SI: 7.1 mmol/d [2.5-7.5 mmol/d])
Serum testosterone (8 AM) = 285 ng/dL (300-900 ng/dL) (SI: 9.9 nmol/L [10.4-31.2 nmol/L])
SHBG, normal
LH = 6.0 mIU/mL (1.0-9.0 mIU/mL) (SI: 6.0 IU/L [1.0-9.0 IU/L])
Prolactin = 6 ng/mL (4-23 ng/mL) (SI: 0.3 nmol/L [0.17-1.00 nmol/L])
PSA = 6.5 ng/mL (<7.0 ng/mL) (SI: 6.5 µg/L [<7 µg/L])

Which of the following treatments should be recommended?

A. Testosterone gel
B. Testosterone gel plus finasteride
C. Hydrochlorothiazide
D. Risedronate
E. Teriparatide

17 A 55-year-old man is referred because of vitamin D deficiency and secondary hyperparathyroidism that were discovered after ankle fracture. His medical history is positive for class 3 obesity and hypertension. Lisinopril is his only medication.

On physical examination, his BMI is 48 kg/m^2 and blood pressure is 120/70 mm Hg. Examination findings are otherwise normal.

Laboratory test results (baseline):

- Serum calcium = 8.9 mg/dL (8.2-10.2 mg/dL) (SI: 2.2 mmol/L [2.1-2.6 mmol/L])
- Albumin = 4.0 g/dL (3.5-5.0 g/dL) (SI: 40 g/L [35-50 g/L])
- Intact PTH = 88 pg/mL (10-65 pg/mL) (SI: 88 ng/L [10-65 ng/L])
- 25-Hydroxyvitamin D = 8 ng/mL (30-80 ng/mL [optimal]) (SI: 20.0 nmol/L [74.9-199.7 nmol/L])
- Urinary calcium = 70 mg/24 h (100-300 mg/24 h) (SI: 1.8 mmol/d [2.5-7.5 mmol/d])
- Tissue transglutaminase antibodies, negative

Which of the following treatments should be recommended for this patient?

A. Cholecalciferol, 400 IU daily
B. Cholecalciferol, 1000 IU daily
C. Cholecalciferol, 4000 IU daily
D. Cholecalciferol, 10,000 IU weekly
E. Calcitriol, 0.5 mcg daily

18 An 82-year-old woman is admitted to the hospital with diffuse bony pain and a pathologic, atraumatic fracture of her left distal radius. She has not had regular medical care. Radiographs reveal widespread lytic and mixed (lytic/sclerotic) lesions throughout the appendicular and axial skeleton. On physical examination, a large breast mass is palpated, and needle biopsy confirms adenocarcinoma of the breast.

Laboratory test results:

- Serum calcium = 12.3 mg/dL (8.2-10.2 mg/dL) (SI: 3.1 mmol/L [2.1-2.6 mmol/L])
- Albumin = 2.8 g/dL (3.5-5.0 g/dL) (SI: 28 g/L [35-50 g/L])
- Creatinine = 6.2 mg/dL (0.6-1.1 mg/dL) (SI: 54.8 µmol/L [53.0-97.2 µmol/L])
- Intact PTH = <10 pg/mL (10-65 pg/mL) (SI: <10 ng/L [10-65 ng/L])
- 25-Hydroxyvitamin D = 8 ng/mL (30-80 ng/mL [optimal]) (SI: 20.0 nmol/L [74.9-199.7 nmol/L])
- Alkaline phosphatase = 320 U/L (50-120 U/L) (SI: 5.3 µkat/L [0.84-2.00 µkat/L])

After 24 hours of vigorous intravenous saline hydration, the following laboratory results are documented:

- Serum calcium = 11.0 mg/dL (SI: 2.8 mmol/L)
- Creatinine = 4.2 mg/dL (SI: 371.3 µmol/L)

The oncology team decides to treat her with a subcutaneous injection of denosumab, 120 mg.

In this patient, which of the following is the most likely adverse effect of this therapy?

A. Worsening renal function
B. Osteonecrosis of the jaw
C. A severe flulike syndrome
D. Impaired fracture healing
E. Severe hypocalcemia

19 A 32-year-old man undergoes total thyroidectomy for papillary thyroid carcinoma and is left with permanent surgical hypoparathyroidism. He takes elemental calcium, 1200 mg 3 times daily with meals; calcitriol, 0.5 mcg twice daily; and levothyroxine, 150 mcg daily. He feels well.

On physical examination, he has a well-healed thyroidectomy scar and negative Chvostek and Trousseau signs.

Laboratory test results 6 months after surgery:

- Serum calcium = 10.0 mg/dL (8.2-10.2 mg/dL) (SI: 2.5 mmol/L [2.1-2.6 mmol/L])
- Albumin = 4.0 g/dL (3.5-5.0 g/dL) (SI: 40 g/L [35-50 g/L])
- Phosphate = 4.9 mg/dL (2.3-4.7 mg/dL) (SI: 1.6 mmol/L [0.7-1.5 mmol/L])
- Urinary calcium = 380 mg/24 h (100-300 mg/24 h) (SI: 9.5 mmol/d [2.5-7.5 mmol/d])

Which of the following should be recommended now?

A. Continue current regimen
B. Decrease calcium supplementation
C. Add sevelamer (oral phosphate binder)
D. Add recombinant human PTH (1-84)
E. Add hydrochlorothiazide

20 A 19-year-old woman presents for follow-up of hypoparathyroidism. She was initially diagnosed at age 9 years after a seizure from severe hypocalcemia and has been maintained on calcium and calcitriol ever since. Over the past several months, she has noted anorexia, 10-lb (4.5-kg) weight loss, weakness, and dizziness.

Physical examination reveals a supine blood pressure of 80/60 mm Hg, pulse rate of 120 beats/min, and dystrophic fingernails and toenails.

Which of the following laboratory measurements is key to the diagnosis?

A. Serum ceruloplasmin
B. Serum iron studies
C. Transglutaminase antibodies
D. Serum cortisol and ACTH
E. Serum TSH

21 A 62-year-old man is referred for evaluation of muscle and bone pain, fatigue, weakness, spontaneous fractures, and difficulty walking. Symptoms began 4 years ago. Physical examination reveals diffuse bony tenderness, proximal muscle weakness, and ataxic gait. DXA documents T-scores of −3 to −4 at all sites.

Laboratory test results:

Chemistry panel, normal
Serum 25-hydroxyvitamin D = 28 ng/mL (30-80 ng/mL [optimal]) (SI: 69.9 nmol/L [62.4-199.7 nmol/L])
Serum 1,25-dihydroxyvitamin D = 12 pg/mL (16-65 pg/mL) (SI: 31.2 pmol/L [41.6-169.0 pmol/L])
PTH = 98 pg/mL (10-65 pg/mL) (SI: 98 ng/L [10-65 ng/L])
Serum phosphate = measurements ranging from 1.1 to 1.3 mg/dL (2.3-4.7 mg/dL) (SI: 0.36 to 0.42 mmol/L [0.74-1.52 mmol/L])
Maximum tubular phosphate reabsorption (phosphorus tubule maximum/glomerular filtration rate), low

Which of the following is the key diagnostic test to order next?

A. FGF-23 measurement
B. 24,25-Dihydroxyvitamin D measurement
C. 24-Hour urine collection for calcium, electrolytes, amino acids, glucose, and creatinine
D. *PHEX* gene testing
E. Sestamibi scan

22 A 61-year-old man is referred for evaluation of possible Paget disease. He was found to have an elevated alkaline phosphatase level on recent laboratory studies done before cataract surgery. He had bariatric surgery 15 years ago and takes cholecalciferol, 2000 IU daily. He has no chronic medical problems and has not been to a physician in the past 5 years. He feels generally well.

Laboratory test results:

Alkaline phosphatase = 220 U/L (50-120 U/L) (SI: 3.7 μkat/L [0.8-2.0 μkat/L])
Serum calcium = 8.6 mg/dL (8.2-10.2 mg/dL) (SI: 2.2 mmol/L [2.1-2.6 mmol/L])
Serum creatinine = 1.3 mg/dL (0.7-1.3 mg/dL) (SI: 114.9 μmol/L [61.9-114.9 μmol/L])
γ-Glutamyltranspeptidase, normal

Which of the following is the best next step in this patient's evaluation?

A. Whole-body bone scan
B. Skeletal survey
C. 25-Hydroxyvitamin D measurement
D. 1,25-Dihydroxyvitamin D measurement
E. Serum C-telopeptide measurement

23 A 57-year-old woman seeks advice regarding osteoporosis and fractures. She entered menopause 5 years ago and has not taken hormone therapy. During childhood, she sustained several long-bone fractures that were attributed to her active lifestyle and participation in sports. Her last childhood fracture was at age 15 years. Since menopause, however, she has sustained fractures at the wrist, humerus, and femur in low-trauma falls. Recent DXA reveals T-scores of −3.0 at the spine, −2.8 at the femoral neck, and −2.7 at the total hip. Her mother was diagnosed with osteoporosis at age 65 years.

On physical examination, she is a well-appearing woman without any dysmorphic features. Her height is 65 in (165.1 cm). Sclerae appear slightly greyish. She has no joint deformities or laxity. Her dentition appears normal. She wears bilateral hearing aids.

Laboratory test results:

- Complete blood cell count, normal
- Electrolytes, normal
- Calcium, normal
- Creatinine, normal
- Liver function tests, normal
- Alkaline phosphatase, normal
- TSH, normal
- 25-Hydroxyvitamin D, normal
- 1,25-Dihydroxyvitamin D, normal
- Intact PTH, normal

Sequencing which of the following genes will establish the diagnosis?

A. Osteoprotegerin gene (*TNFRSF11B*)
B. Type 1 collagen α 1 and 2 genes (*COL1A1*/*COL1A2*)
C. LDL receptor-related protein 5 (*LRP5*)
D. Vitamin D receptor gene (*VDR*)
E. Sclerostin gene (*SOST*)

24 A 57-year-old man has his third episode of nephrolithiasis. Analysis of the stone shows calcium oxalate. Evaluation demonstrates normal serum calcium and PTH levels, with a 24-hour urinary calcium excretion of 335 mg/24 h (100-300 mg/24 h) (SI: 8.4 mmol/d [2.5-7.5 mmol/d]), but normal 24-hour urinary oxalate, uric acid, sodium, and citrate levels. Urine volume is 2600 mL/24 h. His diet contains about 1000 mg of elemental calcium per day.

Which of the following recommendations would provide the greatest reduction in his risk of future calcium oxalate stone disease?

A. Begin hydrochlorothiazide
B. Begin allopurinol
C. Reduce dietary oxalate
D. Reduce dietary calcium
E. Increase fluid intake

25 An emergency department physician calls for advice regarding a 28-year-old woman with a 5-year history of postsurgical hypoparathyroidism. She presented with perioral numbness and tingling and muscle spasms. She has been nonadherent to her regimen of oral calcium and calcitriol. Her weight is 154 lb (70 kg).

Laboratory test results:

- Calcium = 6.5 mg/dL (8.2-10.2 mg/dL) (SI: 1.6 mmol/L [2.1-2.6 mmol/L])
- Albumin = 3.8 g/dL (3.5-5.0 g/dL) (SI: 38 g/L [35-50 g/L])
- Phosphate = 5.3 mg/dL (2.3-4.7 mg/dL) (SI: 1.7 mmol/L [0.7-1.5 mmol/L])
- Magnesium = 1.9 mg/dL (1.5-2.3 mg/dL) (SI: 0.78 mmol/L [0.6-0.9 mmol/L])
- Creatinine = 0.9 mg/dL (0.6-1.1 mg/dL) (SI: 79.6 µmol/L [53.0-97.2 µmol/L])

In addition to restarting treatment with oral calcium and calcitriol, which additional treatment would be best?

A. Intravenous bolus of 100 mg calcium chloride followed by a continuous calcium chloride infusion of 0.5 mg/kg per h
B. Intravenous bolus of 1 g calcium chloride followed by a continuous calcium chloride infusion of 2 mg/kg per h
C. Intravenous bolus of 150 mg calcium gluconate followed by a continuous calcium gluconate infusion of 1 mg/kg per h
D. Intravenous bolus of 150 mg calcium gluconate followed by a continuous calcium gluconate infusion of 1 mg/kg per h, rhPTH (1-84) 100 mcg subcutaneously daily
E. Intravenous bolus of 500 mg calcium gluconate followed by a continuous calcium gluconate infusion to achieve a total dose of 2000 mg calcium over 24 hours

26 A 28-year-old man is referred after an acute episode of renal colic. Imaging studies show bilateral kidney stones. Metabolic evaluation is consistent with primary hyperparathyroidism as illustrated by the following laboratory test results:

Serum calcium = 11.9 mg/dL (8.2-10.2 mg/dL) (SI: 2.98 mmol/L [2.1-2.6 mmol/L])
Serum PTH = 112 pg/mL (10-65 pg/mL) (SI: 112 ng/L [10-65 ng/L])
Urinary calcium excretion = 400 mg/24 h (100-300 mg/24 h) (SI: 10 mmol/d [2.5-7.5 mmol/d])

Following a sestamibi scan demonstrating a "probable" adenoma in the right lower pole, the patient undergoes minimally invasive parathyroidectomy with resection of 1 enlarged parathyroid gland. Pathologic examination confirms a hyperplastic adenoma. Two weeks later, he returns for blood work while taking elemental calcium, 600 mg twice daily.

Laboratory test results 2 weeks after surgery:

Calcium = 11.8 mg/dL (8.2-10.2 mg/dL) (SI: 2.95 mmol/L [2.1-2.6 mmol/L])
Phosphate = 2.2 mg/dL (2.3-4.7 mg/dL) (SI: 0.7 mmol/L [0.7-1.5 mmol/L])
Albumin = 4.2 g/dL (3.5-5.0 g/dL) (SI: 42 g/L [35-50 g/L])
PTH = 120 pg/mL (10-65 pg/mL) (SI: 120 ng/L [10-65 ng/L])
Serum creatinine = 1.0 mg/dL (0.7-1.3 mg/dL) (SI: 88.4 µmol/L [61.9-114.9 µmol/L])

Which of the following is the best next step?

A. Genetic testing for pathogenic variants in the calcium-sensing receptor gene (*CASR*)
B. Genetic testing for pathogenic variants in the multiple endocrine neoplasia type 1 gene (*MEN1*)
C. 4D CT of the neck
D. Repeated sestamibi scan
E. Cessation of calcium supplementation and recheck of laboratory tests in 1 month

27 A 56-year-old woman asks about stopping hormone replacement therapy. She has been taking transdermal estrogen, 0.05 mg twice weekly, and progesterone, 100 mg daily, for relief of vasomotor symptoms for the past 6 years. A recent DXA study showed a T-score of −2.2 at the femoral neck. She wonders what would happen to her bone density if she stops taking estrogen now.

Which of the following describes what will happen to her bone mineral density 1 to 2 years from now if she stops estrogen therapy?

A. Decreases gradually in the spine and hip (1%-2% per year)
B. Decreases rapidly in the spine and hip (3%-5% in the first year)
C. Decreases in the spine but not in the hip
D. Decreases in the hip but not in the spine
E. Remains stable

28 A 67-year-old man with chronic left hip pain was recently diagnosed with Paget disease of bone. His alkaline phosphatase level is 250 mg/dL (40-120 mg/dL) (SI: 4.2 μkat/L [0.7-2.0 μkat/L]), and his γ-glutamyltranspeptidase level is normal. Bone scan shows intense increased uptake in the left ilium, acetabulum, and femoral head. Radiographs show Paget disease in his left hemipelvis and femoral head, as well as moderate degenerative arthritis in the left hip. Treatment of his Paget disease with zoledronic acid is recommended. He wonders what to expect in the next few years.

Which of the following is most likely to occur?

A. Spread of Paget disease to the right hip
B. Hearing loss due to Paget disease
C. Worsening arthritis in the hip
D. Total resolution of all hip pain
E. Osteonecrosis of the femoral neck

Diabetes Mellitus Section 1 Board Review

Serge A. Jabbour, MD

1 A 43-year-old woman is referred for diabetes management. Diabetes was diagnosed at age 22 years, 1 year after she developed dermatomyositis. For a few months, the dermatomyositis was treated with high-dosage steroids, which were then tapered and stopped over a 9-month period. Her diabetes has been difficult to control. Her current treatment regimen consists of 260 units daily of basal and mealtime insulins. She has tried an SGLT-2 inhibitor but could not tolerate it because of recurrent genital mycotic infections. GLP-1 receptor agonists, tried twice, were not effective. Her premeal self-monitoring blood glucose values range between 180 and 300 mg/dL (10.0-16.7 mmol/L).

Her other medical problems include polycystic ovary syndrome, dyslipidemia, hypertension, hypothyroidism, and fatty liver. Her review of systems is notable for some fatigue, mild nocturia, and blurred vision. Her medications include insulin degludec, insulin lispro, metformin, rosuvastatin, fenofibrate, icosapent ethyl, ramipril, levothyroxine, and an oral contraceptive.

On physical examination, her blood pressure is 120/70 mm Hg and BMI is 22 kg/m^2. A photograph of the patient is shown (*see image*).

Laboratory test results:

- Hemoglobin A_{1c} = 9.0% (4.0%-5.6%) (75 mmol/mol [20-38 mmol/mol])
- Serum creatinine = 0.9 mg/dL (0.6-1.1 mg/dL) (SI: 79.6 µmol/L [53.0-97.2 µmol/L])
- Total cholesterol = 185 mg/dL (<200 mg/dL [optimal]) (SI: 4.79 mmol/L [<5.18 mmol/L])
- Triglycerides = 550 mg/dL (<150 mg/dL [optimal]) (SI: 6.22 mmol/L [<1.70 mmol/L])
- TSH = 2.5 mIU/L (0.5-5.0 mIU/L)
- TPO antibodies, positive
- ALT = 84 U/L (10-40 U/L) (SI: 1.40 µkat/L [0.17-0.67 µkat/L])
- Urine albumin-to-creatinine ratio = 240 mg/g creat (<30 mg/g creat)

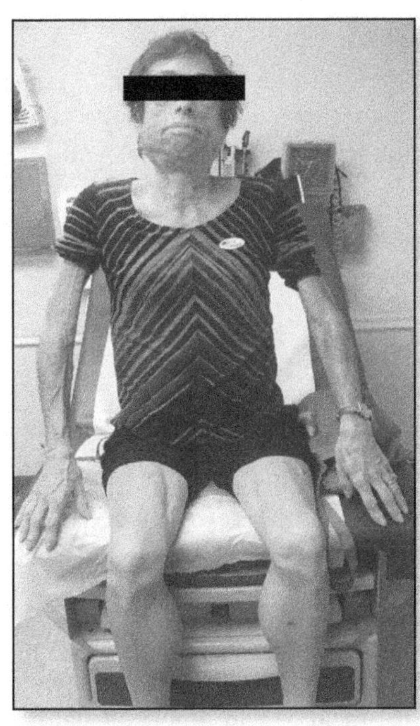

Which of the following should you order next to confirm the diagnosis?

A. Glutamic acid decarboxylase 65 antibody assessment
B. Urinary free cortisol excretion
C. Leptin measurement
D. *HNF1A* gene testing
E. Insulin receptor gene testing

5 A 48-year-old man is self-referred because of concern for metabolic complications due to his progressive weight gain. He has gained a total of 20 lb (9.1 kg) over the past 5 years, since he started antiretroviral therapy for HIV infection. He has a history of hypertension and dyslipidemia. His medications include rosuvastatin, amlodipine, and a combined antiretroviral regimen.

On physical examination, his BMI is 32 kg/m^2 and blood pressure is 135/86 mm Hg. He has truncal obesity and no cushingoid features.

Besides checking his lipid profile and ordering other pertinent tests, which of the following should be measured as the best method to screen him for diabetes?

A. Fructosamine
B. Hemoglobin A_{1c}
C. Fasting glucose
D. Glutamic acid decarboxylase 65 antibodies
E. C-peptide

6 A 65-year-old woman presents for follow-up regarding diabetes management. She is accompanied by her daughter who is very concerned about the patient's worsening gait problem. Type 2 diabetes was diagnosed 15 years ago. She was initially treated with metformin but more antidiabetes agents were added over the years, including basal insulin 4 months ago. Her glucose fingerstick values at home range between 180 and 250 mg/dL (10.0-13.9 mmol/L). She also has a history of hypertension, dyslipidemia, hypothyroidism, and acid reflux.

Her medications include metformin, 1000 mg twice daily; canagliflozin, 300 mg daily; liraglutide, 1.8 mg daily; insulin detemir, 20 units at bedtime; desiccated thyroid, 90 mg daily; atorvastatin, 40 mg daily; losartan, 50 mg daily; esomeprazole, 40 mg daily; biotin, 10 mg daily; and chromium, 1000 mcg daily. Her review of systems is significant for gait imbalance for the past 6 months. She describes it as unsteadiness leading to several near falls when she gets up at night. She also has numbness and weakness in both lower extremities. She has gained 6 lb (2.7 kg) in the past few months.

On physical examination, her blood pressure is 135/85 mm Hg and BMI is 33 kg/m^2. She has a mildly enlarged, firm, and asymmetric thyroid gland with a slightly bigger left lobe. She has muscle atrophy and loss of pinprick sensation in both feet, positive Romberg test, and loss of Achilles reflexes.

Laboratory test results:

Hemoglobin A_{1c} = 7.6% (4.0%-5.6%) (60 mmol/mol [20-38 mmol/mol])
Estimated glomerular filtration rate = 62 mL/min per 1.73 m^2 (>60 mL/min per 1.73 m^2)
TSH = 8.5 mIU/L (0.5-5.0 mIU/L)
ALT = 33 U/L (10-40 U/L) (SI: 0.55 μkat/L [0.17-0.67 μkat/L])
Hemoglobin = 12.2 g/dL (12.1-15.1 g/dL) (SI: 122 g/L [121-151 g/L])
Serum sodium = 140 mEq/L (136-142 mEq/L) (SI: 140 mmol/L [136-142 mmol/L])
Serum potassium = 4.2 mEq/L (3.5-5.0 mEq/L) (SI: 4.2 mmol/L [3.5-5.0 mmol/L])
Serum calcium = 9.4 mg/dL (8.2-10.2 mg/dL) (SI: 2.4 mmol/L [2.1-2.6 mmol/L])
25-Hydroxyvitamin D = 24 ng/mL (30-80 ng/mL [optimal]) (SI: 59.9 nmol/L [74.9-199.7 nmol/L])

Measuring which of the following would provide a diagnosis to explain her gait imbalance?

A. 8-AM serum cortisol
B. Serum magnesium
C. TSH after stopping biotin
D. Serum chromium
E. Serum vitamin B_{12}

7 A 63-year-old man is seeing you for diabetes management. He has a 20-year history of type 2 diabetes complicated by nonproliferative retinopathy and nephropathy. His premeal glucose fingerstick measurements at home are 200 to 225 mg/dL (11.1-12.5 mmol/L) in the morning and 325 to 375 mg/dL (18.0-20.8 mmol/L) in the evening.

His current medications are glimepiride, 2 mg daily; insulin glargine, 24 units at bedtime; rosuvastatin, 20 mg daily; and ramipril, 20 mg daily.

On physical examination, his blood pressure is 126/70 mm Hg and BMI is 32 kg/m². He has loss of pinprick sensation in both feet and 2+ edema in his lower extremities.

Laboratory test results:

Hemoglobin A_{1c} = 8.6% (4.0%-5.6%) (70 mmol/mol [20-38 mmol/mol])
Estimated glomerular filtration rate = 38 mL/min per 1.73 m² (>60 mL/min per 1.73 m²)
TSH = 2.5 mIU/L (0.5-5.0 mIU/L)
ALT = 33 U/L (10-40 U/L) (SI: 0.55 µkat/L [0.17-0.67 µkat/L])
Serum sodium = 138 mEq/L (136-142 mEq/L) (SI: 138 mmol/L [136-142 mmol/L])
Serum potassium = 4.8 mEq/L (3.5-5.0 mEq/L) (SI: 4.8 mmol/L [3.5-5.0 mmol/L])
Spot urinary albumin-to-creatine ratio = 910 mg/g creat (<30 mg/g creat)

In addition to adjusting the insulin glargine dosage and adding mealtime insulin, which of the following agents should be added to reduce the risk of progression of his diabetic nephropathy to end-stage kidney disease?

A. Linagliptin, 5 mg daily
B. Canagliflozin, 100 mg daily
C. Pioglitazone, 15 mg daily
D. Semaglutide, 7 mg daily
E. Pramlintide, 60 mcg 3 times daily

8 A 72-year-old homeless man is admitted to the hospital with severe hypoglycemia. He was found unconscious on the street; when brought to the emergency department, his glucose fingerstick concentration was 36 mg/dL (2.0 mmol/L). Blood was drawn, and intravenous dextrose was administered immediately.

His medical history is unknown, and it is not clear whether he is taking any medications.

Laboratory results:

Plasma glucose = 42 mg/dL (70-99 mg/dL) (SI: 2.3 mmol/L [3.9-5.5 mmol/L])
Plasma insulin = 35 µIU/mL (1.4-14.0 µIU/mL) (SI: 243.1 pmol/L [9.7-97.2 pmol/L])
Plasma C-peptide = 1.2 ng/mL (0.9-4.3 ng/mL) (SI: 0.40 nmol/L [0.30-1.42 nmol/L])
Plasma proinsulin = 88.2 pg/mL (26.5-176.4 pg/mL) (SI: 10 pmol/L [3.0-20.0 pmol/L])
Plasma β-hydroxybutyrate = 12.5 mg/dL (<3.0 mg/dL) (SI: 1201 µmol/L [<288 µmol/L])
Insulin antibodies, negative
Estimated glomerular filtration rate = 85 mL/min per 1.73 m² (>60 mL/min per 1.73 m²)
TSH = 2.5 mIU/L (0.5-5.0 mIU/L)

Which of the following most likely explains the laboratory findings?

A. Glipizide
B. Adrenal insufficiency
C. IGF-2–secreting tumor
D. NPH insulin
E. Hepatic failure

9 A colleague in primary care calls with a question about the diagnosis of diabetes mellitus. She screened an overweight (BMI = 28 kg/m²) 44-year-old man who has a grandmother and sister with diabetes. Neither of his parents has diabetes. Because the patient has sickle-cell disease, hemoglobin A_{1c} was not measured. Instead, a 75-g oral glucose tolerance test was performed and the following results were obtained:

Fasting glucose = 116 mg/dL (SI: 6.4 mmol/L)
1-hour glucose = 224 mg/dL (SI: 12.4 mmol/L)
2-hour glucose = 188 mg/dL (SI: 10.4 mmol/L)

On the basis of these results, which of the following should be recommended now?

A. Another oral glucose tolerance test with measurements of serum insulin to assess insulin resistance
B. Initiation of metformin to treat early type 2 diabetes
C. Weight loss and exercise to prevent type 2 diabetes
D. Another measurement of fasting glucose to exclude type 2 diabetes
E. Genetic screening for pathogenic variants known to cause maturity-onset diabetes of the young

10 A 54-year-old man is referred for management of diabetes. He has had diabetes for 4 years and is treated with metformin, 1000 mg twice daily, and glimepiride, 2 mg twice daily. He also has hypertension treated with ramipril, 10 mg daily, and dyslipidemia treated with atorvastatin, 20 mg daily. Proliferative diabetic retinopathy was diagnosed at his last eye examination 6 months ago, and he underwent panretinal photocoagulation. He has a history of multinodular goiter and benign findings on FNA biopsy 2 years ago. He has no concerns except that he has been unable to lose weight despite trying various diets.

On physical examination, his blood pressure is 130/80 mm Hg and BMI is 32 kg/m^2. He has a goiter with a left dominant nodule of approximately 2 cm.

Laboratory test results:

Hemoglobin A_{1c} = 8.7% (4.0%-5.6%) (72 mmol/mol [20-38 mmol/mol])
Creatinine = 0.7 mg/dL (0.7-1.3 mg/dL) (SI: 61.9 μmol/L [61.9-114.9 μmol/L])
TSH, normal

Once-weekly semaglutide is added.

Which of the following should be done at his follow-up visit, assuming he remains asymptomatic?

A. Amylase and lipase measurement
B. Calcitonin measurement
C. Monofilament testing
D. Creatinine measurement
E. Eye examination

11 A 44-year-old woman is referred for consultation regarding initiation of insulin pump therapy. Gestational diabetes requiring insulin was diagnosed at age 23 years. Type 2 diabetes was not diagnosed until 7 years later at age 30 years, and she was initially treated with metformin and glyburide. Her regimen was then switched to basal and mealtime insulin. Additional medications include flecainide, ramipril, atorvastatin, and coenzyme Q10.

Her medical history is notable for bilateral sensorineural hearing loss, macular pattern dystrophy with retinal pigmentation, Wolff-Parkinson-White syndrome, proteinuria, muscle weakness, and exercise intolerance that improved since she has been taking coenzyme Q10 supplementation. Her family history is notable for a sister who has insulin-dependent diabetes, profound hearing deficit, proteinuria, and renal impairment. Her brother is healthy. The patient has 1 child, a 21-year-old daughter, who is healthy.

On physical examination, her blood pressure is 118/65 mm Hg, and BMI is 22 kg/m^2. She has decreased sensation on monofilament testing of her feet.

Laboratory test results:

Hemoglobin A_{1c} = 7.8% (4.0%-5.6%) (62 mmol/mol [20-38 mmol/mol])
Estimated glomerular filtration rate = 55 mL/min per 1.73 m^2 (>60 mL/min per 1.73 m^2)
Urine albumin-to-creatinine ratio = 265 mg/g creat (<30 mg/g creat)

Which of the following tests is most likely to be positive?

A. Zinc transporter 8 (ZnT8) antibodies
B. Pathogenic variant in the *GCK* gene
C. Glutamic acid decarboxylase 65 antibodies
D. A3243G pathogenic variant in mitochondrial DNA
E. Pathogenic variant in the *HNF1A* gene

12 A 45-year-old woman is referred for discrepancy in her laboratory results. She has had type 2 diabetes for 6 years, hypertension, dyslipidemia, and iron-deficiency anemia.

Her medications include metformin, 1000 mg twice daily; repaglinide, 2 mg with each meal; atorvastatin, 20 mg daily; ramipril, 10 mg daily; iron; cinnamon; and biotin.

On physical examination, her blood pressure is 140/85 mm Hg and BMI is 34 kg/m^2. Examination findings are otherwise unremarkable.

Recent laboratory test results:

- Hemoglobin A_{1c} = 8.0% (4.0%-5.6%) (64 mmol/mol [20-38 mmol/mol])
- Serum 1,5-anhydroglucitol = 5 µg/mL (optimal range for patients with diabetes >10 µg/mL)
- Estimated glomerular filtration rate = 71 mL/min per 1.73 m^2 (>60 mL/min per 1.73 m^2)
- Serum creatinine = 1.1 mg/dL (0.6-1.1 mg/dL) (SI: 97.2 µmol/L [53.0-97.2 µmol/L])
- Hemoglobin = 10.5 g/dL (12.1-15.1 g/dL) (SI: 105 g/L [121-151 g/L])
- Urine albumin-to-creatinine ratio = 125 mg/g creat (<30 mg/g creat)

You add canagliflozin, 100 mg daily, and see her back in 3 months.

Her blood glucose fingerstick measurements are on average 80 to 130 mg/dL (4.4-7.2 mmol/L) fasting in the morning and 120 to 170 mg/dL (6.7-9.4 mmol/L) postprandially.

Laboratory test results:

- Hemoglobin A_{1c} = 6.8% (51 mmol/mol)
- Serum 1,5-anhydroglucitol = 4 µg/mL

Her primary care physician cannot explain why her 1,5-anhydroglucitol level remains less than 10 µg/mL despite her hemoglobin A_{1c} being less than 7.0% (<53 mmol/mol) and her blood glucose fingerstick measurements being at goal.

The laboratory discrepancy is most likely being caused by interference from which of the following?

A. Biotin
B. Iron
C. Undiagnosed sickle-cell trait
D. Cinnamon
E. Canagliflozin

13 A 56-year-old man with a 28-year history of type 1 diabetes has been using an insulin pump for 11 years with a rapid-acting insulin analogue. He has recently been experiencing recurrent high fasting blood glucose values. His diabetes is complicated by proliferative retinopathy, microalbuminuria with a stable creatinine concentration of 1.1 mg/dL (97.2 µmol/L), and peripheral sensory neuropathy. Examination of his logbook documents self-monitored blood glucose levels 4 to 5 times daily before meals. He has a bedtime snack most days. Most mornings, fasting glucose levels are in the high 100s to low 200s (10.0-12.2 mmol/L). He is seeking guidance about achieving better glycemic control. His current hemoglobin A_{1c} level is 7.8% (4.0%-5.6%) (62 mmol/mol [20-38 mmol/mol]).

Which of the following is the best recommendation?

A. Increase the basal insulin rate 2 hours before the time fasting hyperglycemia is occurring
B. Eliminate the bedtime snack
C. Change the method of insulin delivery to multiple daily injections
D. Do overnight basal testing
E. Increase the basal insulin rate overnight

14 A 42-year-old black woman has sickle-cell disease and type 2 diabetes. On point-of-care testing, her hemoglobin A_{1c} level is consistently 4.8% (29 mmol/mol) despite suboptimal control of blood glucose levels on metformin, 1000 mg twice daily, and insulin detemir, 40 units at bedtime. Fasting values on home glucose monitoring are 160 to 190 mg/dL (8.9-10.5 mmol/L).

Which of the following tests should be used to assess the adequacy of her glycemic control?

A. A laboratory-based hemoglobin A_{1c} assay
B. 2-Hour postprandial glucose measurement
C. Urinary glucose testing
D. Fructosamine measurement
E. C-peptide measurement

15 A 69-year-old man with interstitial pulmonary fibrosis is hospitalized with pneumonia and respiratory failure and requires ventilator support in the intensive care unit. There is no history of diabetes. At presentation, his random blood glucose concentration is 183 mg/dL (10.2 mmol/L). After treatment with methylprednisolone, his blood glucose climbs to 402 mg/dL (22.3 mmol/L) and remains in the range of 375 to 399 mg/dL (20.8-22.1 mmol/L).

Which of the following is the best approach to manage this patient's hyperglycemia?

A. Human regular insulin subcutaneously every 4 hours, adjusted to maintain blood glucose between 140 and 180 mg/dL (7.8-10.0 mmol/L)
B. Insulin drip titrated to maintain blood glucose between 140 and 180 mg/dL (7.8-10.0 mmol/L)
C. Insulin drip titrated to maintain blood glucose between 80 and 110 mg/dL (4.4-6.1 mmol/L)
D. Daily insulin glargine plus insulin aspart subcutaneously every 6 hours, adjusted to maintain blood glucose between 140 and 180 mg/dL (7.8-10.0 mmol/L)

16 An 18-year-old woman is seen for erratic blood glucose values. Type 1 diabetes was diagnosed 2 years ago, and a regimen of basal and mealtime insulins was initiated. Her glycemic control has always been adequate, with hemoglobin A_{1c} values around 7.0% (53 mmol/mol). However, a few weeks ago, she started to notice unpredictable blood glucose values with recurrent hypoglycemic episodes (blood glucose 45 to 60 mg/dL [2.5-3.3 mmol/L]). These episodes have occurred mainly after meals and have been accompanied by symptoms. Despite eating more snacks to prevent hypoglycemia, she has lost 4 lb (1.8 kg) in the past 2 weeks. She has no gastrointestinal concerns or dizziness. Her menses are regular. Her current medications are insulins glargine and lispro. Her blood pressure is 110/70 mm Hg, and BMI is 22 kg/m^2.

Physical examination findings are unremarkable.

Laboratory test results:

Hemoglobin A_{1c} = 6.7% (4.0%-5.6%) (50 mmol/mol [20-38 mmol/mol])
Serum cortisol (random) = 11 µg/dL (5-25 µg/dL) (303.5 nmol/L [137.9-689.7 nmol/L])
Electrolytes, normal
Creatinine, normal

Further workup is done.

An elevation in which of the following would most likely explain her hypoglycemia?

A. ACTH
B. Free T_4
C. Tissue transglutaminase IgA antibodies
D. 21-Hydroxylase antibodies
E. Glutamic acid decarboxylase 65 antibodies

17 A 26-year-old woman with an 8-year history of type 1 diabetes is now 6 weeks' pregnant. Her most recent hemoglobin A_{1c} measurement is 6.6% (49 mmol/mol). She is self-monitoring her blood glucose before meals, 1 hour after meals, and at bedtime. She takes insulin detemir, 10 units twice daily, and insulin aspart immediately before meals based on an insulin-to-carbohydrate ratio of 1:12 and a sensitivity (or correction) factor of 1:30, with a target glucose value of 90 mg/dL (5.0 mmol/L). Her blood glucose log for the past few days is shown (*see table*).

Day	Before breakfast	After breakfast	Before lunch	After lunch	Before dinner	After dinner	Bedtime
Day 1	89 mg/dL (SI: 4.9 mmol/L)	187 mg/dL (SI: 10.4 mmol/L)	111 mg/dL (SI: 6.2 mmol/L)	174 mg/dL (SI: 9.7 mmol/L)	85 mg/dL (SI: 4.7 mmol/L)	137 mg/dL (SI: 7.6 mmol/L)	118 mg/dL (SI: 6.5 mmol/L)
Day 2	72 mg/dL (SI: 4.0 mmol/L)	182 mg/dL (SI: 10.1 mmol/L)	68 mg/dL (SI: 3.8 mmol/L)	153 mg/dL (SI: 8.5 mmol/L)	82 mg/dL (SI: 4.6 mmol/L)	149 mg/dL (SI: 8.3 mmol/L)	96 mg/dL (SI: 5.3 mmol/L)
Day 3	89 mg/dL (SI: 4.9 mmol/L)	201 mg/dL (SI: 11.2 mmol/L)	84 mg/dL (SI: 4.7 mmol/L)	181 mg/dL (SI: 10.0 mmol/L)	85 mg/dL (SI: 4.7 mmol/L)	202 mg/dL (SI: 11.2 mmol/L)	88 mg/dL (SI: 4.9 mmol/L)

Which of the following changes would you recommend?

A. Increase the dosage of insulin detemir to 12 units twice daily
B. Allow 15 minutes between the bolus and the meal
C. Change the insulin-to-carbohydrate ratio to 1:15
D. Change the sensitivity factor to 1:20
E. Continue the same regimen

18 A 24-year-old woman without diabetes whose husband has type 1 diabetes is contemplating pregnancy and is inquiring about the risk of type 1 diabetes developing in her child. None of her family members has type 1 diabetes.

Which of the following characterizes the risk of type 1 diabetes developing in this patient's offspring?

A. 0.1%
B. 1.0%
C. 6.0%
D. 20.0%
E. 30.0%

19 A 26-year-old man with a 5-year history of type 1 diabetes is referred because he is interested in insulin pump therapy. He travels often for work, and he has an erratic eating schedule. However, he has good glycemic control, and he no longer wants to be on multiple daily injections. His current insulin regimen consists of insulin glargine, 22 units at bedtime, and insulin lispro, 6 units with each meal (total daily insulin dose: 40 units).

Self-monitoring of blood glucose shows values ranging between 80 and 130 mg/dL (4.4-7.2 mmol/L). He rarely has hypoglycemic events.

On physical examination, his BMI is 24 kg/m^2. Examination findings are unremarkable.

A recent hemoglobin A_{1c} measurement is 6.9% (4.0%-5.6%) (52 mmol/mol [20-38 mmol/mol]).

After he undergoes intensive education (basal/bolus concept, carbohydrate counting, etc), his current injection regimen should be switched to insulin pump therapy (with lispro) with which of the following parameters?

Answer	Basal rate (X units/h)	Carbohydrate ratio (1 unit/X g)	Sensitivity factor (1 unit/X mg/dL)
A.	0.9	20	60
B.	0.6	15	55
C.	1.2	15	45
D.	1.4	10	30
E.	1.0	10	60

20 A 33-year-old man with a 14-year history of type 1 diabetes has been on insulin pump therapy for 3 years. He describes recurrent episodes of mild hypoglycemia in the midafternoon that are characterized by sweating and anxiety. You examine his logbook and see documented hypoglycemic values between 50 and 64 mg/dL (2.8 and 3.6 mmol/L) approximately 5 times per week around 3 to 4 PM. The patient uses insulin glulisine in his pump.

There has been no change in physical activity.

Current pump settings:

Basal rates:

Midnight to 6 AM = 1.2 units/h

6 AM to midnight = 1.4 units/h

Correction (sensitivity) factor = 1 unit: 30 mg/dL glucose

Insulin-to-carbohydrate ratio = 1 unit: 8 g

The patient weighs 156 lb (70.9 kg) (BMI = 26 kg/m^2).

Which of the following is the best next step?

A. Increase his carbohydrate intake at lunch
B. Eat a carbohydrate snack at 2 or 3 PM
C. Change the prelunch carbohydrate ratio to 1:6
D. Perform basal rate testing from breakfast until dinner
E. Lower the basal rate to 1.2 units/h from noon to 6 PM

21 A 69-year-old man with a 15-year history of type 2 diabetes is self-referred to discuss newer therapies with good cardiovascular outcome data. He also has hypertension and dyslipidemia. He experienced a myocardial infarction 1 year ago and an ischemic stroke 4 years ago. His current medications include metformin, pioglitazone, lisinopril, metoprolol, rosuvastatin, and aspirin.

On physical examination, his blood pressure is 133/80 mm Hg and BMI is 35 kg/m^2. His examination findings are otherwise unremarkable.

Laboratory test results:

Hemoglobin A_{1c} = 9.0% (4.0%-5.6%) (75 mmol/mol [20-38 mmol/mol])
Creatinine = 1.2 mg/dL (0.7-1.3 mg/dL) (SI: 106.1 µmol/L [61.9-114.9 µmol/L])
Complete blood cell count, normal
Electrolytes, normal
Liver function tests, normal
TSH, normal

You recommend adding an agent that, besides improving his hemoglobin A_{1c}, has been shown in cardiovascular outcome trials to significantly lower the 3-point major adverse cardiovascular events.

Which of the following agents should be added?

A. Oral semaglutide
B. Once-weekly exenatide
C. Sitagliptin
D. Liraglutide
E. Alogliptin

22 The mechanism of action by which SGLT-2 inhibitors work is to:

A. Block and up-regulate SGLT-2 in the S3 segment of the proximal renal tubule
B. Lower the renal threshold for glucose excretion from 220 mg/dL to 180 mg/dL
C. Down-regulate SGLT-2 in the S1 segment of the distal renal tubule
D. Lower the renal threshold for glucose excretion from 220 mg/dL to less than 100 mg/dL
E. Block SGLT-2 in the distal renal tubule

23 A 20-year-old woman with cystic fibrosis affecting her lungs and liver would like to discuss her risk of having cystic fibrosis–related diabetes (CFRD) and how to screen for it. She has no family history of diabetes. Her BMI is 23 kg/m^2.

Which of the following is the best next step to screen her for CFRD?

A. Hemoglobin A_{1c} measurement
B. Fasting plasma glucose measurement
C. Oral glucose tolerance test
D. Random plasma glucose measurement when symptoms start
E. Fructosamine

24 A 62-year-old man with a 10-year history of type 2 diabetes presents for a follow-up visit. He has a personal history of cardiovascular disease, with a myocardial infarction that occurred at age 58 years. He also has a family history of heart disease. His current medications are lisinopril, 20 mg daily; metformin, 1000 mg daily; insulin lispro, 4 units before each meal; and insulin glargine, 20 units in the morning. He quit smoking 5 years ago after a 20 pack-year history. On physical examination, his seated blood pressure is 140/90 mm Hg and BMI is 30 kg/m^2.

Recent laboratory test results:

Hemoglobin A_{1c} = 6.8% (4.0%-5.6%) (51 mmol/mol [20-38 mmol/mol])
Fasting plasma glucose = 94 mg/dL (70-99 mg/dL) (SI: 5.2 mmol/L [3.9-5.5 mmol/L])
Total cholesterol = 189 mg/dL (<200 mg/dL [optimal]) (SI: 4.90 mmol/L [<5.18 mmol/L])
Triglycerides = 120 mg/dL (<150 mg/dL [optimal]) (SI: 1.36 mmol/L [<1.70 mmol/L])
LDL cholesterol = 135 mg/dL (<100 mg/dL [optimal]) (SI: 3.50 mmol/L [<2.59 mmol/L])
HDL cholesterol = 40 mg/dL (>60 mg/dL [optimal]) (SI: 1.04 mmol/L [>1.55 mmol/L])

Which of the following is the best treatment to address his lipid profile?

A. Pravastatin, 40 mg daily
B. Rosuvastatin, 20 mg daily
C. Lovastatin, 40 mg daily
D. Simvastatin, 20 mg daily
E. Atorvastatin 20 mg daily

25 A 43-year-old woman with a 32-year history of type 1 diabetes is feeling stressed and frustrated because she is having unpredictable hypoglycemia occurring at various times of the day, often within an hour or two after eating. She reports adherence to her insulin regimen (multiple daily injections) and has had nutrition education (carbohydrate counting) in the past and again few months ago. She has a history of diabetic peripheral neuropathy and diabetic retinopathy.

Review of systems reveals blurred vision and fluctuating weight. Her blood pressure is 121/79 mm Hg. A basic metabolic panel is unremarkable. Her glucose meter reveals glucose checks 6 to 7 times daily and highly variable glucose levels ranging from 40 mg/dL to more than 300 mg/dL (2.2-16.7 mmol/L) at various times during the day, with no appreciable pattern.

Which of the following is most likely to uncover the etiology of her hypoglycemia and glycemic variability?

A. Psychiatric evaluation
B. Cosyntropin-stimulation test
C. Gastric emptying study
D. Review of carbohydrate counting skills
E. Abdominal CT

26 A 60-year-old woman sees you for follow-up of type 2 diabetes and is concerned about vision changes. She has had diabetes for 16 years. She has a diagnosis of background retinopathy first noted 18 months ago. For the past month, she has had blurred vision, affecting the near and distant vision of both eyes. Her glucose control is stable with hemoglobin A_{1c} values ranging from 7.6% to 8.2% (60-66 mmol/mol) over the past 2 years. Her blood pressure is 132/78 mm Hg. Visual fields are intact to confrontation, tests of extraocular muscle movements are normal, and nondilated fundoscopic examination shows some microaneurysms and cotton wool spots.

Which of the following is the most likely cause of this woman's vision symptoms?

A. Retinal detachment
B. Macular edema
C. Vitreous hemorrhage
D. Cataracts
E. Mononeuritis of the third cranial nerve

27 A 23-year-old woman with a 15-year history of type 1 diabetes presents with a new skin lesion. She reports a nonpainful sore on her anterior left lower extremity that has enlarged over the past 3 months.

On physical examination, the following lesion is observed (*see image*).

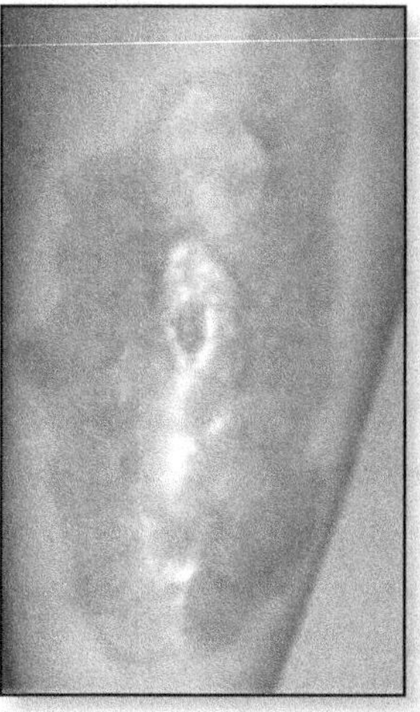

Diabetes-related necrobiosis lipoidica with early ulceration is diagnosed.

Which of the following approaches is most likely to result in complete resolution of this patient's skin lesion?

A. Kidney transplant without a pancreas transplant
B. Dipyridamole
C. Pancreas transplant with or without a kidney transplant
D. Intralesional corticosteroids
E. Topical glucocorticoid

28 An emergency department physician requests an endocrine consult to evaluate a 42-year-old man with a 21-year history of type 1 diabetes, recent hemoglobin A_{1c} value of 9.5% (80 mmol/mol), and a warm, edematous right foot. He has a history of diabetes-related peripheral neuropathy. Foot examination additionally reveals hammer toes without ulcers and a fallen arch on the right foot. Neurologic examination documents loss of protective sensation by monofilament and vibratory perception. He does not have a fever. Complete blood cell count and erythrocyte sedimentation rate are normal. A foot x-ray is shown (*see image*).

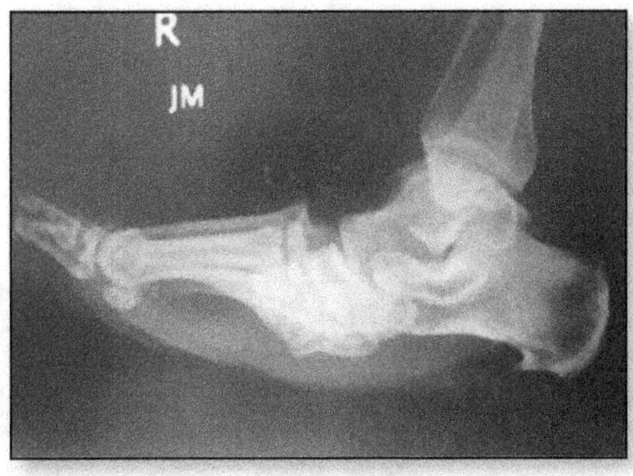

Which of the following does this patient most likely have?

A. Neuropathic arthropathy
B. Osteoarthritis
C. Septic arthritis
D. Pseudogout
E. Cellulitis

Diabetes Mellitus Section 2 Board Review

Michelle F. Magee, MD

29 A 52-year-old woman presents to the emergency department with left lower abdominal and vaginal pain and swelling. She is hospitalized with a new diagnosis of diabetes and has presented in diabetic ketoacidosis. Six days ago, she developed malaise, fever, and myalgias, which she thought was the flu. Four days ago, she had 1 episode of vomiting. Three days ago, she noticed onset of left-labial swelling and pain that has been worsening and now extends up her abdominal wall. She has no known relevant medical history and has not seen a physician in more than 10 years.

On physical examination, she appears unwell. Her temperature is 98.8°F (37.1°C), pulse rate is 130 beats/min, respiratory rate is 24 breaths/min, and blood pressure is 139/85 mm Hg. Lips and oral mucosa are dry. Her abdomen is soft with left lower-quadrant and suprapubic tenderness. There is no rebound or guarding. The left labium is indurated, and erythema extends to the lower abdominal wall. There is no palpable crepitus.

Laboratory test results:

White blood cell count = 19,700/µL (4500-11,000/µL) (SI: 19.7 × 10^9/L [4.5-11.0 × 10^9/L]) (lymphocytes, 7.5%; neutrophil absolute count, 14.3)
Sodium = 130 mEq/L (136-142 mEq/L) (SI: 130 mmol/L [136-142 mmol/L])
Potassium = 3.2 mEq/L (3.5-5.0 mEq/L) (SI: 3.2 mmol/L [3.5-5.0 mmol/L])
Chloride = 95 mEq/L (96-106 mEq/L) (SI: 95 mmol/L [96-106 mmol/L])
Carbon dioxide = 12 mEq/L (22-28 mEq/L) (SI: 12 mmol/L [22-28 mmol/L])
Serum urea nitrogen = 17 mg/dL (8-23 mg/dL) (SI: 6.1 mmol/L [2.9-8.2 mmol/L])
Creatinine = 0.4 mg/dL (0.6-1.1 mg/dL) (SI: 35.4 µmol/L [53.0-97.2 µmol/L])
Estimated glomerular filtration rate = 143 mL/min per 1.73 m^2 (>60 mL/min per 1.73 m^2)
Glucose = 380 mg/dL (70-99 mg/dL) (SI: 21.1 mmol/L [3.9-5.5 mmol/L])
Anion gap = 23
Hemoglobin A_{1c} = 13.9% (4.0%-5.6%) (128 mmol/mol [20-38 mmol/mol])

Abdominal CT is shown (*see images*).

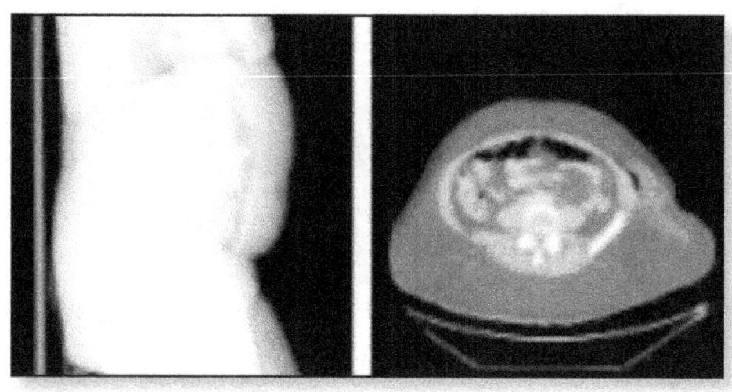

Which of the following diagnoses is most likely responsible for this patient's clinical presentation?

A. Necrotizing cellulitis
B. Cellulitis
C. Fournier gangrene
D. Pyoderma gangrenosum
E. Pyomyositis

30 A 62-year-old woman with a 22-year history of type 2 diabetes presents for routine follow-up. She recently developed unstable angina for which she underwent coronary artery revascularization. She also has hyperlipidemia, hypertension, chronic kidney disease, and congestive heart failure.

She takes insulin degludec U100, 30 units once daily; insulin lispro, 15 units before meals; aspirin,

81 mg daily; clopidogrel; carvedilol; metolazone; and furosemide. She previously took atorvastatin, 80 mg daily, but experienced severe myalgias. The dosage was reduced to 40 mg daily and she is tolerating this well. She is concerned about her new diagnosis of coronary artery disease and asks whether she should be taking any other medications to reduce risk for heart attack or stroke.

On physical examination, her BMI is 31 kg/m^2. Her blood pressure is 124/81 mm Hg, and pulse rate is 86 beats/min. Lungs are clear on auscultation, and the rest of her examination findings are normal except for mild reduction in sensation bilaterally in the feet.

Laboratory test results:

- Hemoglobin A_{1c} = 9.7% (4.0%-5.6%) (83 mmol/mol [20-38 mmol/mol])
- AST, normal
- ALT, normal
- Estimated glomerular filtration rate = 47 mL/min per 1.73 m^2 (>60 mL/min per 1.73 m^2)
- Total cholesterol = 135 mg/dL (<200 mg/dL) (SI: 3.50 mmol/L [<5.18 mmol/L])
- HDL cholesterol = 37 mg/dL (>60 mg/dL) (SI: 0.96 mmol/L [>1.55 mmol/L])
- LDL cholesterol = 78 mg/dL (<100 mg/dL) (SI: 2.02 mmol/L [<2.59 mmol/L])
- Triglycerides = 100 mg/dL (<150 mg/dL) (SI: 1.13 mmol/L [<1.70 mmol/L])

This woman is at very high risk for future atherosclerotic cardiovascular disease events. From the glycemic control perspective, she is advised to start taking a GLP-1 receptor agonist, which has been shown to reduce risk for adverse cardiac events based on large cardiovascular disease outcome trials.

According to the current American Diabetes Association and American College of Cardiology secondary atherosclerotic disease prevention recommendations, which agent should be added as the best next step to reduce this patient's risk of a future cardiovascular event?

A. Icosapent ethyl
B. Evolocumab
C. Coenzyme Q10
D. Colchicine
E. Ezetimibe

31 A 58-year-old man with longstanding type 2 diabetes and a kidney transplant has insulin resistance. He is taking U500 insulin via an insulin pump and uses continuous glucose monitoring. He follows a low-fat, consistent-carbohydrate diet. His weight is 277.2 lb (126 kg), and his hemoglobin A_{1c} level is 9.7% (83 mmol/mol).

Pump settings:

- Blood glucose target = 140 mg/dL (SI: 7.8 mmol/L)
- Basal rates: 12 PM-3 AM = 0.6 units/h
  - 3 AM-8 AM 0.8 units/h
  - 8 AM-12 PM 1.1 units/h
- Insulin-to-carbohydrate ratio = 1:9; delivered 30 minutes before meals
- Insulin sensitivity factor = 1:50
- Active insulin time = 6 hours

His continuous glucose monitoring report is shown (*see image*).

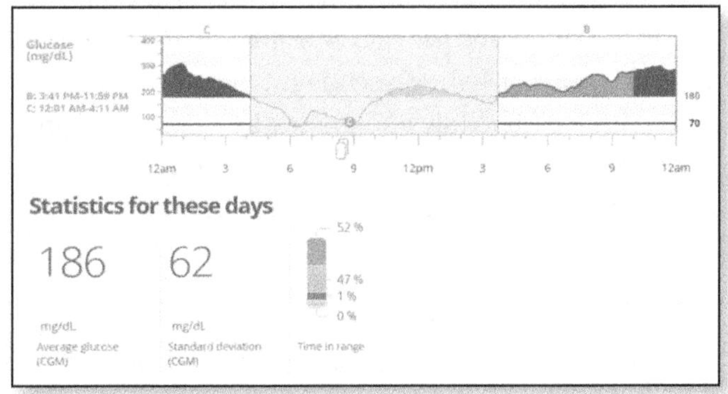

His 12 AM to 3 AM basal rate has been lowered several times in an effort to attenuate his nocturnal hypoglycemia, and progressive reductions in his insulin-to-carbohydrate ratio have been made to correct the hyperglycemia he is experiencing postprandially and during the first part of the night.

As a next step, which of the following single adjustments to his insulin pump regimen led to the improvement in the data shown on the follow-up continuous glucose monitoring report (see image)*?*

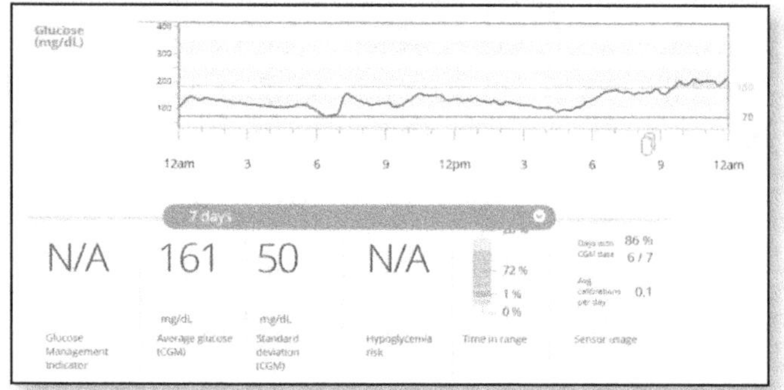

A. A meal bolus 45 minutes before meals
B. An increase in the insulin-to-carbohydrate ratio
C. An increase in basal insulin from 4 PM to 12 AM
D. A change in mealtime insulin to faster-acting insulin aspart injections
E. A reduction in basal insulin from 3 AM to 8 AM

32 A 28-year-old woman who is 14 weeks pregnant has had type 1 diabetes since age 11 years. She has hypoglycemia unawareness. She has an erratic schedule and misses 1 or more insulin doses at least 3 to 4 days each week. This leads to hyperglycemia necessitating correction doses of insulin. She was found unconscious by her 3-year-old son who alerted his grandmother. When emergency medical technicians arrived at her home, her blood glucose was undetectable and D50 was administered with limited response. In the emergency department, her blood glucose concentration was 117 mg/dL (6.5 mmol/L), but it subsequently dropped to 53 mg/dL (2.9 mmol/L).

Her home regimen consists of insulin glargine, 30 units daily, and insulin lispro, 12 units with meals. She recalls beginning to prepare a late breakfast at home and having marked nausea. The next thing she remembers is regaining consciousness in the emergency department.

Her medical history includes labile glycemic control with recurrent severe hypoglycemic episodes (including during 7 previous pregnancies), spontaneous abortions, and preeclampsia.

Hemoglobin A_{1c} = 9.2% (4.0%-5.6%)
(77 mmol/mol [20-38 mmol/mol])
Creatinine = 1.9 mg/dL (0.6-1.1 mg/dL)
(SI: 168.0 μmol/L [53.0-97.2 μmol/L])

Results from her blood glucose monitoring and insulin dosing record are shown (*see table*).

She is provided survival skills diabetes education, including guidance for a consistent carbohydrate diet.

Day	Overnight	Prebreakfast	2 hours after breakfast	Lunch	2 hours after lunch	Dinner	2 hours after dinner	Bedtime
1	No check	202 mg/dL (SI: 11.2 mmol/L) +5u +2c	**50*** mg/dL (SI: 2.8 mmol/L) f/up 109 mg/dL (SI: 6.0 mmol/L)	131 mg/dL (SI: 7.3 mmol/L)	154 mg/dL (SI: 8.5 mmol/L) +5u	**70*** mg/dL (SI: 3.9 mmol/L) +5u	132 mg/dL (SI: 7.3 mmol/L)	158 mg/dL (SI: 8.8 mmol/L) 18 units glargine
2	**40*** mg/dL (SI: 2.2 mmol/L) f/up 171 mg/dL (SI: 9.5 mmol/L)	147 mg/dL (SI: 8.2 mmol/L) +5u	147 mg/dL (SI: 8.2 mmol/L)	80-**61*** mg/dL (SI: 4.4-3.4 mmol/L) +5u	112 mg/dL (SI: 6.2 mmol/L)	117 mg/dL (SI: 11.2 mmol/L) +5u	202 mg/dL (SI: 11.2 mmol/L) +2c	127 mg/dL (SI: 7.0 mmol/L) 14 units glargine
3		**60*** mg/dL (SI: 3.3 mmol/L) f/up 143 mg/dL (SI: 7.9 mmol/L) +5u	**48*** mg/dL (SI: 2.7 mmol/L) f/up 85 mg/dL (SI: 4.7 mmol/L)	151 mg/dL (SI: 2.7 mmol/L) +5u				

* Treated for hypoglycemia. + Denotes rapid-acting insulin analogue dose where +u = scheduled dose and +c = correction dose; f/u = follow-up blood glucose.

Answer	Hemoglobin A_{1c} target	Blood glucose targets	Glargine dose	Prandial dose	Correction factor
A.	<6.0%	Fasting blood glucose <95 mg/dL; 2-hour postprandial <120 mg/dL	12 units	I:C = 1:12	1/50 if >95 mg/dL
B.	<7.0%	Fasting blood glucose <95 mg/dL; 2-hour postprandial <120 mg/dL	7 units	I:C = 1:10	1/60 if >120 mg/dL
C.	<6.0%	Fasting blood glucose <120 mg/dL; 2-hour postprandial <150 mg/dL	14 units	3 units	1/50 if >150 mg/dL
D.	<7.0%	Fasting blood glucose <120 mg/dL; 2-hour postprandial <150 mg/dL	12 units	3 units	1/60 if >150 mg/dL
E.	<8.0%	Fasting blood glucose <140 mg/dL; 2-hour postprandial <180 mg/dL	7 units	2 units	1/70 if >180 mg/dL

Which of the above regimens would should be recommended for this pregnant woman with type 1 diabetes upon hospital discharge (see table*)?*

33 A 42-year-old woman has type 1 diabetes that was diagnosed at age 14 years, hypertension, end-stage renal disease (on hemodialysis), coronary artery disease with percutaneous coronary intervention (× 2), and hyperlipidemia. She presents with pain, edema, and discomfort over the right thigh adjacent to her femoral permanent dialysis catheter insertion site. The discomfort has progressively worsened over the past 1 to 2 weeks.

On physical examination, she is in no acute distress. Her oral temperature is 98.1°F (36.7°C), pulse rate is 92 beats/min, respiratory rate is 17 breaths/min, and blood pressure is 150/71 mm Hg. The arteriovenous graft in the left upper extremity has no thrill or bruit present. There is no localized inflammation or exudate at the site of the femoral permanent dialysis catheter. There is a diffuse well-demarcated area of swelling over the upper two-thirds of the thigh in a mediolateral distribution that is tender and without erythema. She has no pedal edema or foot lesions, and pedal pulses are 1+ and equal bilaterally.

Laboratory test results:

White blood cell count = 9900/μL (4500-11,000/μL) (SI: 9.9×10^9/L [$4.5\text{-}11.0 \times 10^9$/L])
Hemoglobin = 7.8 g/dL (12.1-15.1 g/dL) (SI: 78 g/L [121-151 g/L])
Hematocrit = 25.8% (35%-45%) (SI: 0.258 [0.35-0.45])
Platelet count = 402×10^3/μL ($150\text{-}450 \times 10^3$/μL) (SI: 402×10^9/L [$150\text{-}450 \times 10^9$/L])
Glucose = 119 mg/dL (70-99 mg/dL) (SI: 6.6 mmol/L [3.9-5.5 mmol/L])
Hemoglobin A_{1c} = 10.6% (4.0%-5.6%) (92 mmol/mol [20-38 mmol/mol])

MRI without contrast of the right lower extremity is shown (*see images*).

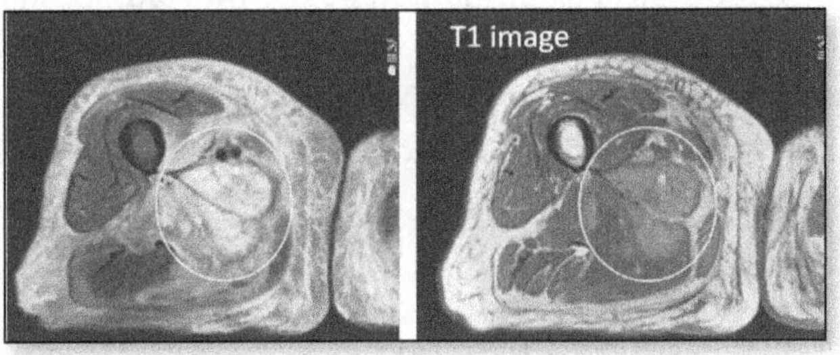

Which of the following is the most likely etiology of the thigh swelling and pain in this patient with type 1 diabetes?

A. Diabetes-related muscle infarction
B. Hematoma
C. Gangrenous myositis
D. Muscle denervation
E. Infectious myositis/pyomyositis

34 A 41-year-old man with a history of cardiomyopathy, heart failure with reduced ejection fraction (ejection fraction = 25%-30%), hypertension, morbid obesity, type 2 diabetes, chronic kidney disease, and a venous stasis ulcer has been admitted to the hospital with an acute heart failure exacerbation. His care is being managed by the advanced heart failure team who asks for an endocrine consultation because his hemoglobin A_{1c} level is 11.0% (97 mmol/mol) and estimated glomerular filtration rate is 25 mL/min per 1.73 m^2. The team would like an opinion on starting an SGLT-2 inhibitor in view of the encouraging results of recent large cardiovascular outcome trials that have demonstrated reduction in hospitalizations for heart failure.

His most recent insulin regimen at home consisted of insulin glargine, 25 units in the morning, and insulin aspart, 10 units with meals. He reports often missing his mealtime insulin doses and eating poorly as he travels a lot for work.

On physical examination, he has morbid obesity (BMI = 42 kg/m^2), jugular venous distension to the midneck, 2+ to 3+ lower-extremity edema, a left ankle stasis ulcer, and reduced 10-g monofilament sensation below the knee.

Laboratory test results:

- Sodium = 143 mEq/L (136-142 mEq/L)
  (SI: 143 mmol/L [136-142 mmol/L])
- Potassium = 4.3 mEq/L (3.5-5.0 mEq/L)
  (SI: 4.3 mmol/L [3.5-5.0 mmol/L])
- Chloride = 109 mEq/L (96-106 mEq/L)
  (SI: 109 mmol/L [96-106 mmol/L])
- Bicarbonate = 25 mEq/L (21-28 mEq/L)
  (SI: 25 mmol/L [21-28 mmol/L])
- Serum urea nitrogen = 25 mg/dL (8-23 mg/dL)
  (SI: 8.9 mmol/L [2.9-8.2 mmol/L])
- Creatinine = 2.5 mg/dL (0.7-1.3 mg/dL)
  (SI: 221 μmol/L [61.9-114.9 μmol/L])
- Estimated glomerular filtration rate = 29 mL/min per 1.73 m^2 (>60 mL/min per 1.73 m^2)
- Glucose = 154 mg/dL (70-99 mg/dL)
  (SI: 8.5 mmol/L [3.9-5.5 mmol/L])

While in the hospital, his treatment regimen consists of insulin glargine, 25 units nightly, and linagliptin, 5 mg daily, with blood glucose values ranging from 148 to 202 mg/dL (8.2-11.2 mmol/L).

Which of the following should be recommended for combination therapy with basal insulin as the safest medication that has the potential to positively influence this patient's cardiovascular outcomes?

A. Dapagliflozin
B. Dulaglutide
C. Saxagliptin
D. Linagliptin
E. Metformin

35 A 53-year-old woman with an 18-year history of type 2 diabetes, hypertension complicated by chronic kidney disease, proliferative retinopathy, peripheral neuropathy, peripheral vascular disease, and toe amputation has been admitted to the hospital following several syncopal episodes. An endocrine consult is requested to assess whether dysautonomia could have a role in her presentation and, if so, to recommend how to manage her supine hypertension.

She is recovering from a recent viral syndrome and describes 2 episodes before hospital admission that occurred after she attempted to get up and ambulate. She became lightheaded, had palpitations, and fell to the ground. For several years, she has been having lightheadedness if she gets up quickly, especially in the morning. She has blunted hypoglycemia awareness. She has not noticed early satiety. She has a tendency to be constipated. She reports often eating fast food, and home meals include processed and canned foods. She does not exercise.

Medications include insulin detemir, insulin aspart with meals, metoprolol extended release, losartan, atorvastatin, and aspirin.

On physical examination, she is in no acute distress. She is obese (BMI = 30 kg/m^2). Her temperature is 98.2°F (36.8°C), pulse rate is 92 beats/min, and blood pressure is 176/84 mm Hg supine. When standing, her blood pressure drops 49 mm Hg systolic and 22 mm Hg diastolic. Her heart rate does not increase concomitantly with the fall in blood pressure. Findings on head and neck examination are normal. Findings on cardiorespiratory examination are normal. There is markedly decreased sensation in both feet to 10 g monofilament.

Laboratory test results:

- Blood glucose = ranges from 101-140 mg/dL (70-99 mg/dL) (SI: ranges from 5.6-7.8 mmol/L [3.9-5.5 mmol/L])
- Hemoglobin A_{1c} = 10.3% (4.0%-5.6%) (89 mmol/mol [20-38 mmol/mol])
- Creatinine (at admission) = 2.1 mg/dL (0.6-1.1 mg/dL) (SI: 185.6 μmol/L [53.0-97.2 μmol/L])
- Creatinine (current) = 1.4 mg/dL (0.6-1.1 mg/dL) (SI: 123.8 μmol/L [53.0-97.2 μmol/L])
- Urine albumin-to-creatinine ratio = 1654.7 mg/g (<30 mg/g creat)
- Hemoglobin = 9.8 g/dL (12.1-15.1 g/dL) (SI: 98 g/L [121-151 g/L])
- Hematocrit = 32.3% (35%-45%) (SI: 0.323 [0.35-0.45])

Despite requiring fluids and discontinuing all antihypertensive agents upon hospital admission, systolic blood pressures are around 180 mm Hg while recumbent, coupled with overt orthostatic hypotension with persistent drop in systolic blood pressure greater than 20 mm Hg and drop in diastolic blood pressure greater than 10 mm Hg upon standing. Echocardiography demonstrates normal left ventricular ejection fraction and evidence of diastolic dysfunction. Autonomic neuropathy with orthostatic hypotension and marked supine hypertension are diagnosed.

In addition to avoiding the supine position during the day and raising the head of her bed, which pharmacologic intervention should be recommended at bedtime to treat her supine hypertension?

A. Clonidine
B. Propranolol
C. Hydralazine
D. Ibuprofen
E. Midodrine

36 An 80-year-old man with longstanding type 2 diabetes, hypertension, and hyperlipidemia presents for a routine follow-up visit. He has been missing some mealtime insulin boluses and "lets his sugars stay over 200 mg/dL" in view of his history of severe hypoglycemia. He has been wearing his continuous glucose monitor on the right side and administering most of his injections in the left lower side of his abdomen. When he injects into other sites, he reports that he is more likely to become hypoglycemic. He frequently reuses his insulin pen needles.

Medications include insulin detemir, 30 units daily; insulin lispro, 12 to 16 units with meals; canagliflozin; enalapril; and rosuvastatin.

The continuous glucose sensor insertion site in the right upper abdominal quadrant is clear, and his most common insulin injection site in the left lower quadrant is shown in the photograph (*see image*).

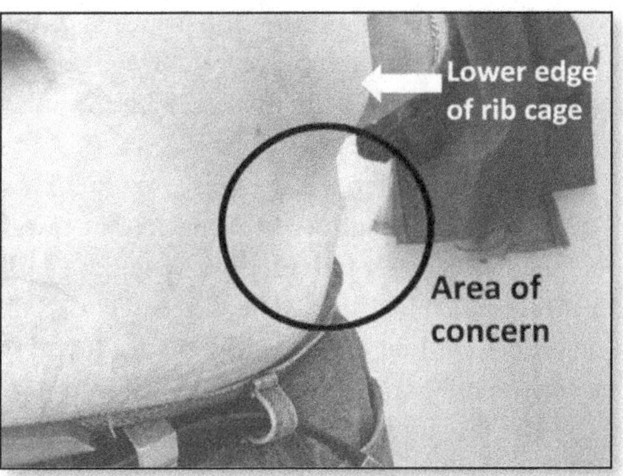

A similar area of depression is also seen to a lesser extent in the right lower quadrant of his abdomen.

His hemoglobin A_{1c} level is 8.4% (68 mmol/mol), and the percentage of time his blood glucose is in the desired target range is 72%.

Which of the following treatment strategies is most likely to address the underlying pathophysiologic process taking place at his insulin injection sites?

A. Rotating insulin injection sites
B. Applying topical cromolyn
C. Avoiding reuse of needles
D. Adding dexamethasone to the insulin
E. Injecting anabolic steroid into the site

37 A 46-year-old woman asks whether she should be screened for diabetes, as both of her older siblings have it. She has no symptoms, and does not have hypertension, dyslipidemia, or a personal history of cardiovascular disease. Her only medication is a daily multivitamin. She does not smoke cigarettes and walks for exercise most days.

On physical examination, her blood pressure is 124/78 mm Hg and BMI is 22 kg/m^2. The rest of her examination findings are unremarkable.

When should this patient be screened for diabetes?

A. Now
B. At age 50 years
C. Only if she develops hypertension
D. If her BMI increases to greater than 25 kg/m^2
E. If her triglyceride concentration is greater than 150 mg/dL (>1.70 mmol/L)

38 A 31-year-old man with type 1 diabetes diagnosed 3 months ago presents with episodes of recurrent hypoglycemia. He is on a regimen of multiple daily insulin injections. His current hemoglobin A_{1c} level is 6.3% (45 mmol/mol), which has decreased from 9.2% (77 mmol/mol) at diagnosis. He checks fingerstick blood glucose values 4 to 6 times daily (before and/or after meals and at bedtime). The past few weeks, his blood glucose values after meals have frequently been between 70 and 80 mg/dL (3.9-4.4 mmol/L). He also has fasting hypoglycemia (50-70 mg/dL [2.8-3.9 mmol/L]) once or twice weekly.

How should this patient be advised patient regarding the best course of action now?

A. Reduce basal insulin doses by 10% to 20%
B. Reduce all insulin doses by 10% to 20%
C. Reduce premeal insulin by 10% to 20%
D. Increase carbohydrate intake to at least 50 g with each meal

39 A 43-year-old woman presents for follow-up of type 2 diabetes, which was diagnosed 3 months ago. At diagnosis, her hemoglobin A_{1c} level was 8.7% (72 mmol/mol). Her BMI at that time was 35 kg/m^2. She enrolled in a commercial weight-loss program with prepackaged meals and is exercising 5 days a week. She has lost 10 lb (4.5 kg). She is taking metformin monotherapy, 1500 mg daily.

Laboratory test results from today's visit:

Hemoglobin A_{1c} = 7.9% (4.0%-5.6%)
(63 mmol/mol [20-38 mmol/mol])
Fasting blood glucose = 146 mg/dL (70-99 mg/dL)
(SI: 8.1 mmol/L [3.9-5.5 mmol/L])

Which of the following is the best next step to improve her glycemic control?

A. Stop metformin; begin insulin glargine
B. Continue metformin; add dulaglutide
C. Increase the metformin dosage
D. Stop metformin; begin empagliflozin
E. Continue metformin; add sitagliptin

40 Diabetes mellitus was recently diagnosed in a 56-year-old woman when she was found to have a fasting plasma glucose concentration of 147 mg/dL (8.2 mmol/L) at her annual physical. She has no symptoms of hyperglycemia.

Other abnormal laboratory values:

AST = 119 U/L (20-48 U/L) (SI: 2.0 μkat/L [0.33-0.80 μkat/L])
ALT = 134 U/L (10-40 U/L) (SI: 2.3 μkat/L [0.17-0.67 μkat/L])
Hemoglobin A_{1c} = 6.9% (4.0%-5.6%)
(52 mmol/mol [20-38 mmol/mol])

She has no family history of diabetes. Several of her relatives have had liver disease, but she does not know the cause. She has had oligomenorrhea for several years and has not had a period for more than 4 months.

On physical examination, she has a mildly enlarged, nontender liver. There is no ascites or other signs of chronic liver disease, and she does not have pedal edema. Liver ultrasonography shows a mildly enlarged liver without masses, no evidence of steatosis, and no biliary disease. Hepatitis (A, B, C) serologies are negative.

Which of the following tests is most likely to reveal the etiology of her diabetes?

A. *HNF1A* genetic testing
B. Zinc transporter 8 (ZnT8) antibody measurement
C. Transferrin saturation
D. Serum ceruloplasmin measurement
E. Mitochondrial antibody titers

41 A 51-year-old African American woman is admitted to hospital. She presented to the emergency department with abdominal pain and vomiting. She had gestational diabetes during each of 2 pregnancies and has otherwise been well. Her father, an older brother, aunt, and several of her grandparents developed type 2 diabetes in their late 50s. She binge drank alcohol in the past but has not been drinking alcohol recently. She has lost 15 to 20 lb (6.8-9.1 kg) over the last 2 months and has had polyuria, nocturia, and polydipsia for about 2 to 3 weeks.

On physical examination, her BMI is 31 kg/m^2. Her pulse rate is 92 beats/min, and respiratory rate is 18 breaths/min. Findings on funduscopic and abdominal examination are normal. There are no signs of neuropathy.

Laboratory test results:

- Blood glucose = 617 mg/dL (70-99 mg/dL) (SI: 34.2 mmol/L [3.9-5.5 mmol/L])
- Hemoglobin A_{1c} = 10.7% (4.0%-5.6%) (93 mmol/mol [20-38 mmol/mol])
- Bicarbonate = 20 mEq/L (21-28 mEq/L) (SI: 20 mmol/L [21-28 mmol/L])
- Creatinine = 1.7 mg/dL (0.7-1.3 mg/dL) (SI: 150.3 µmol/L [61.9-114.9 µmol/L])
- Triglycerides = 750 mg/dL (<150 mg/dL [optimal]) (SI: 8.48 mmol/L [<1.70 mmol/L])
- Lipase = 70 U/L (10-73 U/L) (SI: 1.17 µkat/L [0.17-1.22 µkat/L])
- Amylase = 55 U/L (26-102 U/L) (SI: 0.92 µkat/L [0.43-1.70 µkat/L])
- pH = 7.23 (7.35-7.45)

Which of the following is the most likely diagnosis?

A. Latent autoimmune diabetes
B. Ketosis-prone diabetes
C. Maturity-onset diabetes of the young
D. Alcoholic ketoacidosis
E. Pancreatitis

42 A 63-year-old man with type 2 diabetes had Roux-en-Y gastric bypass 18 months ago. He is admitted to the hospital following a seizure. His wife called 911 when she found him confused. Blood glucose measured by the emergency medical technicians was 23 mg/dL (1.3 mmol/L), and he responded to treatment with D50.

After gastric bypass, he lost 50 lb (22.7 kg), but he was not able to stop insulin therapy. For about 2 months, he has been feeling "funny" and not thinking clearly for approximately 2 hours after meals, particularly after those with more carbohydrates than usual. Juice relieves the symptoms. He checks fingerstick blood glucose infrequently.

Continuous glucose monitoring is initiated, and the results are shown (*see image*):

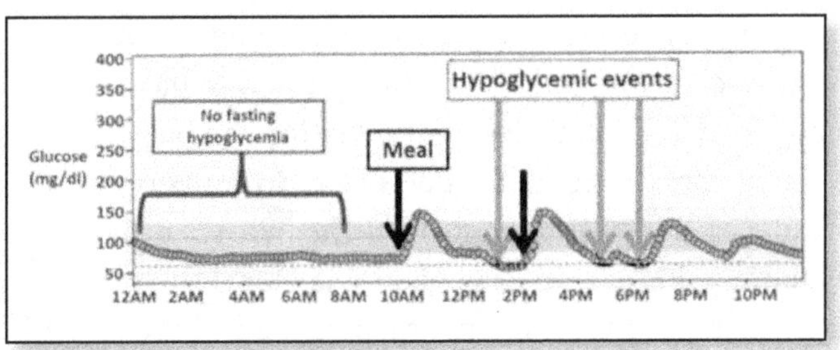

These patterns are typical of glycemic excursions in the setting of postbariatric hypoglycemia.

In conjunction with a controlled portion, low–glycemic index carbohydrate diet (<30 g/meal, 15 g per snack), which addition to her diabetes medication regimen should be considered as a next step for hypoglycemia management?

A. Octreotide
B. Diazoxide
C. Acarbose
D. Liraglutide
E. Metformin

43 A 31-year-old man with type 2 diabetes has a hemoglobin A_{1c} level of 9.2% (77 mmol/mol) on therapy with triple oral agents. Initiation of insulin therapy is recommended. After some discussion, he agrees to start once-daily basal insulin. His job requires frequent travel across time zones, and he wonders if it will be a problem to time the basal insulin injections when he travels to Australia or Latin America. He is concerned about the risk of hypoglycemia while traveling.

Formulary issues aside, which of the following regimens should be recommended for this patient?

A. NPH insulin at bedtime; give it at the same time when traveling
B. Insulin detemir at bedtime; decrease the insulin dose by half when traveling
C. U300 insulin glargine; give at the same time as he would take it at home
D. Insulin degludec; take it at his convenience once daily

44 A 29-year-old woman (G3P2) with type 1 diabetes who is at 14 weeks' gestation presents to the emergency department with vomiting and abdominal pain. She has vomited several times every day for the past few weeks. She takes insulin detemir, 40 units once daily, and insulin aspart, 15 units before meals. Diabetic ketoacidosis is diagnosed, and she is admitted to the intensive care unit and treated with intravenous hydration and an insulin drip.

Twenty-four hours later, she has improved clinically. However, she vomited an hour ago and has some residual abdominal pain.

Laboratory test results now show the following:

Serum glucose = 132 mg/dL (70-99 mg/dL)
(SI: 7.3 mmol/L [3.9-5.5 mmol/L])
Anion gap = 9
Albumin = 1.8 g/dL (3.5-5.0 g/dL)
(SI: 18 g/L [35-50 g/L])
Serum β-hydroxybutyrate, negative

The intensive care unit team seeks advice on transitioning the patient's regimen to subcutaneous insulin. For the last 6 hours, the hourly rate of her insulin drip has been 4 units/h.

Which of the following is the best advice now?

A. Transition to insulin glargine, 38 units daily and start insulin lispro, 12 units with meals
B. Transition to insulin detemir, 38 units daily, and start insulin lispro, 12 units with meals
C. Transition to insulin degludec, 38 units daily, and start insulin lispro, 12 units with meals
D. Continue the intravenous insulin drip, allow the patient to eat, and start insulin aspart with meals
E. Continue the intravenous insulin drip and maintain nothing-by-mouth-status

45 A 71-year-old man has had type 2 diabetes for 47 years. His hemoglobin A_{1c} level has been maintained in the range of 6.5% to 7.0% (48-53 mmol/mol), and he has no microvascular or macrovascular complications. For several months, his wife has been giving him candy or juice when he seems to be thinking less clearly, which is often several times daily. He can become quite confused. She is worried he is developing dementia.

He took insulin glargine, 38 units each evening, and premeal insulin aspart with each meal until 2 months ago when his endocrinologist reduced the glargine dosage to 20 units after documenting a hemoglobin A_{1c} level of 6.2% (44 mmol/mol). He does not write down his meal insulin doses, but he takes up to 12 units of insulin aspart with a meal.

Laboratory test results:

Hemoglobin A_{1c} = 7.3% (4.0%-5.6%)
(56 mmol/mol [20-38 mmol/mol])
Fructosamine = 330 μmol/L (200-285 μmol/L)
C-peptide = <0.1 ng/mL (0.9-4.3 ng/mL)
(SI: <0.03 nmol/L [0.30-1.42 nmol/L])

A cosyntropin-stimulation test reveals a baseline cortisol value of 18.0 μg/dL (496.6 mmol/L) and a 30-minute value of 22.8 μg/dL (629.0 mmol/L).

Diagnostic continuous glucose monitor testing is ordered, the results of which are shown (*see image*).

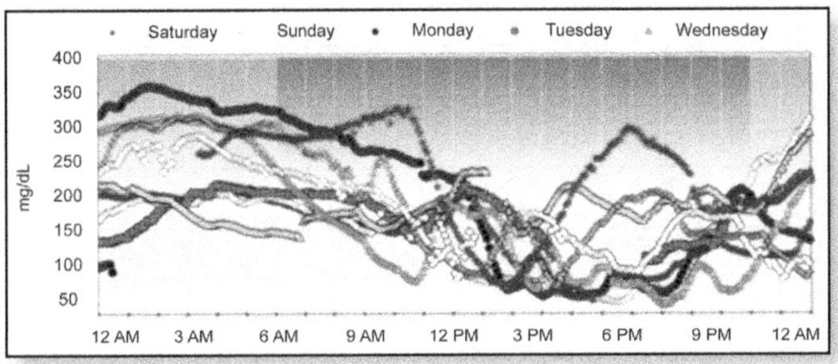

Which of the following simplification strategies should be recommended to adjust the insulin regimen for this patient?

A. Replace the sliding scale with a fixed and reduced dose of insulin with each meal
B. Replace the mealtime insulin with once-daily noninsulin agents to control postprandial glycemia
C. Move basal insulin to the morning and titrate the dose up to control fasting hyperglycemia
D. Coordinate with his wife to assist the patient when he seems to be thinking less clearly
E. Prescribe insulin pump therapy

46 A 19-year-old woman with type 1 diabetes who uses an insulin pump wants to train for a "Tough Mudder" endurance event. She is planning to do cross-training, including jogging, weight lifting, and stair training. She is concerned about her risk of hypoglycemia and asks for advice on how to minimize this possibility.

Which of the following should this patient do in addition to monitoring blood glucose before, during, and after exercise?

A. Consider lifting weights for a short period before jogging to reduce the chance of hypoglycemia
B. Raise her basal rate during jogging to avoid postexercise hyperglycemia that can occur with aerobic activity
C. Not worry about hypoglycemia during jogging as long as her glucose level is greater than 150 mg/dL (>8.3 mmol/L) before she begins her run
D. Minimize aerobic activity if she wants to avoid hypoglycemia

47 A 31-year-old woman with a 22-year history of type 1 diabetes was recently told by her ophthalmologist that she has early nonproliferative diabetic retinopathy. She is concerned about progression and losing her vision and asks what she can do to help prevent progression of this complication.

In addressing her concern, you explain that the amount of vision loss due to diabetic retinopathy that can be prevented at this early nonproliferative stage with targeted glycemic, blood pressure, and lipid control is expected to be:

A. <10%
B. 20%-30%
C. 50%
D. 75%
E. >90%

48 A 59-year-old man with suboptimally controlled type 2 diabetes and longstanding hypertension presents to the emergency department because he is worried that he has shingles. He has noticed drooping and pain on the left side of his face and some trouble speaking. He has no other symptoms. He has a history of retinopathy and distal somatosensory neuropathy.

On physical examination, he has a right facial droop and some tenderness in the affected area. There is no rash present. His ear canal and tympanic membrane look normal. The rest of the neurologic examination findings are normal, except for reduced sensation in the lower extremities to the mid-shin.

Laboratory test results:

Hemoglobin A_{1c} = 9.3% (4.0%-5.6%) (78 mmol/mol [20-38 mmol/mol])
Complete blood cell count and chemistries, normal

Head CT without contrast is unremarkable.

Which of the following is the most likely cause of his facial palsy?

A. Diabetic radiculopathy
B. Diabetic autonomic neuropathy
C. Herpes zoster
D. Otitis media
E. Stroke

49 A 61-year-old woman with a history of hypertension and gout presents with a painful swollen lower extremity, and deep venous thrombosis is diagnosed. She is extremely fatigued, has lost more than 20 lb (9.1 kg), and has polydipsia and polyuria. Her blood glucose concentration is 253 mg/dL (14.0 mmol/L), and new-onset diabetes mellitus is diagnosed.

On physical examination, she is a thin woman with a swollen, tender right calf and a rash scattered across her feet and ankles (*see image*).

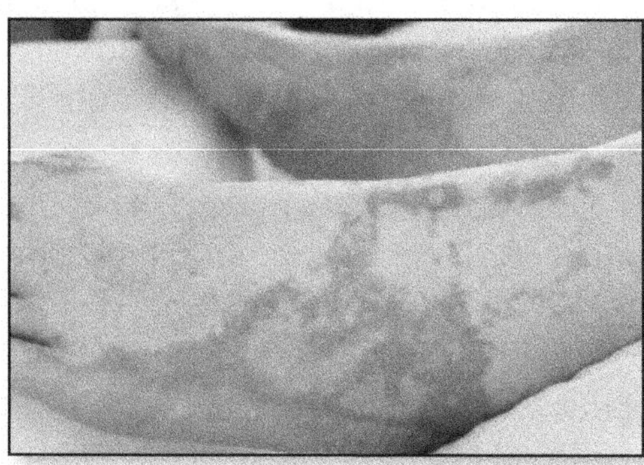

Which of the following is the most likely etiology of her diabetes?

A. Acromegaly
B. Rabson-Mendenhall syndrome
C. Glucagonoma syndrome
D. Cushing disease
E. Latent autoimmune diabetes

50 A 26-year-old man with type 1 diabetes who is on a regimen of multiple daily insulin injections recently returned from a ski trip in the Swiss Alps. During his trip, he experienced frequent, unusually high fingerstick blood glucose readings not explained by food or activity changes.

Which of the following factor(s) may have impacted the accuracy of his blood glucose meter readings during his trip?

Answer	Temperature	Altitude
A.	+	+
B.	–	–
C.	–	+
D.	+	–

51 A 21-year-old woman with a 2-year history of type 1 diabetes comes to the emergency department after experiencing 1 week of polyuria, weight loss, and blurred vision. Her blood glucose values have been ranging between 200 and 300 mg/dL (11.1-16.7 mmol/L) for several days, and she has been administering many correction doses of insulin lispro. She had onset of nausea and vomiting this morning.

She is following a multiple daily insulin injection regimen. She has gained 25 lb (11.4 kg) since her diabetes diagnosis, mostly in the past 6 months. She is very upset by this. She has depression, which has been treated with olanzapine for the past year. She takes an oral contraceptive pill and is feeling extremely stressed due to preparation for final exams at her university next month.

On physical examination, her BMI is 27 kg/m^2. She has moderate midepigastric tenderness to palpation, but her examination findings are otherwise normal.

Initial laboratory test results:

Serum glucose = 146 mg/dL (70-99 mg/dL)
(SI: 8.1 mmol/L [3.9-5.5 mmol/L])
Hemoglobin A_{1c} = 9.2% (4.0%-5.6%)
(77 mmol/mol [20-38 mmol/mol])
Bicarbonate = 14 mEq/L (21-28 mEq/L)
(SI: 14 mmol/L [21-28 mmol/L])
Serum pH = 7.2 (7.35-7.45)
Serum urea nitrogen = 34 mg/dL (8-23 mg/dL)
(SI: 12.1 mmol/L [2.9-8.2 mmol/L])

Serum creatinine = 1.9 mg/dL (0.6-1.1 mg/dL) (SI: 168.0 μmol/L [53.0-97.2 μmol/L])
Serum potassium = 5.3 mEq/L (3.5-5.0 mEq/L) (SI: 5.3 mmol/L [3.5-5.0 mmol/L])
Urinalysis = 4+ glucose, large ketones, few white blood cells, no red blood cells, no blood

On the basis of her clinical history, which of the following is the most likely cause of diabetic ketoacidosis in this patient?

A. Acute kidney injury
B. Olanzapine
C. Nonadherence to insulin therapy
D. Early pregnancy

52 A 34-year-old Asian man with a history of Graves disease reports episodes of diaphoresis, tachycardia, and tremor over the past 6 months. These episodes typically occur when he skips a meal or during exercise and are reversed with ingestion of sugary beverages. He is brought to the emergency department after losing consciousness while out jogging. His hyperthyroidism has been treated with methimazole, and his TSH levels have been normal over the past year. He has no other notable medical history. He has no family members with diabetes or hypoglycemia.

On physical examination, he is lethargic and diaphoretic. His blood pressure is 148/92 mm Hg, and his pulse rate is 108 beats/min. Vitiligo is noted. His thyroid is nonpalpable. The rest of the examination findings are normal.

A blood glucose measurement is documented to be 37 mg/dL (2.1 mmol/L). Results of other routine laboratory tests are normal, including those assessing renal and hepatic function.

Although all of the following tests may appropriately be part of the evaluation for hypoglycemia, which test is most likely to demonstrate the cause of this patient's hypoglycemic syndrome?

A. Insulin autoantibody assessment
B. Urinary sulfonylurea screen
C. Cortisol measurement
D. Insulinlike growth factor 2 measurement
E. Metanephrine measurement

53 A 51-year-old man with type 2 diabetes presents to the emergency department with symptomatic hyperglycemia and blurry vision. He started insulin 2 months ago and has been measuring fingerstick blood glucose 4 times daily. He has called his endocrinologist every 2 weeks for insulin dosage titration. Glucose readings have been ranging from 300 to 400 mg/dL (16.7-22.2 mmol/L). He is now taking 95 units of insulin glargine twice daily and 30 units of insulin aspart with each meal (total daily insulin dose = 288 units). His BMI is 26 kg/m^2.

Laboratory test results:

Random blood glucose = 466 mg/dL (SI: 25.9 mmol/L)
Hemoglobin A_{1c} = >13% (4.0%-5.6%) (>119 mmol/mol [20-38 mmol/mol])

He receives intravenous hydration and insulin aspart per emergency department protocol, and his blood glucose decreases to less than 240 mg/dL (<13.2 mmol/L) over 4 to 6 hours.

How should the emergency department team be advised to manage his uncontrolled type 2 diabetes?

A. Admit him to the hospital for management of uncontrolled hyperglycemia
B. Stop both insulin glargine and insulin aspart and begin U500 regular insulin
C. Ask him to demonstrate how he self-administers insulin injections
D. Increase the doses of insulin glargine and insulin aspart by 30% each

54 Consultation is requested to provide insulin management recommendations for a 49-year-old man who has type 2 diabetes. He has sustained multiple injuries in a car accident. He has been in the intensive care unit for 6 days and is ready to be transferred to a surgical unit. In the intensive care unit, he was managed with an insulin drip and his rate over the last 24 hours has been stable at 2 units/h (total daily dose 48 units). It is anticipated that while he will make a full recovery, it will be at least a few weeks until he can eat. Continuous enteral nutrition will be initiated.

Which of the following insulin regimens will best match his physiologic basal-bolus insulin needs to enable glycemic control during continuous enteral tube feeding?

A. NPH U100 insulin, 8 units at 11 PM plus rapid-acting insulin every 4 hours
B. Insulin glargine U100, 8 units twice daily plus regular insulin every 6 hours
C. Regular U100 insulin every 4 hours
D. Insulin glargine U300, 22 units once daily plus rapid-acting insulin every 4 hours

55 A 63-year-old man with longstanding type 2 diabetes, nonproliferative diabetes-related retinopathy, hypertension, dyslipidemia, and chronic kidney disease presents for a follow-up visit. His last appointment was more than a year ago. He notes that when he does his daily walk, his right leg feels "tired" after a few blocks.

His medications are metformin, empagliflozin, insulin glargine, lisinopril, hydrochlorothiazide, aspirin, and simvastatin.

On physical examination, his blood pressure is 132/78 mm Hg, pulse rate is 84 beats/min, and BMI is 24 kg/m^2. He does not have ankle edema. He has reduced pedal pulses. There is no hair on his toes, and the toenails are thickened. His ankle brachial index is 1.4 (normal range, 0.91-1.30).

Laboratory test results:

Estimated glomerular filtration rate = 53 mL/min per 1.73 m^2 (>60 mL/min per 1.73 m^2)
Hemoglobin A_{1c} = 7.1% (4.0%-5.6%) (54 mmol/mol [20-38 mmol/mol])

Which of the following should be the next step to evaluate for the presence of peripheral arterial disease in this patient?

A. Transcutaneous oxygen pressure in the foot
B. Vascular segmental pressures and pulse volume recordings
C. Systolic toe pressure
D. Treadmill functional testing
E. Percutaneous angiography of the affected leg

56 A 20-year-old woman (G1P0) presents at 10 weeks' gestation after being referred by her obstetrician. She has a normal menstrual cycle history, had no difficulty conceiving, and has an otherwise unremarkable medical history. She is not taking any medications except a prenatal vitamin. Her family history is notable for diabetes mellitus in her father and several uncles and aunts, but she does not know which type it is.

On physical examination, her BMI is 21 kg/m^2. Her examination findings are unremarkable.

Laboratory test results obtained at her obstetrics visit:

Fasting plasma glucose = 115 mg/dL (70-99 mg/dL) (SI: 6.4 mmol/L [3.9-5.5 mmol/L])
Hemoglobin A_{1c} = 6.7% (4.0%-5.6%) (50 mmol/mol [20-38 mmol/mol])

On the basis of the presented information, which of the following is the most likely underlying etiology of her diabetes?

A. Type 1 diabetes
B. Type 2 diabetes
C. Gestational diabetes
D. Maturity-onset diabetes of the young
E. Latent autoimmune diabetes in adults

Female Reproduction Board Review

Kathryn A. Martin, MD

1 A 28-year-old woman seeks evaluation for polycystic ovary syndrome. She has oligomenorrhea, hirsutism, and acne. Transvaginal ultrasonography shows polycystic ovary morphology. She is eager to start treatment for her acne and hirsutism. An estrogen-progestin contraceptive (ethinyl estradiol, 20 mcg, with norethindrone acetate, 1 mg) is prescribed. Eight months later, the patient returns for follow-up evaluation. Her acne has improved, but she reports that she has not had any bleeding during the placebo week for the past 4 cycles. Several home pregnancy tests have been negative. She has not missed a single pill, and she takes no other medications. Her BMI is 22 kg/m^2. She wonders whether the pill has "stopped working."

Which of the following is the best next step in this patient's management?

A. Serum prolactin measurement
B. Serum FSH measurement
C. Reassurance; no evaluation needed
D. Monthly serum hCG measurements
E. Endometrial biopsy

2 A 25-year-old woman presents to discuss the results of the evaluation from her first visit. She sought evaluation for irregular menstrual periods that occur approximately every 60 to 70 days. She has also been concerned about facial hair on her upper lip, chin, and neck that has been present since age 18 years but is now gradually worsening. Laboratory testing was ordered at the first visit. She previously had documentation of normal TSH, prolactin, and day 3 FSH.

On physical examination, her BMI is 28 kg/m^2 and blood pressure is 120/70 mm Hg. She has increased coarse terminal hair on the upper lip, chin, neck, and in the midsternal area. Her modified Ferriman-Gallwey score is 9 (a modified Ferriman-Gallwey score >8 is considered to be "mild" hirsutism).

Laboratory test results (sample drawn on day 50 of her last cycle):

Serum prolactin = 18 ng/mL (4-23 ng/mL) (SI: 0.78 nmol/L [0.17-1.00 nmol/L])
Serum total testosterone = 66 ng/dL (8-60 ng/dL) (SI: 2.3 nmol/L [0.3-2.1 nmol/L])
Serum 17-hydroxyprogesterone = 40 ng/dL (<80 ng/dL) (SI: 1.2 nmol/L [<2.42 nmol/L])
Hemoglobin A_{1c} = 5.2% (4.0%-5.6%) (33 mmol/mol [20-38 mmol/mol])

Which of the following additional tests is required to make a diagnosis in this patient?

A. No further testing needed
B. Serum free testosterone measurement
C. Serum LH and FSH measurements
D. Serum antimullerian hormone measurement
E. Transvaginal ultrasonography

3 A 38-year-old woman with a history of polycystic ovary syndrome presents for management of hirsutism. She also desires contraception. She has periods approximately every 3 months, sometimes with heavy bleeding. An endometrial biopsy done by her gynecologist because of her infrequent menses and heavy bleeding showed proliferative endometrium. She was given a 10-day course of medroxyprogesterone acetate, 10 mg.

She has longstanding hirsutism and has developed some alopecia over the past 2 years. She is not obese and has no history of hypertension, diabetes mellitus, migraines, or dyslipidemia.

On physical examination, her Ferriman-Gallwey score is 14, BMI is 23 kg/m^2, and she has mild scalp hair loss.

Laboratory test results:

Testosterone = 62 ng/dL (8-60 ng/dL)
(SI: 2.2 nmol/L [0.3-2.1 nmol/L])
Day 3 FSH = 9.0 mIU/mL (2.0-12.0 mIU/mL)
(SI: 9.0 IU/L [2.0-12.0 IU/L])
LH = 8.0 mIU/mL (1.0-18.0 mIU/mL)
(SI: 8.0 IU/L [1.0-18.0 IU/L])

Which of the following is the best therapy to manage her symptoms and provide contraception?

A. Oral estrogen-progestin contraceptive (ethinyl estradiol, 50 mcg/norgestrel, 0.5 mg)
B. Levonorgestrel-releasing intrauterine device and laser hair removal
C. Spironolactone, 100 mg twice daily, and barrier contraception
D. Oral estrogen-progestin contraceptive (ethinyl estradiol, 20 mcg/norethindrone acetate, 1 mg)
E. Levonorgestrel-releasing intrauterine device and flutamide

4 An 18-year-old woman requests evaluation for primary amenorrhea. She was a healthy baby and experienced normal growth and development during early childhood. Pubic hair appeared at age 9 years and breast development started at age 11 years, but she has never menstruated. She is not sexually active.

On physical examination, her height is 65 in (165 cm) and weight is 132 lb (60 kg) (BMI = 22 kg/m^2). Mild acne is noted on her face and back. Several dark hairs are present on her upper lip and chest. The patient has Tanner stage 5 breasts and stage 5 pubic hair.

Laboratory test results:

Serum LH = 8.0 mIU/L (1.0-18.0 mIU/L)
(SI: 8.0 IU/L [1.0-18.0 IU/L])
FSH = 6.0 mIU/mL (2.0-12.0 mIU/mL)
(SI: 6.0 IU/L [2.0-12.0 IU/L])
Serum prolactin = 8 ng/mL (4-23 ng/mL)
(SI: 0.35 nmol/L [0.17-1.00 nmol/L])
Serum estradiol = 60 pg/mL (10-180 pg/mL)
(SI: 220.3 pmol/L [36.7-660.8 pmol/L])
Serum testosterone = 29 ng/dL (8-60 ng/dL)
(SI: 1.0 nmol/L [0.3-2.1 nmol/L])

Pelvic ultrasonography reveals absence of a uterus.

Which of the following is this patient's most likely karyotype?

A. 45,X
B. 46,XX
C. 46,XY
D. 47,XXY

5 A 29-year-old woman is referred for evaluation of infertility. She and her husband have been trying to conceive for the past year. The patient reports that she has always had regular monthly menses until several years ago when they became irregular (every 2 to 3 months). She has also developed some night sweats that come and go. She finds them bothersome enough to seek medical attention.

On physical examination, her BMI is 22 kg/m^2 and blood pressure is 110/70 mm Hg. She has no acne or hirsutism.

Laboratory test results:
Day 3 of cycle:

Serum TSH = 1.6 mIU/L (0.5-5.0 mIU/L)
(SI: 1.6 mIU/L [0.5-5.0 mIU/L])
Serum FSH = 42.0 mIU/mL (2.0-12.0 mIU/mL [follicular]) (SI: 42.0 IU/L [2.0-12.0 IU/L])
Serum LH = 30.0 mIU/L (1.0-18.0 mIU/L [follicular]) (SI: 30.0 mIU/L [1.0-18.0 mIU/L)
Serum prolactin = 12 ng/mL (4-23 ng/mL)
(SI: 0.52 nmol/L [0.17-1.00 nmol/L])
Serum estradiol = 19 pg/mL (10-180 pg/mL [follicular]) (SI: 69.7 pmol/L [36.7-660.8 pmol/L])

Additional testing:

Karyotype = 46,XX
Fragile X premutation, negative
Serum adrenal cortical and 21-hydroxylase antibodies, negative

Her husband's semen analysis is normal.

Which of the following therapies is most likely to help this patient become pregnant?

A. Clomiphene citrate
B. Low-dosage estradiol therapy
C. GnRH agonist followed by exogenous gonadotropins
D. In vitro fertilization with donor oocytes
E. Letrozole therapy

6 A 30-year-old transgender man is referred to start gender-affirming hormonal therapy (testosterone). You review treatment goals and expectations, the risks and benefits of therapy, and the potential impact on future fertility. He is obese (BMI = 32 kg/m^2), but has no history of hypertension, dyslipidemia, type 2 diabetes, or venous thromboembolism. Testosterone cypionate, 200 mg intramuscularly every 2 weeks, is prescribed.

Which of the following clinical changes is he most likely to see in the first 6 months of hormone therapy?

A. Increase in oily skin
B. Deepening of the voice
C. Breast growth
D. Weight loss
E. Increased muscle strength

7 A 38-year-old woman seeks evaluation of hormonal symptoms that are becoming increasingly difficult to manage. She has always had minor mood changes before her periods. However, for the past 2 years, she has experienced premenstrual anger, irritability, and tearfulness that lasts for 1 to 2 weeks at a time. These symptoms are accompanied by bloating, night sweats, and fatigue, and she now is having difficulty functioning at work. The patient's menstrual cycles occur approximately once monthly.

On physical examination, the patient appears anxious, but her examination findings are otherwise unremarkable. Her BMI is 24 kg/m^2, pulse rate is 88 beats/min, and blood pressure is 130/80 mm Hg.

Which of the following is the best next step to confirm her diagnosis?

A. Daily prospective symptom diary for 2 cycles
B. Serum TSH measurement
C. Serum antimullerian hormone measurement
D. Day 3 serum FSH measurement
E. Depression screening

8 A 50-year-old woman presents with concerns of scalp hair loss and facial hair. Menarche was at age 12 years, and she had regular menses during her reproductive years. Her final menstrual period was 2 years ago. Over the past 18 months, she has developed facial hair and rapidly progressive loss of scalp hair. She has also noticed increased libido.

On physical examination, her BMI is 27 kg/m^2 and blood pressure is 150/90 mm Hg. She is very muscular. She has terminal hairs on her chin in a full-beard distribution, as well as hair on her upper abdomen, lower back, and sternum with a Ferriman-Gallwey score of 12 (>8 considered to be abnormal). Her clitoris measures 11 mm × 5 mm (upper normal limit is a clitoral index of 35 mm^2).

Laboratory test results:

Testosterone = 350 ng/dL (8-60 ng/dL)
(SI: 12.1 nmol/L [0.3-2.1 nmol/L])
DHEA-S = 120 µg/dL (15-200 µg/dL)
(SI: 3.3 µmol/L [0.41-5.42 µmol/L])
FSH = 19.0 mIU/mL (>30.0 mIU/mL [postmenopausal]) (SI: 19.0 IU/L [>30.0 IU/L])
LH = 8.0 mIU/mL (>30.0 mIU/mL [postmenopausal]) (SI: 8.0 IU/L [>30.0 IU/L])

Which of the following is the best next test to evaluate this patient?

A. Transvaginal ultrasonography
B. Dexamethasone-suppression test
C. Serum inhibin measurement
D. Adrenal CT
E. Serum 17-hydroxyprogesterone measurement

9 A 45-year-old woman seeks evaluation for night sweats, hot flashes during the day, and 1 year of irregular periods. She also desires contraception. She is having menses every 6 to 8 weeks, sometimes with heavy flow. Her symptoms and lack of sleep are interfering with her ability to perform well at work. She is otherwise in good health with no history of cigarette smoking, hypertension, dyslipidemia, venous thromboembolism, or diabetes mellitus. She has no family history of venous thromboembolism or coronary disease. Her BMI is 22 kg/m^2.

Which of the following treatments should be suggested for this patient?

A. Transdermal estradiol, 0.025 mg patch, with oral micronized progesterone, 100 mg daily
B. Combined estrogen-progestin contraceptive (ethinyl estradiol, 20 mcg, with norethindrone, 1 mg, given continuously [ie, no placebos])
C. Levonorgestrel-releasing intrauterine device and gabapentin, 300 mg orally at bedtime
D. Medroxyprogesterone acetate, 10 mg for 10 days every other month
E. Levonorgestrel-containing intrauterine device

10 An 18-year-old woman presents with primary amenorrhea and short stature. Her blood pressure is 140/90 mm Hg. Her height is 56 in (142.2 cm) (BMI = 28 kg/m^2). She has absent breast development and scant pubic and axillary hair.

Laboratory test results:

FSH = 35.0 mIU/mL (2.0-12.0 mIU/mL)
(SI: 35.0 IU/L [2.0-12.0 IU/L])
LH = 28.0 mIU/mL (1.0-18.0 mIU/mL)
(SI: 28.0 IU/L [1.0-18.0 IU/L])
Estradiol = <10 pg/mL (10-180 pg/mL)
(SI: <36.7 pmol/L [36.7-660.8 pmol/L])
Karyotype = 45,X

Which of the following is the most important test in her subsequent evaluation?

A. Transvaginal ultrasonography
B. Hemoglobin A_{1c} measurement
C. TSH measurement
D. Thyroid ultrasonography
E. Cardiac MRI

11 A 28-year-old woman presents with a history of irregular menses and then amenorrhea. Menarche was at age 14 years; her periods were irregular for the first 18 months, then regular every 28 days. She had a miscarriage 6 months ago when she was 12 weeks pregnant, which required a dilatation and curettage. Since that time, she has had no menstrual bleeding. She runs 5 miles 3 days a week. Her BMI is 20 kg/m^2.

Laboratory test results:

hCG = <3.0 mIU/mL (<3.0 mIU/mL)
(SI: <3.0 IU/L [<3.0 IU/L])
LH = 4.0 mIU/mL (1.0-18.0 mIU/mL)
(SI: 4.0 IU/L [1.0-18.0 IU/L])
FSH = 5.0 mIU/mL (2.0-12.0 mIU/mL)
(SI: 5.0 IU/L [2.0-12.0 IU/L])
Estradiol = 70 pg/mL (10-180 pg/mL)
(SI: 257.0 pmol/L [36.7-660.8 pmol/L]
TSH = 5.2 mIU/L (0.5-5.0 mIU/L)
Prolactin = 32 ng/mL (4-30 ng/mL)
(SI: 1.39 nmol/L [0.17-1.30 nmol/L])

Which of the following is the most likely cause of her amenorrhea?

A. Prolactinoma
B. Functional hypothalamic amenorrhea
C. Intrauterine adhesions (Asherman syndrome)
D. Hypothyroidism
E. Primary ovarian insufficiency

12 A 51-year-old woman would like to try hormone therapy for her menopausal symptoms. She has been experiencing severe hot flashes and night sweats for the past year (her final menstrual period was 18 months ago). Her medical history includes hypothyroidism and nephrolithiasis. Her gynecologic history includes G0P0, menarche at age 9 years, and final menstrual period at age 49 years. She has a paternal uncle with Parkinson disease and a maternal aunt with breast cancer (diagnosed at age 70 years).

Which of the following factors is the most important when deciding whether she is a candidate for menopausal hormone therapy?

A. Family history of Parkinson disease
B. Maternal aunt with postmenopausal breast cancer
C. Reproductive history, including age at menarche and age at first pregnancy
D. History of autoimmune thyroid disease
E. History of kidney stones

13 A 41-year-old woman seeks advice on treatment of menopausal symptoms. Six months ago, she underwent total abdominal hysterectomy and bilateral salpingo-oophorectomy for a history of leiomyomata. Since her surgery, she has had intractable hot flashes at night, as well as during the day. She is otherwise in excellent health and has no contraindications to menopausal hormone therapy.

Which of the following should be suggested for her hot flashes?

A. Oral 17β-estradiol, 2 mg daily
B. Gabapentin, 300 to 900 mg daily
C. Venlafaxine, 75 mg daily
D. Low-dosage oral contraceptives (ethinyl estradiol, 20 mcg/norethindrone acetate, 1 mg)

14 A 20-year-old college student presents with a 4-month history of amenorrhea. Her menarche was at age 14 years (normal, age 12 years). She played sports in high school and occasionally missed a period. During college, her menses were every 30 to 35 days. She attributes this to stress related to her schoolwork. She has mild acne, but no hirsutism. She has no headaches or vision symptoms.

Laboratory test results:
FSH = 1.0 mIU/mL (2.0-12.0 mIU/mL)
(SI: 1.0 IU/L [2.0-12.0 IU/L])
LH = 2.0 mIU/L (1.0-18.0 mIU/mL)
(SI: 2.0 IU/L [1.0-18.0 IU/L])
Estradiol = 520 pg/mL (10-180 pg/mL)
(SI: 1909 pmol/L [36.7-660.8 pmol/L])
Prolactin = 68 ng/mL (4-30 ng/mL)
(SI: 2.96 nmol/L [0.17-1.30 nmol/L])

Which of the following is the most likely diagnosis in this patient?

A. Pregnancy
B. Polycystic ovary syndrome
C. Nonclassic congenital adrenal hyperplasia due to 21-hydroxylase deficiency
D. Primary ovarian insufficiency
E. Prolactinoma

15 A 32-year-old woman with polycystic ovary syndrome presents to discuss fatigue. Over the past 3 years, she has gained approximately 40 lb (18.2 kg) (from 160 to 200 lb [73 to 91 kg]). In addition, she has been unusually tired at work and sometimes finds it hard to stay awake in meetings. She had menarche at age 11 years, hirsutism and acne since age 13 years, and has been on a combined estrogen-progestin contraceptive for the past 10 years. She has a family history of hypertension and type 2 diabetes. A recent hemoglobin A_{1c} measurement was normal.

On physical examination, her blood pressure is 130/90 mm Hg and BMI is 30 kg/m^2.

Which of the following is the best next step in this patient's evaluation?

A. 24-Hour urinary free cortisol measurement
B. Oral glucose tolerance test
C. Sleep study
D. Serum total testosterone measurement
E. TSH measurement

16 A 46-year-old perimenopausal woman presents with persistent symptoms despite taking menopausal hormone therapy. Two years ago, she developed severe hot flashes, night sweats, and irritability. She also described "not feeling like herself." She was prescribed transdermal estradiol, 25 mcg twice weekly. She had a levonorgestrel-releasing intrauterine device inserted 2 years ago. Her hot flashes improved dramatically when her estradiol dosage was increased to 37.5 mcg twice weekly. However, other bothersome symptoms persist (eg, lack of energy and not feeling like herself). A recent TSH measurement was normal. She is otherwise in excellent health.

On physical examination, her blood pressure is 105/70 mm Hg and BMI is 21 kg/m^2.

Which of the following should be suggested next in this patient's management?

A. Increase the estrogen dosage to a 50-mcg patch
B. Start escitalopram, 10 mg daily
C. Switch to a low-dosage estrogen-progestin oral contraceptive
D. Start a tricyclic antidepressant
E. Refer for cognitive behavioral therapy

17 A 46-year-old woman seeks evaluation for irregular menses. Since menarche at age 12 years, she had regular 28- to 30-day cycles until about 6 months ago when her intermenstrual interval shortened to 24 to 25 days. Now her cycles are unpredictable (anywhere from every 24 to 90 days). She exercises daily for 30 minutes. She has no hot flashes, but she is not sleeping well and has been experiencing mild aches and pains (without swelling) since her periods became irregular. She has no galactorrhea or headaches. A recent TSH measurement was normal and hCG was negative. She would like to know what is causing her irregular periods.

On physical examination, her blood pressure is 90/65 mm Hg and BMI is 19.5 kg/m^2.

Which of the following tests should be ordered to determine the cause of this patient's problem?

A. Prolactin measurement
B. FSH measurement
C. Antimullerian hormone measurement
D. Serum estradiol measurement
E. No testing required

18 A 22-year-old woman with a 4-year history of functional hypothalamic amenorrhea comes to clinic for follow-up. She has a history of excessive exercise and restricted eating. Her BMI at her initial visit was 17 kg/m^2, and she had low bone mineral density (Z-score at femoral neck = −2.2). She understands that her low bone mineral density is related to her nutrition and excessive exercise, as evaluation for secondary causes has been negative. Eighteen months ago, she decided to implement lifestyle changes by moderating her exercise and improving her nutrition. Her weight has increased, and her BMI is now 18.5 kg/m^2. She is pleased that she has been able to make these changes but is disappointed that her periods have not returned. She wonders whether something else is wrong.

Laboratory test results:

hCG = <3.0 mIU/mL (<3.0 mIU/mL)
(SI: <3.0 IU/L [<3.0 IU/L])
TSH = 1.9 mIU/L (0.5-5.0 mIU/L)
Prolactin = 15 ng/mL (4-30 ng/mL)
(SI: 0.65 nmol/L [0.17-1.30 nmol/L])
Estradiol = 110 pg/mL (10-180 pg/mL)
(SI: 403.8 pmol/L [36.7-660.8 pmol/L])
LH = 6.0 mIU/mL (1.0-18.0 mIU/mL)
(SI: 6.0 IU/L [1.0-18.0 IU/L])
FSH = 8.0 mIU/mL (2.0-12.0 mIU/mL)
(SI: 8.0 IU/L [2.0-12.0 IU/L])
Progesterone = 7.0 ng/mL (≤1.0 ng/mL)
(SI: 22.3 nmol/L [≤3.2 nmol/L])

Which of the following should be recommended now?

A. Start transdermal 17β-estradiol patch with cyclic micronized progesterone
B. Start alendronate, 70 mg weekly
C. Start a low-dosage combined estrogen-progestin oral contraceptive
D. No treatment

Male Reproduction Board Review

Frances J. Hayes, MB BCh, BAO

1 A 67-year-old man seeks evaluation for an inability to ejaculate. He reports a normal libido and is sexually active with his wife. He has noticed that it takes a little longer to get an erection than in the past, but he can still get and maintain one that is adequate for intercourse. He generally reaches orgasm but is concerned that there is no longer an ejaculate. His history is notable for hypertension and benign prostatic hyperplasia for which he takes hydrochlorothiazide, 12.5 mg daily, and tamsulosin, 0.4 mg daily.

On physical examination, his BMI is 31 kg/m^2 and blood pressure is 125/80 mm Hg. He is well virilized. Testes measure 15 mL bilaterally. Rectal examination reveals mild prostate enlargement. His morning testosterone concentration is 325 ng/dL (11.3 nmol/L).

Which of the following strategies is most likely to help his ejaculatory dysfunction?

A. Substitute finasteride for tamsulosin
B. Initiate testosterone replacement
C. Start a phosphodiesterase-5 inhibitor
D. Substitute eplerenone for hydrochlorothiazide

2 A 19-year-old biologic male patient is referred to discuss transgender hormone therapy. Preferred pronouns are female (she/her/hers). She has disclosed her gender dysphoria to family and close friends and is seeing a therapist. For the past year, she has experimented with wearing make-up and dressing in feminine clothes on the weekends. She uses gender-neutral bathrooms at work. Her medical history is notable for heterozygosity for a factor V Leiden pathogenic variant identified on screening after her mother had an unprovoked pulmonary embolism. She does not smoke cigarettes and takes no medications. Her BMI is 22 kg/m^2, and blood pressure is 110/70 mm Hg. Her therapist is supportive of her decision to start hormone therapy to alleviate her dysphoria.

Which of the following would be the most appropriate initial hormone regimen for this patient?

A. Leuprolide, 3.75 mg intramuscularly, plus estradiol, 2 mg orally
B. Leuprolide, 3.75 mg intramuscularly, plus estradiol, 50 mcg by transdermal patch
C. Low-dosage birth control pill containing 20 mcg of ethinyl estradiol and drospirenone plus spironolactone, 100 mg orally
D. Spironolactone, 100 mg, and finasteride, 5 mg orally

3 A 21-year-old transgender woman who had been managed by her primary care physician is referred because of a documented estradiol concentration of 550 pg/mL (2019 pmol/L). She admits to having adjusted her dosage of estrogen because of frustration with the slow rate of breast growth. She now reports breast tenderness and nausea. Physical examination is notable for Tanner stage 3 breast development. Hormone data obtained on the day of her consultation confirm the following:

Estradiol = 630 pg/mL (10-180 pg/mL)
(SI: 2313 pmol/L [36.7-660.8 pmol/L])
Gonadotropins, undetectable
Testosterone = 20 ng/dL (8-60 ng/dL)
(SI: 0.7 nmol/L [0.3-2.1 nmol/L])

Based on the patient's hormone profile, which of the following forms of estrogen is she most likely taking?

A. Conjugated equine estrogens, 2.5 mg by mouth daily
B. 17β-estradiol, 4 mg by mouth daily
C. Ethinyl estradiol, 30 mcg by mouth daily
D. Estradiol valerate, 40 mg intramuscularly weekly

4 An 18-year-old man arrives to clinic with both parents to discuss his recent diagnosis of Klinefelter syndrome. He was noted to have small testes during a routine physical examination by his pediatrician and was found to have a 47,XXY karyotype. On physical examination, his height is 72 in (182.9 cm). He has no gynecomastia and has normal facial, axillary, and pubic hair. His testes measure 4 mL bilaterally.

Laboratory test results:
Total testosterone = 306 ng/dL (300-900 ng/dL)
(SI: 10.6 nmol/L [10.4-31.2 nmol/L])
Free testosterone = 4.2 ng/dL (9.0-30.0 ng/dL)
(SI: 0.15 nmol/L [0.31-1.04 nmol/L])
LH = 33.7 mIU/mL (1.0-9.0 mIU/mL)
(SI: 33.7 IU/L [1.0-9.0 IU/L])
FSH = 58.1 mIU/mL (1.0-13.0 mIU/mL)
(SI: 58.1 IU/L [1.0-13.0 IU/L])

His mother asks if the diagnosis of Klinefelter syndrome means that he can never father a child.

Which of the following options is most likely to help this patient achieve biologic paternity?

A. No treatment is needed as he has a high likelihood of having sperm in his ejaculate
B. hCG injections
C. Microdissection testicular sperm extraction followed by intracytoplasmic sperm injection
D. Clomiphene citrate

5 A 25-year-old man is concerned about recent-onset breast tenderness and swelling associated with fatigue, irritability, and insomnia. He is not taking any medications and reports no use of anabolic steroids or recreational drugs.

On physical examination, his BMI is 23 kg/m^2. His pulse rate is 100 beats/min. His thyroid gland is diffusely enlarged. He has normal facial, axillary, and pubic hair. He has bilateral breast enlargement, which is tender to palpation. His testes measure 20 mL bilaterally and there are no palpable masses.

Laboratory test results:
TSH = <0.01 mIU/L (0.5-5.0 mIU/L)
Free T_4 = 6.6 ng/dL (0.8-1.8 ng/dL)
(SI: 84.9 pmol/L [10.30-23.17 pmol/L])
Total T_3 = 540 ng/dL (70-200 ng/dL)
(SI: 8.32 nmol/L [1.08-3.08 nmol/L])

Which of the following hormone profiles would be expected in this patient with gynecomastia?

Answer	Total testosterone	Free testosterone	Estradiol	LH
A.	Low	Low	High	Low
B.	High	Low or low-normal	High	Normal
C.	Normal	Normal	High	Low
D.	High	High	High	High

6 An 18-year-old man is referred for further evaluation of congenital hypogonadotropic hypogonadism. He has no sense of smell, which was confirmed by quantitative smell testing. There is no history of deafness. There is no family history of anosmia, delayed puberty, or hypogonadism.

On physical examination, his height is 67 in (170.2 cm) (BMI = 22 kg/m^2), and arm span is 70 in (177.8 cm). He has slight axillary hair and Tanner stage 2 pubic hair but no facial or chest hair. He has a normal phallus, and his testes measure 2 mL bilaterally. There is no evidence of synkinesia. Musculoskeletal examination shows syndactyly of the fingers and toes.

Laboratory test results:
Total testosterone = 52 ng/dL (300-900 ng/dL)
(SI: 1.8 nmol/L [10.4-31.2 nmol/L]
Gonadotropins, undetectable

IGF-1, low
Prolactin, normal
TSH, normal
Free T_4, normal
ACTH, normal
Pituitary MRI shows no structural abnormality.

A pathogenic variant in which of the following genes most likely underlies his presentation?

A. *GNRHR*
B. *FGFR1*
C. *PROP1*
D. *CHD7*
E. *NR0B1*

7 A 35-year-old man is referred for evaluation of infertility as his wife has not conceived after 12 months of regular, unprotected intercourse. He reports normal libido and erections. He is taking no medications and does not use recreational drugs. His wife is 32 years old, has a 4-year-old daughter from a previous relationship, and is ovulating according to basal body temperature measurements. On physical examination, he has normal secondary sexual characteristics and no gynecomastia. Testicular volume is 25 mL bilaterally.

Evaluation shows the following:

Total testosterone = 500 ng/dL (300-900 ng/dL)
(SI: 17.4 nmol/L [10.4-31.2 nmol/L])
FSH = 4.4 mIU/mL (1.0-13.0 mIU/mL)
(SI: 4.4 IU/L [1.0-11.0 IU/L])
LH = 6.1 mIU/mL (1.0-9.0 mIU/mL)
(SI: 6.1 IU/L [1.0-9.0 IU/L])

Seminal fluid analysis shows a volume of 1.3 mL (normal >1.5 mL) and pH of 6.8 (normal >7.2). No sperm are present. A repeated analysis confirms azoospermia.

Which of the following is the most likely cause of this patient's infertility?

A. Anabolic steroid use
B. Congenital bilateral absence of the vas deferens
C. Y-chromosome microdeletions
D. Mosaic Klinefelter syndrome
E. Partial androgen insensitivity syndrome

8 A 30-year-old man reports a 6-month history of increasing breast tenderness. He takes no medications or supplements and states that he does not use recreational drugs. He otherwise feels well with good appetite and stable weight.

On physical examination, his blood pressure is 120/80 mm Hg, pulse rate is 60 beats/min, and BMI is 23 kg/m^2. He is well virilized and muscular. His thyroid and abdominal examination are normal. He has 4-cm, slightly tender bilateral gynecomastia. His testes are 15 mL bilaterally, and there are no palpable testicular masses.

Laboratory test results:

Total testosterone = 725 ng/dL (300-900 ng/dL)
(SI: 25.2 nmol/L [10.4-31.2 nmol/L])
Estradiol = 145 pg/mL (10-40 pg/mL)
(SI: 532.3 pmol/L [36.7-146.8 pmol/L])
FSH = 1.0 mIU/mL (1.0-13.0 mIU/mL)
(SI: 1.0 IU/L [1.0-11.0 IU/L])
LH = <0.5 mIU/mL (1.0-9.0 mIU/mL)
(SI: <0.5 IU/L [1.0-9.0 IU/L])
Prolactin = 40 ng/mL (4-23 ng/mL)
(SI: 1.74 nmol/L [0.17-1.00 nmol/L])

Which of the following is the most likely diagnosis?

A. Hyperprolactinemia
B. Estrogen-producing Leydig-cell tumor
C. Abuse of a nonaromatizable androgen
D. hCG-producing germ-cell tumor
E. Hyperthyroidism

9 A 45-year-old man presents with an 18-month history of increasing fatigue, decreasing libido, and erectile dysfunction. He underwent normal puberty and has 2 biologic children. His medical history includes hepatitis C infection but no head or testicular trauma. He states that he does not use androgens.

On physical examination, the patient is normally virilized. His blood pressure is 110/70 mm Hg. BMI is 27 kg/m^2. He has bilateral nontender gynecomastia. He has no striae or ecchymoses. His phallus is normal. Testes are 15 mL bilaterally.

Laboratory test results:

Total testosterone (8 AM) (by liquid chromatography tandem mass spectrometry) = 650 ng/dL (300-900 ng/dL) (SI: 22.6 nmol/L [10.4-31.2 nmol/L]) (repeated measurement = 750 ng/dL [26.0 nmol/L])
LH = 7.7 mIU/mL (1.0-9.0 mIU/mL) (SI: 7.7 IU/L [1.0-9.0 IU/L])
FSH = 6.1 mIU/mL (1.0-13.0 mIU/mL) (SI: 6.1 IU/L [1.0-13.0 IU/L])
TSH = 2.2 mIU/L (0.5-5.0 mIU/L)
Cortisol (10 AM) = 19.8 μg/dL (5-25 μg/dL) (SI: 546.2 nmol/L [137.9-689.7 nmol/L])

Which of the following is the best next diagnostic step in this patient's evaluation?

A. Measure free testosterone
B. Determine the urinary testosterone-to-epitestosterone ratio
C. Screen for pathogenic variants in the androgen receptor gene
D. Measure late-night salivary cortisol

10 A 69-year-old man is referred by his primary care physician for further management of hypogonadism diagnosed when he presented with decreased energy and libido. At baseline, he had 2 morning testosterone values in the hypogonadal range (190 and 215 ng/dL [6.6 and 7.5 nmol/L]) and a hematocrit measurement of 50% (0.50). He has received intramuscular injections of testosterone cypionate, 200 mg every 2 weeks, for the past 6 months. His libido has improved on this regimen, but he continues to feel tired and sometimes takes an afternoon nap. He does not smoke cigarettes.

On physical examination, his BMI is 36 kg/m^2. He is well virilized, he has normal findings on testicular exam, and his lungs are clear to auscultation. A trough testosterone level drawn before his next injection is 310 ng/dL (10.7 nmol/L), and his hematocrit is now 54% (0.54).

Which of the following is the best next step in this patient's management?

A. Schedule a sleep study
B. Switch from testosterone cypionate to enanthate at the current dosage
C. Continue his current testosterone regimen but arrange for him to have monthly phlebotomy
D. Increase the testosterone dosage to 250 mg every 2 weeks

11 A 60-year-old African American man is referred by his primary care physician to discuss testosterone replacement therapy. During workup for decreased libido and erectile dysfunction, hypogonadism was diagnosed and he is eager to start therapy. He has no lower urinary tract symptoms. He had a myocardial infarction 10 years earlier and is taking an extended-release formulation of isosorbide mononitrate on which he has no angina.

On physical examination, his BMI is 32 kg/m^2 and blood pressure is 125/80 mm Hg. He is well virilized and has normal testes. His prostate feels slightly enlarged but no nodules are palpable.

Laboratory test results:

Testosterone (8 AM) = 150 ng/dL (300-900 ng/dL) (SI: 5.2 nmol/L [10.4-31.2 nmol/L]) (repeated measurement = 180 ng/dL [6.2 nmol/L])
LH = 6.8 mIU/mL (1.0-9.0 mIU/mL) (SI: 6.8 IU/L [1.0-9.0 IU/L])
FSH = 9.5 mIU/mL (1.0-13.0 mIU/mL) (SI: 9.5 IU/L [1.0-13.0 IU/L])
Hematocrit = 47% (41%-50%) (SI: 0.47 [0.41-0.50]
Prolactin = 11 ng/mL (4-23 ng/mL) (SI: 0.48 nmol/L [0.17-1.00 nmol/L])
PSA = 3.3 ng/mL (<3.8 ng/mL) (SI: 3.3 μg/L [<3.8 μg/L]) (repeated measurement = 3.1 ng/mL [3.1 μg/L])

Which of the following is the best next step in this patient's management?

A. Start a phosphodiesterase-5 inhibitor
B. Start testosterone replacement therapy
C. Measure free testosterone
D. Refer him to a urologist

12 A 29-year-old man is referred for evaluation of hypogonadism 2 months after sustaining a head injury after being knocked off his motorcycle. MRI of his brain was normal. He has made good progress since his accident but still has some problems with short-term memory and strength. His libido, which had been quite low when he was discharged from hospital, has begun to improve and he gets spontaneous erections a few times per week. He is married and would like to start a family in the next 1 to 2 years.

On physical examination, his BMI is 23 kg/m^2. He has normal secondary sexual characteristics and normal testicular size. His neurologic examination reveals no focal deficits.

Laboratory test results:

Total testosterone = 180 ng/dL (300-900 ng/dL) (SI: 6.2 nmol/L [10.4-31.2 nmol/L])
LH = 3.9 mIU/mL (1.0-9.0 mIU/mL) (SI: 3.9 IU/L [1.0-9.0 IU/L])

Which of the following is the most appropriate next step in this patient's management?

A. Start treatment with hCG
B. Start testosterone replacement
C. Reevaluate his hypothalamic-pituitary-gonadal axis in 6 months
D. Start a phosphodiesterase-5 inhibitor

13 A 70-year-old man is referred for evaluation of hypogonadism because he has been experiencing low mood, decreased energy levels, and decreased libido. He was recently hospitalized for treatment of pneumonia. At a follow-up visit with his primary care physician 1 week ago, his serum testosterone concentration was low.

On physical examination, his BMI is 25.5 kg/m^2. He has a few bibasilar crackles. He is well virilized, he has no gynecomastia, and his testes are normal in size.

Laboratory test results (sample drawn in the early morning):

Total testosterone = 220 ng/dL (300-900 ng/dL) (SI: 7.6 nmol/L [10.4-31.2 nmol/L])
Repeat testosterone drawn fasting in the early morning of today's clinic visit = 235 ng/dL (SI: 8.2 nmol/L)
Serum LH = 6.2 mIU/mL (1.0-9.0 mIU/mL) (SI: 6.2 IU/L [1.0-9.0 IU/L])

Which of the following is the best next diagnostic test to order?

A. Free testosterone measurement
B. Transferrin saturation
C. Serum prolactin measurement
D. Serum total testosterone measurement in 3 months
E. Pituitary MRI

14 A 40-year-old man is found to have a low testosterone level during an extensive laboratory evaluation performed as part of an executive health screen. He reports normal energy levels and sexual function and has no history of headaches or vision problems.

On physical examination, his BMI is 26 kg/m^2. He has no gynecomastia. He has normal facial, axillary, and pubic hair. His testes measure 12 mL bilaterally.

Laboratory test results:

Testosterone = 45 ng/dL (300-900 ng/dL) (SI: 1.6 nmol/L [10.4-31.2 nmol/L])
LH = <1.0 mIU/mL (1.0-9.0 mIU/mL) (SI: <1.0 IU/L [1.0-9.0 IU/L])
FSH = <1.0 mIU/mL (1.0-13.0 mIU/mL) (SI: <1.0 IU/L [1.0-13.0 IU/L])
Hematocrit = 52% (41%-50%) (SI: 0.52 [0.41-0.50])
Prolactin = 24 ng/mL (4-23 ng/mL) (SI: 1.0 nmol/L [0.17-1.00 nmol/L])

Pituitary MRI shows a 5-mm hypoenhancing lesion.

Which of the following is this patient's most likely diagnosis?

A. Congenital hypogonadotropic hypogonadism
B. Anabolic steroid use
C. Hyperprolactinemia
D. Opioid use
E. Hereditary hemochromatosis

15 A 70-year-old man was prescribed testosterone therapy by his primary care physician to treat hypogonadism. He had several questions about the risks and benefits of his treatment that his primary care physician was not able to answer to his satisfaction, so he requested a referral to a specialist. He has a history of well-controlled hypertension but is otherwise in good health. He reports nocturia once nightly but no other lower urinary tract symptoms.

On physical examination, his blood pressure is 130/80 mm Hg and his BMI is 29 kg/m^2. Rectal examination reveals a mildly enlarged, smooth prostate without nodules on examination.

Laboratory test results:

Hematocrit = 44% (41%-50%) (SI: 0.44 [0.41-0.50])
PSA = 1.7 ng/mL (<5.3 ng/mL) (SI: 1.7 µg/L [<5.3 µg/L])

Which of the following adverse effects should the patient be counseled is most likely to occur if treated with testosterone?

A. Increased aggression
B. Acute urinary retention
C. PSA elevation above 4 ng/mL (>4 µg/L)
D. Erythrocytosis
E. Abnormal liver function test results

16 A 32-year-old man and his 30-year-old wife would like to have a child. The man has a history of a nonfunctional pituitary macroadenoma that was resected at age 28 years. Preoperative and postoperative hormone testing confirmed secondary hypogonadism and hypothyroidism. He has been treated with testosterone and levothyroxine since then. He has no other medical problems. His wife is healthy, has regular menstrual cycles, and is ovulating according to ovulation predictor kits. His current medications are 1% testosterone gel, 5 g daily, and levothyroxine, 150 mcg daily.

On physical examination, he has normal secondary sexual characteristics. His testicular volume is 15 mL bilaterally.

Laboratory test results:

Total testosterone = 450 ng/dL (300-900 ng/dL) (SI: 15.6 nmol/L [10.4-31.2 nmol/L])
FSH = 0.2 mIU/mL (1.0-13.0 mIU/mL) (SI: 0.2 IU/L [1.0-13.0 IU/L])
LH = 0.3 mIU/mL (1.0-9.0 mIU/mL) (SI: 0.3 IU/L [1.0-9.0 IU/L])
Free T_4 = 1.6 ng/dL (0.8-1.8 ng/dL) (SI: 20.6 pmol/L [10.30-23.17 pmol/L])

Seminal fluid analysis showed azoospermia with normal volume and pH.

In addition to stopping testosterone therapy, which of the following is the most appropriate initial treatment option?

A. GnRH
B. hCG
C. hCG plus rhFSH
D. Clomiphene
E. Referral to assisted reproductive technology specialist for testicular biopsy and sperm harvesting

17 A 22-year-old man is referred by his oncologist to discuss options for fertility preservation because he was recently diagnosed with Hodgkin lymphoma. He is scheduled to start chemotherapy with cyclophosphamide in the coming week. The patient is currently single but would like to have children in the future.

On physical examination, his testicular volume is 25 mL bilaterally. His testosterone concentration is 290 ng/dL (300-900 ng/dL) (SI: 10.1 nmol/L [10.4-31.2 nmol/L]).

A semen analysis documents a sperm concentration of 10 million/mL.

Which of the following should be offered to this patient for fertility preservation?

A. Treatment with an aromatase inhibitor during chemotherapy
B. Treatment with a GnRH agonist during chemotherapy
C. Cryopreservation of spermatogonial stem cells before chemotherapy for future transplant
D. Sperm cryopreservation before chemotherapy
E. Initiation of testosterone replacement

18 A 73-year-old man wishes to discuss treatment options for newly diagnosed hypogonadism. He is not keen on the idea of having to apply a testosterone gel or patch daily and expresses a preference for injections. However, he has a history of depression and is worried that testosterone injections may negatively affect his mood. He has read about the long-acting depot formulation of testosterone undecanoate. He likes the fact that the injection must only be administered every 10 weeks and asks for additional information about its safety profile.

Which of the following is a potential adverse effect that this patient might experience as a result of this regimen?

A. Significant fluctuations in energy levels and mood
B. Jaundice
C. Cough and shortness of breath following the injection
D. Skin irritation
E. Flu-like illness

Obesity & Lipids Board Review

Andrea D. Coviello, MD

1 A 42-year-old woman seeks advice on weight loss. She weighed 123 lb (55.9 kg) when she graduated high school. She describes gradual weight gain after the birth of her second child at age 34 years. Her current BMI is 38 kg/m^2. She has a strong family history of hyperlipidemia and heart disease, with family members being affected in their 50s and early 60s. Both of her parents and 1 older sibling take statin medications. She has been told that she also has high cholesterol, but she has not started lipid-lowering therapy. She would like to start a "keto-diet" but would like to know the likely impact on her cholesterol.

Baseline lipid profile:

Total cholesterol = 252 mg/dL (SI: 6.53 mmol/L)
LDL cholesterol = 151 mg/dL (SI: 3.91 mmol/L)
HDL cholesterol = 42 mg/dL (SI: 1.09 mmol/L)
Triglycerides = 296 mg/dL (SI: 3.34 mmol/L)

Which of the following is the most likely effect that following a low-carbohydrate ketogenic diet will have on this patient's cholesterol profile?

A. Decreased HDL cholesterol
B. Decreased LDL cholesterol
C. Increased triglycerides
D. Increased LDL cholesterol
E. No change

2 A 56-year-old man is referred for preoperative assessment in preparation for bariatric surgery. He has class III obesity with a BMI of 48 kg/m^2 and has had type 2 diabetes for 11 years. He was initially treated with metformin and glipizide and progressed to require basal and mealtime insulin, which he states had made losing weight difficult. He was treated with semaglutide weekly and lost 15 lb (6.8 kg), but his weight has now plateaued. He would now like to pursue bariatric surgery.

Which bariatric procedure should be recommended to him?

A. Gastric banding
B. Sleeve gastrectomy
C. Roux-en-Y gastric bypass
D. Intragastric balloon placement

3 A 74-year-old man had an ischemic stroke 6 months ago with residual right-sided weakness of his arm and leg. His medical history is notable for hypertension, hyperlipidemia, prediabetes, and fatty liver disease. He is a former cigarette smoker. He has no history of coronary artery disease or peripheral vascular disease. At hospital discharge, he was started on atorvastatin, 80 mg daily, but he developed myalgias, which prompted a lowering of his dosage to 40 mg daily.

Laboratory test results:

Total cholesterol = 155 mg/dL (SI: 4.01 mmol/L)
LDL cholesterol = 89 mg/dL (SI: 2.31 mmol/L)
HDL cholesterol = 37 mg/dL (SI: 0.96 mmol/L)
Triglycerides = 145 mg/dL (SI: 1.64 mmol/L)
ALT = 64 U/L (10-40 U/L) (SI: 1.07 μkat/L [0.17-0.67 μkat/L])
AST = 58 U/L (20-48 U/L) (SI: 0.97 μkat/L [0.33-0.80 μkat/L])

Which of the following is the best next step for the management of this patient's high cholesterol?

A. Change atorvastatin to pitavastatin
B. Add niacin
C. Add fenofibrate
D. Add ezetimibe
E. Stop atorvastatin and start a PCSK9 inhibitor

4 A 78-year-old woman would like to discuss treatment of her hyperlipidemia. She had a heart attack at age 75 years and started taking atorvastatin, 40 mg daily. She tells you that she "felt terrible" on atorvastatin and "hurt all over." She then tried low-dosage rosuvastatin and simvastatin with the same complaint of diffuse muscle aches. Ezetimibe is recommended as a next step, but she would also like an opinion about supplements that may lower cholesterol. She brought a list of options with her.

Given her statin intolerance, which of the following supplements should she avoid taking?

A. Red yeast rice
B. Berberine
C. Coenzyme Q10
D. Folate

5 A 55-year-old female fitness instructor is concerned about her high cholesterol. Menopause occurred 3 years ago. She does not have diabetes or cardiovascular disease. However, she is concerned because her father had a myocardial infarction at age 45 years. He was treated aggressively with atorvastatin, 80 mg daily, and ezetimibe, 10 mg daily, and is doing well at age 85 years. The patient's fasting lipid profile is notable for a total cholesterol concentration of 252 mg/dL (6.53 mmol/L) and an LDL-cholesterol concentration of 169 mg/dL (4.38 mmol/L). Measurements of TSH and fasting glucose are normal. Her 10-year cardiovascular disease risk estimate is 6.3%. She does not want to take a statin. She undergoes a CT scan to determine her coronary artery calcium score, which returns as "0." She elects to follow a vegan diet rich in olive oil and low in saturated fat. Six months later, her LDL-cholesterol value is 123 mg/dL (3.19 mmol/L) (*see table*).

Analyte	Baseline	After change to vegan diet	Reference ranges
Total cholesterol	252 mg/dL (SI: 6.53 mmol/L)	239 mg/dL (SI: 6.19 mmol/L)	<200 mg/dL (SI: <5.18 mmol/L)
LDL cholesterol	169 mg/dL (SI: 4.38 mmol/L)	123 mg/dL (SI: 3.19 mmol/L)	<100 mg/dL (SI: <2.59 mmol/L)
HDL cholesterol	47 mg/dL (SI: 1.22 mmol/L)	41 mg/dL (SI: 1.06 mmol/L)	>60 mg/dL (SI: >1.55 mmol/L)
Triglycerides	214 mg/dL (SI: 2.42 mmol/L)	374 mg/dL (SI: 4.23 mmol/L)	<150 mg/dL (SI: <1.70 mmol/L)

Which of the following is the best next test to assess her risk of cardiovascular disease?

A. Non–HDL-cholesterol measurement
B. Lipoprotein (a) measurement
C. Apolipoprotein B measurement
D. Chylomicron measurement
E. Nuclear magnetic resonance spectroscopy

6 A 39-year-old woman who recently moved to the area seeks assistance to manage low cholesterol. She was diagnosed with low cholesterol as an infant and was on parenteral nutrition until age 12 years. Since then, she has been treated with daily high-dosage vitamin supplements A, D, E, and K and with intravenous lipid infusions 3 times weekly. She has a history and osteoporosis for which she takes alendronate and anemia. Both of her parents have normal cholesterol. Baseline blood tests are ordered and she is referred to ophthalmology and neurology.

Physical examination findings are notable for a blood pressure of 111/81 mm Hg and weight of 105.5 lb (48 kg) (BMI = 21 kg/m^2).

Laboratory test results:

Total cholesterol = 22 mg/dL (SI: 0.57 mmol/L)
HDL cholesterol = 16 mg/dL (SI: 0.41 mmol/L)
Triglycerides = 12 mg/dL (SI: 0.14 mmol/L)
LDL cholesterol = <10 mg/dL (SI: <0.26 mmol/L)
Apolipoprotein B = <3 mg/dL (50-110 mg/dL) (SI: 0.03 g/L [0.5-1.1 g/L])
Hemoglobin = 14.0 g/dL (12.1-15.1 g/dL) (SI: 140 g/L [121-151 g/L])

Hematocrit = 42% (35%-45%) (SI: 0.42 [0.35-0.45])
ALT = 29 U/L (10-40 U/L) (SI: 0.48 μkat/L [0.17-0.67 μkat/L])
AST = 44 U/L (20-48 U/L) (SI: 0.73 μkat/L [0.33-0.80 μkat/L])

This patient most likely has a genetic variant in which of the following genes?

A. Lipoprotein lipase (*LPL*)
B. Microsomal triglyceride transfer protein (*MTTP*)
C. Apolipoprotein CII (*APOC2*)
D. Apolipoprotein A1 (*APOA1*)
E. Cholesterol ester transfer protein (*CETP*)

7 A 31-year-old woman is referred by her obstetrician-gynecologist because of very high cholesterol. She has no history of cardiovascular disease but notes that multiple family members have been diagnosed with coronary artery disease in their 40s and 50s. She has never been on lipid-lowering therapy. Her only medical problems are infertility and abnormal uterine bleeding. She delivered a healthy baby 5 months ago and plans to breastfeed for 1 year.

Measurement	Prepregnancy	Current
Total cholesterol	361 mg/dL (SI: 9.35 mmol/L)	364 mg/dL (SI: 9.43 mmol/L)
LDL cholesterol	300 mg/dL (SI: 7.77 mmol/L)	301 mg/dL (SI: 7.80 mmol/L)
HDL cholesterol	41 mg/dL (SI: 1.06 mmol/L)	53 mg/dL (SI: 1.37 mmol/L)
Triglycerides	99 mg/dL (SI: 1.12 mmol/L)	49 mg/dL (SI: 0.55 mmol/L)
TSH	0.72 mIU/L	...
Free T_4	0.83 ng/dL (SI: 10.7 pmol/L)	...
Fasting glucose	100 mg/dL (SI: 5.55 mmol/L)	...

Which of the following should be added as the best next step in this patient's management?

A. Simvastatin
B. Pitavastatin
C. Evolocumab
D. Atorvastatin
E. Colesevelam

8 A 55-year-old woman with type 2 diabetes, sleep apnea, hypertension, degenerative arthritis, and hyperlipidemia seeks help with weight loss. She expresses interest in bariatric surgery and asks which type of surgery would be best.

Which of the following procedures is most likely to result in the greatest degree of weight loss in this woman?

A. Sleeve gastrectomy
B. Roux-en-Y gastric bypass
C. Laparoscopic banding procedure
D. Biliopancreatic diversion
E. Endoscopically placed dual balloon device

9 The mother of an 18-year-old girl is concerned about her daughter's weight and long-term health risks. She tells you that her daughter was always the tallest kid in her class. She gained weight quickly as an infant and toddler and her weight was greater than the 95th percentile by the age of 2 years. She was hungry all the time as a child and struggled with obesity despite being very physically active and playing sports. She performed well academically and had many friends. She went through puberty at age 11 years and has always had regular menses. Her BMI is 36 kg/m^2.

A pathogenic variant in which of the following genes is the most likely cause of obesity in this young woman?

A. Melanocortin 4 receptor (*MC4R*)
B. Leptin (*LEP*)
C. Leptin receptor (*LEPR*)
D. Proopiomelanocortin (*POMC*)
E. Fat mass and obesity-associated protein (*FTO*)

10 A 54-year-old postmenopausal women presents for medically supervised weight loss with a meal replacement program. Her height is 66 in (167.5 cm), and weight is 188 lb (85.5 kg) (BMI = 30 kg/m^2). She has seasonal allergies treated with cetirizine, asthma treated with fluticasone, hypertension treated with atenolol, type 2 diabetes treated with metformin and glipizide, and hyperlipidemia treated with atorvastatin. Physical examination findings are notable for central adiposity. A review of her current medications reveals that she is on multiple weight-promoting medications.

Of the patient's medications, which of the following is considered weight neutral?

A. Atenolol
B. Glipizide
C. Cetirizine
D. Atorvastatin
E. Fluticasone

11 A 42-year-old woman with polycystic ovary syndrome is referred for weight management. Polycystic ovary syndrome was diagnosed at age 15 years. She gained weight through college and during her first job, which was very sedentary. She had a baby at age 36 years with the assistance of clomiphene but had difficulty losing weight after delivery. She has lost 18 lb (8.2 kg) over the last 6 months by participating in a commercial weight-loss program and exercising regularly, but her weight has plateaued. She has prediabetes, fatty liver, and depression. Current medications include metformin and a selective serotonin reuptake inhibitor. She also has gallstones, which were noted on abdominal ultrasonography 6 months ago. Her BMI is 38 kg/m^2.

Which of the following should be recommended for continued weight loss?

A. Naltrexone/bupropion
B. Liraglutide, 3.0 mg daily
C. Phentermine/topiramate
D. Semaglutide

12 A 62-year-old man is referred by his cardiologist for help with weight loss. His medical history is notable for hypertension, type 2 diabetes, familial combined hyperlipidemia, and coronary artery disease. He had a myocardial infarction 6 months ago complicated by tachyarrhythmias initially but with preserved cardiac function according to transthoracic echocardiography. He just completed a cardiac rehabilitation program. His cardiologist would like him to lose weight to reduce his risk of a second cardiovascular event.

On physical examination, his blood pressure is 156/92 mm Hg and pulse rate is 76 beats/min. His BMI is 63 kg/m^2. Lungs are clear to auscultation, with no rales. Cardiovascular examination reveals an increased heart rate but no murmurs. He has bilateral edema with a woody quality consistent with venous stasis.

In addition to a diet and exercise program, which of the following medications should be recommended?

A. Liraglutide
B. Phentermine extended-release
C. Phentermine/topiramate
D. Naltrexone/bupropion
E. Diethylpropion

13 A 36-year-old woman with a peak lifetime BMI of 46 kg/m^2 had a laparoscopic gastric bypass operation in another state 8 weeks ago. She initially did well, but over the last 3 weeks she has begun to experience episodes of vomiting. Over the last 5 days, she has been vomiting almost everything she eats. Over the last 2 days, her husband says that she has become increasingly confused, dysarthric, and unsteady on her feet. On neurologic examination, she is clearly confused, has nystagmus, is unsteady on standing, has decreased sensation on her lower extremities, and has a right third nerve palsy.

This patient most likely has a deficiency of which of the following?

A. Vitamin B_{12}
B. Vitamin D (severe)
C. Thiamine
D. Folate
E. Zinc

14 A 32-year-old woman is referred because of "low" blood cholesterol levels. She had a bout of abdominal pain several weeks ago and her physician ordered right upper-quadrant ultrasonography, which revealed a fatty liver. She was previously healthy and takes no medications. Her BMI is 25 kg/m^2. Her physical examination findings are unremarkable. Given her fatty liver disease, her physician ordered a cholesterol panel and a hemoglobin A_{1c} measurement.

Laboratory test results:

- Hemoglobin A_{1c} = 5.5% (4.0%-5.6%) (37 mmol/mol [20-38 mmol/mol])
- Total cholesterol = 56 mg/dL (SI: 1.45 mmol/L)
- HDL cholesterol = 24 mg/dL (SI: 0.62 mmol/L)
- LDL cholesterol = 24 mg/dL (SI: 0.62 mmol/L)
- Triglycerides = 38 mg/dL (SI: 0.43 mmol/L)
- Hepatic profile, within normal limits

Which of the following is the most likely diagnosis?

A. Hypobetalipoproteinemia
B. Abetalipoproteinemia
C. Dysbetalipoproteinemia
D. Hypoalphalipoproteinemia

15 A patient with HIV infection who is currently treated with a protease inhibitor and antiviral medications is referred after developing mild lipoatrophy. His lipid panel is as follows:

- Total cholesterol = 280 mg/dL (SI: 7.25 mmol/L)
- LDL cholesterol = 180 mg/dL (SI: 4.66 mmol/L)
- HDL cholesterol = 30 mg/dL (SI: 0.78 mmol/L)
- Triglycerides = 350 mg/dL (SI: 3.96 mmol/L)

Treatment is started with atorvastatin, 10 mg daily, and his LDL-cholesterol concentration decreases to 120 mg/dL (3.11 mmol/L).

Which of the following is most likely to occur and prevent the use of a higher statin dosage in this patient?

A. Diabetes mellitus
B. Myositis
C. Inhibition of antiviral agents
D. Drug interaction with antibiotics
E. Hepatitis

16 A 58-year-old man is referred for treatment of high cholesterol in the setting of progressive coronary artery disease despite lipid-lowering therapy after his first myocardial infarction at age 48 years. He has hypertension and type 2 diabetes and is a former cigarette smoker. His father had his first myocardial infarction at age 52 years, another at 58 years, and a fatal myocardial infarction at 63 years. The patient has been taking atorvastatin, 80 mg daily, but he developed anginal symptoms 3 months ago and had 2 stents placed. His last LDL-cholesterol measurement was 108 mg/dL (2.80 mmol/L). He wants to know what he can do to decrease his risk of another cardiovascular event.

- Total cholesterol = 160 mg/dL (SI: 4.14 mmol/L)
- LDL cholesterol = 109 mg/dL (SI: 2.82 mmol/L)
- HDL cholesterol = 30 mg/dL (SI: 0.78 mmol/L)
- Triglycerides = 105 mg/dL (SI: 1.19 mmol/L)

Which of the following is the best management strategy?

A. No further treatment
B. Add icosapent ethyl
C. Add niacin
D. Add evolocumab
E. Perform lipopheresis

17 A 43-year-old man seeks help addressing high cholesterol. After experiencing an episode of angina, he had a positive treadmill stress test. On physical examination, he has a firm papulonodular rash on both elbows and orange-yellow linear xanthomas of his palmar creases.

Fasting lipid panel:

- Total cholesterol = 325 mg/dL (SI: 8.42 mmol/L)
- Triglycerides = 340 mg/dL (SI: 3.84 mmol/L)
- HDL cholesterol = 30 mg/dL (SI: 0.78 mmol/L)
- LDL cholesterol = 227 mg/dL (SI: 5.88 mmol/L)

Which of the following abnormalities does this man most likely have?

A. ABCA1 deficiency
B. LDL-receptor deficiency
C. Apolipoprotein *E2/E2*
D. Apolipoprotein CII deficiency
E. Lipoprotein lipase deficiency

18 A 64-year-old woman is referred for hyperlipidemia. She has a history of primary biliary cirrhosis, and ursodeoxycholic acid was prescribed 10 months ago. She currently has no signs or symptoms of coronary artery disease, but there is a strong history of cardiovascular disease in her family.

Laboratory test results:

Alkaline phosphatase = 820 U/L (50-120 U/L) (SI: 13.7 µkat/L [0.74-2.00 µkat/L])
Total bilirubin = 1.1 mg/dL (0.3-1.2 mg/dL) (SI: 18.1 µmol/L [5.1-20.5 µmol/L])
Total cholesterol = 487 mg/dL (SI: 12.61 mmol/L)
Triglycerides = 286 mg/dL (SI: 3.23 mmol/L)
HDL cholesterol = 38 mg/dL (SI: 0.98 mmol/L)
LDL cholesterol = 392 mg/dL (SI: 10.15 mmol/L)

Which of the following is the most likely explanation for her lipid profile?

A. Accumulation of lipoprotein (a)
B. A complication of ursodeoxycholic acid treatment
C. Lecithin-cholesterol acyltransferase (LCAT) deficiency
D. Liver disease causing increased apolipoprotein B production
E. Accumulation of lipoprotein X

19 A 30-year-old woman with systemic lupus erythematosus and the following lipid profile is referred for evaluation:

Total cholesterol = 300 mg/dL (SI: 7.77 mmol/L)
HDL cholesterol = 30 mg/dL (SI: 0.78 mmol/L)
Triglycerides = 1000 mg/dL (SI: 11.30 mmol/L)

LDL cholesterol cannot be estimated. Her current medications include prednisone, 20 mg daily; hydrochlorothiazide; lisinopril; metoprolol; and infliximab.

There is concern that medications could be contributing to her dyslipidemia. Which of the following adjustments should be recommended?

A. Switch prednisone to dexamethasone
B. Switch metoprolol to amlodipine
C. Switch infliximab to apremilast
D. Switch hydrochlorothiazide to chlorthalidone
E. Discontinue lisinopril

20 A 35-year-old Japanese-American woman with the following lipid panel is referred for evaluation:

Total cholesterol = 245 mg/dL (SI: 6.35 mmol/L)
LDL cholesterol = 110 mg/dL (SI: 2.85 mmol/L)
HDL cholesterol = 120 mg/dL (SI: 3.11 mmol/L)
Triglycerides = 75 mg/dL (SI: 0.85 mmol/L)

Which of the following is the most likely cause of this lipid profile?

A. Cholesterol ester transfer protein (CETP) deficiency
B. Lecithin cholesterol acyltransferase (LCAT) deficiency
C. Hepatic lipase deficiency
D. Scavenger receptor B1 (SR-B1) deficiency
E. ABCA1 deficiency

21 A 22-year-old male college student is referred for severe hypertriglyceridemia (>1500 mg/dL [>17.0 mmol/L]). He has a history of pancreatitis. His height is 67 in (170.2 cm), and weight is 185 lb (84.1 kg) (BMI = 29 kg/m^2). He reports that much of this weight gain has occurred in the past 3 years, as he weighed 145 lb (65.9 kg) (BMI = 23 kg/m^2) when he graduated from high school. He usually eats in the school food court—pizzas, burgers, and fries. He does not take any medications or supplements.

Which of the following is the most important immediate lifestyle change to recommend?

A. Avoid omega-3 saturated fats
B. Reduce intake of noncomplex carbohydrates
C. Avoid alcohol
D. Drink more fruit juice
E. Reduce intake of fried foods

22 A 58-year-old woman with type 2 diabetes, hyperlipidemia, and hypertension is referred to you for treatment of her cholesterol. Her American Heart Association 10-year risk of cardiovascular disease is 11.5%. She also has chronic hepatitis C infection with mildly elevated transaminases (<2 times the upper normal limit). She is concerned about starting a statin because of possible liver injury. Her LDL-cholesterol concentration is 164 mg/dL (4.25 mmol/L) and fasting triglyceride concentration is 225 mg/dL (2.54 mmol/L).

Which of the following treatments is the best approach in this patient's management?

A. Start a statin
B. Diet alone until after treatment of hepatitis C
C. Start fenofibrate
D. Start ezetimibe
E. Start niacin

23 A 38-year-old man with an 8-year history of coronary artery disease and multiple hospitalizations for coronary artery stent placements is referred for evaluation. The patient's family has a strong history of heart disease: his father and 2 paternal uncles died before age 50 years. The patient has been taking atorvastatin, 80 mg daily for the last 5 years.

Laboratory test results:

Total cholesterol = 210 mg/dL (SI: 5.44 mmol/L)
LDL cholesterol = 150 mg/dL (SI: 3.89 mmol/L)
HDL cholesterol = 40 mg/dL (SI: 1.04 mmol/L)
Triglycerides = 100 mg/dL (SI: 1.13 mmol/L)

On physical examination, you should look for which of the following findings?

A. Lipemia retinalis
B. Corneal arcus
C. Eruptive xanthomas
D. Palmar xanthomas
E. Arthropathy

24 A 28-year-old woman has lipid levels drawn at a health fair. She is found to have a triglyceride concentration of 525 mg/dL (5.93 mmol/L) and an HDL-cholesterol concentration of 82 mg/dL (2.12 mmol/L). Her LDL-cholesterol level cannot be calculated. She is asymptomatic and has no personal or family history of coronary disease, pancreatitis, or known lipid disorders. She is currently taking oral contraceptives.

Which of the following is the most likely explanation for her lipid levels?

A. Lipoprotein lipase deficiency
B. Apolipoprotein C2 deficiency
C. Oral contraceptive use
D. Cholesteryl ester transfer protein deficiency
E. Soy isoflavones

25 An 18-year-old man is referred by an ophthalmologist after documentation of abnormal cholesterol levels. The patient describes progressive fatigue over the last 4 years. When his parents noticed clouding of his corneas, they took him to see an ophthalmologist who ordered the following laboratory tests (fasting):

HDL cholesterol = 6 mg/dL (SI: 0.16 mmol/L)
LDL cholesterol = 190 mg/dL (SI: 4.92 mmol/L)
Triglycerides = 290 mg/dL (SI: 3.28 mmol/L)

On physical examination, he is a thin, ill-appearing young man. His tonsils are of normal color and size and he has no tendinous xanthomas. Additional laboratory testing documents 3+ proteinuria and a serum creatinine concentration of 2.8 mg/dL (247.5 μmol/L).

Which of the following abnormalities does he most likely have?

A. ATP-binding cassette A1 (ABCA1) deficiency
B. Surreptitious testosterone abuse
C. Defective apolipoprotein B
D. Lipoprotein lipase deficiency
E. Lecithin-cholesterol acyltransferase deficiency

26 A 44-year-old man recently presented with new-onset angina and a positive exercise stress test. He reports no history of hypertension, diabetes mellitus, or cigarette smoking. He follows no specific diet but exercises regularly. His father died of a myocardial infarction at age 45 years, and his brother underwent a revascularization procedure at age 46 years. His father and brother had lipid abnormalities characterized by high triglyceride levels and low HDL-cholesterol levels. The patient's physical examination findings are normal.

Fasting lipid levels:

Total cholesterol = 270 mg/dL (SI: 6.99 mmol/L)
Triglycerides = 300 mg/dL (SI: 3.39 mmol/L)
HDL cholesterol = 30 mg/dL (SI: 0.78 mmol/L)
LDL cholesterol = 180 mg/dL (SI: 4.66 mmol/L)

Which of the following best explains his lipid profile?

A. Familial hypercholesterolemia
B. Lipoprotein lipase deficiency
C. Familial defective apolipoprotein B
D. Familial combined hyperlipidemia
E. Apolipoprotein A1 deficiency

27 A 70-year-old woman is referred for lipid management. She has moderately well-controlled type 2 diabetes with a hemoglobin A_{1c} level of 7.8% (62 mmol/mol). She has a history of several episodes of pancreatitis, as well as a myocardial infarction at age 68 years. After her heart attack, she started atorvastatin, 40 mg daily, which brought her LDL-cholesterol concentration down from 158 mg/dL (4.09 mmol/L) to 88 mg/dL (2.28 mmol/L), but her fasting triglycerides are persistently elevated at 760 mg/dL (8.59 mmol/L). She had been prescribed gemfibrozil but has not yet started it.

Which of the following is the best next step in managing her cholesterol?

A. Stop atorvastatin and start gemfibrozil
B. Continue atorvastatin and add gemfibrozil
C. Stop atorvastatin and start fenofibrate
D. Continue atorvastatin and add fenofibrate
E. Continue atorvastatin and add niacin

Pituitary Board Review

Laurence Katznelson, MD

1 A 24-year-old woman is referred for endocrine evaluation. Her parents report that she received GH injections since age 1 year for growth retardation and GH deficiency. Her growth rate was appropriate while on treatment. Menarche occurred at age 11 years. At age 12 years, she developed fatigue and weight gain, and laboratory tests revealed the following:

TSH = 0.2 mIU/L (0.5-5.0 mIU/L)
Free T_4 = 0.3 ng/dL (0.8-1.8 ng/dL)
(SI: 3.7 pmol/L [10.30-23.17 pmol/L])

Levothyroxine was initiated at that time. She stopped taking GH when she completed growth at age 18 years. She has no polyuria or polydipsia. Of note, 1 month ago she fell off a chair and struck her head; she is not sure whether she lost consciousness.

Laboratory test results (ordered by the referring physician):

Prolactin = 2 ng/mL (4-30 ng/mL)
(SI: 0.09 nmol/L [0.17-1.30 nmol/L])
Free T_4 = 1.3 ng/dL (0.8-1.8 ng/dL)
(SI: 16.7 pmol/L [10.30-23.17 pmol/L])
LH = 13.0 mIU/mL (1.0-18.0 mIU/L [follicular])
(SI: 13.0 IU/L [1.0-18.0 IU/L])
FSH = 21.0 mIU/mL (2.0-12.0 mIU/L [follicular])
(SI: 21.0 IU/L [1.0-13.0 IU/L])

A 250-mcg intravenous cosyntropin-stimulation test results in a 60-minute serum cortisol value of 23 µg/dL (635 nmol/L). Brain MRI reveals a slight reduction in sellar contents.

On physical examination, she has normal vital signs and she appears euthyroid.

Which of the following is the most likely cause of these biochemical findings?

A. Pathogenic variant in the *PROP1* gene
B. Pathogenic variant in the *POU1F1* gene
C. Pathogenic variant in the *TBX19(TPIT)* gene
D. Langerhans cell histiocytosis
E. Hypopituitarism following brain injury

2 A 65-year-old man has a history of renal cell cancer with metastases to the lung. He has been undergoing adjuvant chemotherapy, including treatment with nivolumab. Over the past 3 weeks, he has noted abrupt onset of frequent urination and increased thirst, along with new headaches. MRI is performed, which documents a 1.5-cm hypoenhancing sellar mass.

On physical examination, he is a tired-appearing man. His blood pressure is 98/66 mm Hg, pulse rate is 92 beats/min, and BMI is 21.1 kg/m^2.

Laboratory test results:

Serum sodium = 152 mEq/L (136-142 mEq/L)
(SI: 152 mmol/L [136-142 mmol/L])
Prolactin = 53 ng/mL (4-30 ng/mL)
(SI: 2.3 nmol/L [0.17-1.30 nmol/L])
Plasma glucose = 89 mg/dL (70-99 mg/dL)
(SI: 4.9 mmol/L [3.9-5.5 mmol/L])
Free T_4 = 0.9 ng/dL (0.8-1.8 ng/dL)
(SI: 11.6 pmol/L [10.30-23.17 pmol/L])
TSH = 0.8 mIU/L (0.5-5.0 mIU/L)

Which of the following is the most likely diagnosis?

A. Clinically nonfunctioning pituitary adenoma
B. Prolactinoma
C. Nivolumab-induced hypophysitis
D. Metastasis
E. Histiocytosis

3 A 42-year-old man reports fatigue, weight gain, and decreased strength. He describes worsening short-term memory recall, and he has felt slightly more depressed than usual. He has a known history of a pituitary adenoma, and he underwent transsphenoidal surgery 3 years ago. Since the operation, he has had normal thyroid and adrenal function. He has had some difficulty maintaining an erection over the past year. On physical examination, he appears overweight, with an increase in abdominal girth.

Laboratory test results:

- Complete blood cell count, normal
- Fasting blood glucose = 123 mg/dL (70-99 mg/dL) (SI: 6.8 mmol/L [3.9-5.5 mmol/L])
- TSH = 1.2 mIU/L (0.5-5.0 mIU/L)
- Free T_4 = 1.5 ng/dL (0.8-1.8 ng/dL) (SI: 19.3 pmol/L [10.30-23.17 pmol/L])
- Cortisol (8 AM) = 16 µg/dL (5-25 µg/dL) (SI: 441.4 nmol/L [137.9-689.7 nmol/L])
- Total testosterone (8 AM) = 250 ng/dL (300-900 ng/dL) (SI: 8.7 nmol/L [10.4-31.2 nmol/L])
- IGF-1 = 95 ng/mL (98-261 ng/mL) (SI: 12.4 nmol/L [12.8-34.2 nmol/L])

Which of the following tests should be performed to determine the cause of his signs and symptoms?

A. Morning GH measurement
B. Glucagon-stimulation test with measurement of GH
C. IGFBP-3 measurement
D. Cosyntropin-stimulation test
E. No testing is necessary

4 A 38-year-old woman presents with weight loss, tremor, palpitations, and sweating that have been progressive over the past 4 months. She has had mild frontal headaches, and her menses are irregular.

On physical examination, her blood pressure is 150/95 mm Hg and pulse rate is 96 beats/min. She has no proptosis. She has an enlarged, nontender thyroid gland. Her skin is moist and warm.

Laboratory test results:

- Free T_4 = 2.8 ng/dL (0.8-1.8 ng/dL) (SI: 36.0 pmol/L [10.30-23.17 pmol/L])
- Total T_3 = 413 ng/dL (70-200 ng/dL) (SI: 6.36 nmol/L [1.08-3.08 nmol/L])
- TSH = 1.9 mIU/L (0.5-5.0 mIU/L)
- Prolactin = 28 ng/mL (4-30 ng/mL) (SI: 1.21 nmol/L [0.17-1.30 nmol/L])

A radioiodine scan reveals 50% uptake in a homogeneous pattern in the thyroid gland.

Which of the following is the best next step to confirm this patient's diagnosis?

A. Response of TSH to a trial of cabergoline
B. α-Subunit measurement
C. Assessment for a pathogenic variant in the thyroid hormone receptor gene
D. Administration of thyroid hormone
E. Thyroid-stimulating immunoglobulin measurement

5 A 33-year-old woman has had partial hypopituitarism for 10 years after successful resection of a corticotroph pituitary adenoma. She has been treated with hydrocortisone, levothyroxine, and a low-dosage oral contraceptive pill. Given progressive fatigue, she undergoes testing for GH reserve, and she is found to have GH deficiency. She opts to start GH replacement.

Which of the following may occur after initiation of GH replacement in this patient?

A. A need to reduce the levothyroxine dosage
B. A need to reduce the oral contraceptive pill dosage
C. A need to increase the hydrocortisone dosage
D. An increase in serum prolactin
E. A decrease in blood glucose

6 A 44-year-old woman undergoes transsphenoidal surgery for a clinically nonfunctioning pituitary macroadenoma. Immediately following surgery, she is found to have normal adrenal function, and she is discharged home on day 3 without evidence of diabetes insipidus. On day 8, she calls the clinic and describes nausea and fatigue. On day 9, she has laboratory tests and is admitted to the intensive care unit after the following results are documented:

Serum sodium = 118 mEq/L (136-142 mEq/L) (SI: 118 mmol/L [136-142 mmol/L])
Urine osmolality = 373 mOsm/kg (150-1150 mOsm/kg) (SI: 373 mmol/kg [150-1150 mmol/kg])

On physical examination, her blood pressure is 125/84 mm Hg and pulse rate is 84 beats/min. Her weight is 130 lb (59 kg). She is fatigued but answers questions appropriately. Her volume status appears normal.

Which of the following is the most rapid and effective method to correct her serum sodium?

A. Restrict free water intake to less than 1500 mL/24 h
B. Start demeclocycline
C. Start tolvaptan
D. Start hypertonic saline at a rate of 5 mL/h
E. Start intravenous normal saline at a rate of 200 mL/h

7 Acromegaly is diagnosed in a 63-year-old woman. Initial MRI shows a 1.3-cm pituitary tumor with minimal extension superiorly and laterally. After transsphenoidal surgery, she still has some residual tumor in the left cavernous sinus. She has persistent, unremitting frontal headaches, and her arthralgias are painful. Hypertension persists following surgery. Her postoperative GH level is 3.0 ng/mL (3.0 μg/L) and it does not suppress with hyperglycemia after a glucose load. Her IGF-1 level is 624 ng/mL (72-207 ng/mL) (SI: 81.7 nmol/L [9.4-27.1 nmol/L]).

Which of the following treatment options should be recommended now?

A. Stereotactic radiosurgery to address the residual tumor
B. Lanreotide depot monthly
C. Another transsphenoidal surgery
D. Pegvisomant weekly
E. Cabergoline

8 A 41-year-old woman presents with amenorrhea and galactorrhea and is found to have a prolactin level of 152 ng/mL (4-23 ng/mL) (SI: 6.6 nmol/L [0.17-1.00 nmol/L]). MRI documents a 24-mm pituitary adenoma that abuts the optic chiasm. While taking bromocriptine, 2.5 mg daily, her prolactin level decreases to 38 ng/mL (1.7 nmol/L), menses return but are irregular, and galactorrhea improves but persists. She asks if this management is sufficient for long-term care.

Which of the following should be the next management step?

A. Increase the bromocriptine dosage
B. Switch bromocriptine to cabergoline
C. Discuss surgery
D. Perform pituitary-directed MRI in 6 months
E. Administer octreotide long-acting release

9 A 37-year-old woman with amenorrhea and galactorrhea is found to have a prolactin concentration of 1593 ng/mL (69.3 nmol/L) and a 2.6-cm pituitary macroadenoma on MRI. With cabergoline, 0.5 mg twice weekly, prolactin levels normalize and the tumor size decreases to 7 mm. Over the next 18 months (while taking her medication regularly), her prolactin level increases to 284 ng/mL (12.3 nmol/L) and her tumor grows to 1.4 cm. Despite a gradual increase in the cabergoline dosage to 2 mg daily over the next year, her prolactin level rises to 4513 ng/mL (196.2 nmol/L) and her tumor grows to 3.2 cm and involves the local parenchyma. She subsequently undergoes a 2-stage transsphenoidal/transcranial near-total resection and stereotactic radiosurgery. Over the ensuing 2 years, the tumor continues to grow and she is losing vision.

Which of the following treatments is the best choice now?

A. Temozolomide
B. Another craniotomy
C. Conventional radiotherapy
D. Pasireotide
E. Octreotide long-acting release

10 A 68-year-old man with metastatic melanoma being treated with chemotherapy is admitted to the hospital with lethargy, altered mental status, and hypotension. He takes levothyroxine for hypothyroidism (thyroidectomy was performed to treat thyroid cancer many years ago). In addition to melanoma therapy, medications include iron for anemia.

Laboratory test results:

Random cortisol = 0.9 µg/dL (2-14 µg/dL) (SI: 24.8 nmol/L [55.2-386.2 nmol/L])
ACTH = <5 pg/mL (10-60 pg/mL) (<1.1 pmol/L [2.2-13.2 pmol/L])
Testosterone = 23 ng/dL (300-900 ng/dL) (SI: 0.8 nmol/L [10.4-31.2 nmol/L])
LH = 0.3 mIU/mL (1.0-9.0 mIU/L) (SI: 0.3 IU/L [1.0-9.0 IU/L])
FSH = 2.0 mIU/mL (1.0-13.0 mIU/L) (SI: 2.0 IU/L [1.0-13.0 IU/L])
IGF-1 = 35 ng/mL (67-195 ng/mL) (SI: 4.6 nmol/L [8.8-25.5 nmol/L])
Prolactin = 0.8 ng/mL (4-23 ng/mL) (SI: 0.03 nmol/L [0.17-1.00 nmol/L])
TSH = 0.2 mIU/L (0.5-5.0 mIU/L)
Free T_4 = 0.6 ng/dL (0.8-1.8 ng/dL) (SI: 7.7 pmol/L [10.30-23.17 pmol/L])

MRI shows homogeneous enlargement of the pituitary and stalk, which was not present on MRI 2 months ago.

Which of the following medications is the most likely cause of these pituitary abnormalities?

A. Prednisone
B. Ipilimumab
C. Temozolomide
D. Sunitinib
E. Iron administration

11 A 42-year-old man is found to have a 2.4-cm sellar mass on CT performed in the emergency department following minor head trauma. His physical examination findings are normal, as are his laboratory test results, aside from a mild prolactin elevation of 31 ng/dL (1.3 nmol/L). Following surgery for what turns out to be a gonadotroph adenoma, his pituitary function is normal, but the 3-month postoperative MRI clearly shows residual tumor present in the cavernous sinus. The patient is very concerned about the persistence of the tumor.

Which of the following treatments is most likely to prevent further growth of the residual adenoma?

A. Radiotherapy
B. Pegvisomant
C. Repeated surgery
D. GnRH antagonist
E. Pasireotide

12 A 57-year-old woman with acromegaly has a GH level of 11.7 ng/mL (11.7 µg/L) and an IGF-1 level of 631 ng/mL (78-220 ng/mL) (SI: 82.7 nmol/L [10.2-28.8 nmol/L]) after surgery. As one of the complications of acromegaly, she has difficult-to-control diabetes mellitus (hemoglobin A_{1c} = 8.4% [68 mmol/mol]). She is very concerned about the type of adjunctive medical therapy she should have.

Which of the following medications is most likely to worsen her diabetes control?

A. Octreotide LAR
B. Lanreotide depot
C. Pegvisomant
D. Cabergoline
E. Pasireotide

13 A 28-year-old woman has had amenorrhea for 4 years and is found to have a serum prolactin level of 48.3 ng/mL (2.1 nmol/L). Evaluation documents normal thyroid, renal, and hepatic function and a negative pregnancy test. MRI reveals a 4-mm hypointense area in the pituitary compatible with a microadenoma. Although she is sexually active, she is not planning to get pregnant for at least 4 to 5 years. She has poor health insurance and is concerned about the cost of medications.

Which of the following is the best treatment plan for this patient?

A. Transsphenoidal surgery
B. Bromocriptine
C. Cabergoline
D. Oral contraceptives
E. Reassurance and observation

14 Cushing disease is diagnosed in a 48-year-old woman. Preoperative laboratory test results:

Cortisol (8 AM) = 26.7 μg/dL (5-25 μg/dL) (SI: 736.6 nmol/L [137.9-689.7 nmol/L])
ACTH (8 AM) = 109 pg/mL (10-60 pg/mL) (SI: 24.0 pmol/L [2.2-13.2 pmol/L])

MRI shows a 4-mm pituitary lesion. Glucocorticoids are withheld after surgery. Twenty-four hours after transsphenoidal surgery, her morning cortisol level is 11 μg/dL (303.5 nmol/L). Seventy-two hours after surgery, her morning cortisol level is 10.2 μg/dL (281.4 nmol/L), and she is discharged home. One week postoperatively, her morning cortisol level is 13 μg/dL (358.6 nmol/L).

Which of the following is the best management recommendation?

A. Another transsphenoidal surgery
B. Hydrocortisone daily
C. Medical therapy for persistent Cushing disease
D. Stereotactic radiosurgery
E. Cosyntropin-stimulation test to determine whether maintenance hydrocortisone treatment is needed

15 A 37-year-old man has had recurrence of his Cushing disease 5 years after what appeared to be a curative resection of a pituitary adenoma. A late-night salivary cortisol measurement was elevated on annual screening, and he subsequently began to develop facial rounding, erythema, and increased abdominal fat. He again became hyperglycemic with a hemoglobin A_{1c} level of 6.8% (51 mmol/mol).

Laboratory test results:

Urinary free cortisol = 110 μg/24 h (4-50 μg/24 h) (SI: 303.6 nmol/d [11-138 nmol/d])
Cortisol (AM) = 21.3 μg/dL (5-25 μg/dL) (SI: 587.6 nmol/L [137.9-689.7 nmol/L])
ACTH = 83 pg/mL (10-60 pg/mL) (SI: 18.3 pmol/L [2.2-13.2 pmol/L])

However, MRI shows no evidence of tumor regrowth. After discussion of therapeutic options, he begins taking mifepristone, 300 mg daily, increasing to 600 mg daily. Over the next several months, his symptoms resolve and he feels normal. However, the following laboratory test results are documented:

Urinary free cortisol = 230 μg/24 h (SI: 634.8 nmol/d)
Cortisol (AM) = 35.1 μg/dL (SI: 968.3 nmol/L)
ACTH = 253 pg/mL (SI: 55.7 pmol/L)

Which of the following should be the next step in this patient's management?

A. Increase the mifepristone dosage to 900 mg daily
B. Continue the mifepristone dosage at 600 mg daily
C. Decrease the mifepristone dosage to 300 mg daily
D. Add pasireotide LAR, 20 mg every 4 weeks
E. Refer for stereotactic radiosurgery

16 A 48-year-old man with a history of hypopituitarism after surgical removal of a nonfunctioning pituitary tumor is interested in fertility. His growth and development were normal, and he fathered 2 children who are now 12 and 14 years old. The 1.3-cm pituitary tumor was found incidentally at age 39 years when head CT was performed after a motorcycle crash. He currently takes hormone replacement with levothyroxine, hydrocortisone, GH, and transdermal testosterone. He states he has normal libido and erectile function. On physical examination, he is well virilized with 20-mL testes bilaterally that have normal consistency.

Which of the following should be the next step in this patient's management?

A. Switch from testosterone to hCG injections, 3 times weekly
B. Switch from testosterone to hCG injections, 3 times weekly, and FSH injections, twice weekly
C. Refer for microdissection testicular sperm extraction
D. Obtain a semen analysis
E. Suggest he consider adoption

17 The parents of an 18-year-old man ask if he should continue taking GH when he goes to college. Isolated idiopathic GH deficiency was diagnosed at age 9 years, and the patient experienced a substantial increase in height when he started GH treatment. His growth rate slowed to less than 1 cm/y for the past 2 years.

How should you advise them?

A. Perform a GH-stimulation test one month after stopping GH
B. Measure IGF-1 one month after stopping GH
C. Discontinue GH therapy because growth has been completed
D. Continue GH therapy but decrease the dosage to a more typical adult dosage
E. Measure morning GH one week after stopping GH

18 A 33-year-old woman has developed Cushing syndrome during her 16th week of pregnancy. She has hypertension, diabetes mellitus, hirsutism, and wide, purple striae on her abdomen.

Laboratory test results:

Serum cortisol (8 AM) = 37 µg/dL (5-25 µg/dL) (SI: 1020.8 nmol/L [137.9-689.7 nmol/L])
ACTH = 129 pg/mL (10-60 pg/mL) (SI: 28.4 pmol/L [2.2-13.2 pmol/L])
Urinary free cortisol = 475 µg/24 h (4-50 µg/24 h) (SI: 1311 nmol/d [11-138 nmol/d])

MRI shows a 6-mm pituitary adenoma.

Which of the following treatment options is the most appropriate to control her Cushing disease?

A. Transsphenoidal surgery after delivery
B. Transsphenoidal surgery now
C. Mifepristone
D. Pasireotide
E. Cabergoline

19 A 34-year-old woman has been diagnosed with a 2.5-cm clinically nonfunctioning pituitary macroadenoma that has caused chiasmal compression. Her preoperative evaluation reveals no evidence of acromegaly, Cushing disease, or salt and water imbalance. She undergoes transsphenoidal surgery, which is uneventful. Twenty hours after surgery, she develops marked increase in thirst and polyuria.

Laboratory test results:

Serum sodium = 152 mEq/L (136-142 mEq/L) (SI: 152 mmol/L [136-142 mmol/L])
Urine osmolality = 110 mOsm/kg (150-1150 mOsm/kg) (SI: 110 mmol/kg [150-1150 mmol/kg])

Which of the following treatment options should be initiated?

A. DDAVP, 0.1 mg orally as needed for polyuria and hypernatremia
B. Tolvaptan
C. 1 L fluid restriction
D. DDAVP, scheduled dosing, 0.2 mg orally twice daily
E. Intranasal DDAVP, 10 mcg nightly

20 A 32-year-old man is referred for fatigue and weakness. Nine months ago, he was in a motor vehicle crash and had a severe brain injury, resulting in cerebral hemorrhage and edema. He was in a coma for 10 days, followed by prolonged inpatient and then outpatient rehabilitation. Over the past 2 months, he has had progressive fatigue, as well as reduction in muscle mass. He is frustrated by the lack of successful rehabilitation despite physical therapy. He has gained 12 lb (5.5 kg) over the past 3 months.

On physical examination, he has reduced skeletal muscle mass and increased abdominal girth.

Laboratory test results:

Morning cortisol = 12 μg/dL (2-14 μg/dL)
(SI: 331.1 nmol/L [55.2-386.2 nmol/L])
ACTH = 9 pg/mL (10-60 pg/mL)
(SI: 2.0 pmol/L [2.2-13.2 pmol/L])
LH = 5.3 mIU/mL (1.0-9.0 mIU/L)
(SI: 5.3 IU/L [1.0-9.0 IU/L])
FSH = 4.0 mIU/mL (1.0-13.0 mIU/L)
(SI: 4.0 IU/L [1.0-13.0 IU/L])
Testosterone = 275 ng/dL (300-900 ng/dL)
(SI: 9.5 nmol/L [10.4-31.2 nmol/L])
IGF-1 = 95 ng/mL (113-297 ng/mL)
(SI: 12.4 nmol/L [14.8-38.9 nmol/L])
Prolactin = 1.8 ng/mL (4-23 ng/mL)
(SI: 0.08 nmol/L [0.17-1.00 nmol/L])
Free T_4 = 1.0 ng/dL (0.8-1.8 ng/dL)
(SI: 12.9 pmol/L [10.30-23.17 pmol/L])
TSH = 0.6 mIU/L (0.5-5.0 mIU/L)

Which of the following is the most likely cause of his progressive fatigue?

A. Testosterone deficiency
B. GH deficiency
C. Adrenal insufficiency
D. Hypothyroidism
E. Hypoprolactinemia

21 A 33-year-old woman seeks evaluation for an 18-month history of galactorrhea and a 12-month history of amenorrhea. Her prolactin level is 530 ng/mL (23.0 nmol/L), and MRI shows a 22-mm pituitary macroadenoma that abuts the chiasm. Bromocriptine is started at a dosage of 5 mg orally daily, and her prolactin level after 1 month of therapy is 72 ng/mL (3.1 nmol/L). Amenorrhea persists. Her regimen is switched to cabergoline, and at a dosage of 1.0 mg twice weekly there is no further change in either her serum prolactin level or the MRI findings. She has never been pregnant and is interested in fertility.

Which of the following is the best next step in this patient's management?

A. Switch cabergoline back to bromocriptine
B. Recommend radiation therapy
C. Refer for transsphenoidal surgery
D. Start clomiphene
E. Start temozolomide

22 A 30-year-old woman develops progressive, severe headaches, nausea, vomiting, and fatigue during her 33rd week of pregnancy. She has no notable medical history and was able to become pregnant within 2 months of trying. Her pregnancy course has been smooth until now.

Physical examination findings are normal for 33 weeks' gestation. Her obstetrician persuades the radiologist to perform a noncontrast MRI of her head, and she is found to have a diffusely enlarged pituitary gland with suprasellar extension to the optic chiasm, but without compression of the chiasm.

Laboratory test results:

Total T_4 = 13.0 μg/dL (5.5-12.5 μg/dL)
(SI: 167.3 nmol/L [70.8-160.9 nmol/L])
TSH = 1.3 mIU/L (0.5-5.0 mIU/L)
Cortisol (8 AM) = 9.0 μg/dL (5-25 μg/dL)
(SI: 248.3 nmol/L [137.9-689.7 nmol/L])
Prolactin = 137 ng/mL (4-30 ng/mL)
(SI: 6.0 nmol/L [0.17-1.30 nmol/L])

Which of the following is the most likely diagnosis of the mass?

A. Pituitary adenoma
B. Histiocytosis
C. Lymphocytic hypophysitis
D. Rathke cyst
E. Metastasis

Thyroid Board Review

Jacqueline Jonklaas, MD, PhD, MPH

1 A 54-year-old woman has been treated for hypothyroidism for many years. While taking a levothyroxine dosage of 112 mcg daily, she has maintained a stable serum TSH concentration of 1 to 4 mIU/L. She is hospitalized for abdominal pain and diagnosed with an aortic aneurysm. During recovery from her surgery, continuous enteral tube feeding is initiated. Her hypothyroidism treatment regimen is maintained with levothyroxine, 112 mcg daily (tablet given orally at 6 AM). Her hospitalization is prolonged because she develops pneumonia. Serum TSH is measured and is found to be elevated at 32 mIU/L.

Which of the following would be the most cost-effective change in the patient's therapeutic regimen to normalize her serum TSH?

A. Discontinue enteral feeding
B. Increase the levothyroxine dosage to 125 mcg daily
C. Switch the levothyroxine tablets to liquid levothyroxine delivered in a gel capsule
D. Switch the levothyroxine tablets to intravenous levothyroxine
E. Hold enteral feeding from 5:30 AM to 7:30 AM daily

2 A 31-year-old man with a diagnosis of schizophrenia was admitted to the hospital after a suicide attempt. He had attempted strangulation using a noose but was rescued by a family member. Although found unconscious, he quickly regained consciousness. He was admitted to the hospital for psychiatric evaluation and treatment. Six days later, the patient has now become increasingly agitated and anxious. When examined, he has evidence of a large contusion across his neck. His pulse rate is 120 beats/min, and his patellar deep tendon reflexes are brisk. Thyroid function tests are ordered.

Which of the following is the most likely pattern of thyroid function test results in this patient (see table)?

	TSH	**Free T_4**	**Total T_3**	**Thyroglobulin**
Answer	**Reference range: 0.5-5.0 mIU/L**	**Reference range: 0.8-1.8 ng/dL (SI: 10.30-23.17 pmol/L)**	**Reference range: 70-200 ng/dL (SI: 1.08-3.08 nmol/L)**	**Reference range: 3-42 ng/mL (SI: 3-42 µg/L)**
A.	10 mIU/L	0.6 ng/dL (SI: 7.7 pmol/L)	80 ng/dL (SI: 1.2 nmol/L)	25 ng/mL (SI: 25 µg/L)
B.	8 mIU/L	2.1 ng/dL (SI: 27.0 pmol/L)	200 ng/dL (SI: 3.1 nmol/L)	80 ng/mL (SI: 80 µg/L)
C.	0.01 mIU/L	2.5 ng/dL (SI: 32.2 pmol/L)	210 ng/dL (SI: 3.2 nmol/L)	100 ng/mL (SI: 100 µg/L)
D.	0.1 mIU/L	1.4 ng/dL (SI: 18.0 pmol/L)	290 ng/dL (SI: 4.5 nmol/L)	60 ng/mL (SI: 60 µg/L)
E.	2.5 mIU/L	1.1 ng/dL (SI: 14.2 pmol/L)	90 ng/dL (SI: 1.4 nmol/L)	39 ng/mL (SI: 39 µg/L)

3 A previously healthy 23-year-old man is admitted to the hospital with weight loss, tremors, palpitations, generalized weakness, and right-sided abdominal pain. On physical examination, he has a slightly enlarged thyroid gland without nodules or tenderness to palpation, tachycardia with a prominent precordial impulse, brisk deep tendon reflexes, and a 6-cm right testicular mass. Further imaging of the chest and abdomen suggests metastatic disease to his liver, abdomen, and retroperitoneum. A biopsy of one of the patient's liver lesions stains positive for hCG, and stage IIIC metastatic nonseminomatous germ-cell tumor (choriocarcinoma) is diagnosed.

Laboratory test results:

Serum TSH = <0.001 mIU/L (0.5-5.0 mIU/L)
Free T_4 = 5.1 ng/dL (0.8-1.8 ng/dL)
(SI: 65.6 pmol/L [10.30-23.17 pmol/L])
Total T_3 = 365 ng/dL (70-200 ng/dL)
(SI: 5.6 nmol/L [1.08-3.08 nmol/L])

Assuming that the etiology of this patient's hyperthyroidism is linked to his testicular tumor, which of the following would you expect upon further evaluation?

A. Thyroid ultrasonography showing reduced vascularity
B. Positive TSH-receptor antibodies
C. An hCG value of 6000 mIU/mL
D. An hCG value greater than 6,000,000 mIU/mL
E. A biopsy showing choriocarcinoma metastatic to the thyroid gland

4 A 36-year-old woman has hypothyroidism treated with levothyroxine. She had been taking a 112-mcg tablet of levothyroxine every morning with excellent adherence and almost never forgets a dose. She has consistently maintained normal serum TSH values and generally feels well. She is scrupulous in following instructions for administration of her levothyroxine. Her previous routine was to take it first thing in the morning and delay her breakfast until arriving at work in order to have a full hour elapse between taking her dose and eating.

She now has a new job as an emergency medical technician and has found it impossible to eat breakfast while working. Therefore, she sets her alarm for 5 AM each morning to take her levothyroxine. She tries to go back to sleep for an hour, eats breakfast at 6 AM, and arrives at work by 7 AM. She generally does not eat the same food for breakfast each morning. She has a very regular work, meal, and sleep schedule. She asks for advice about when to take levothyroxine. She is anxious to take the medication as prescribed but is finding it difficult to sleep between 5 AM and 6 AM and feels more tired than usual. Her serum TSH concentration is 1.3 mIU/L.

Which of the following is the best advice to give this patient to facilitate adherence and maintain euthyroidism?

A. Take 7 tablets (112 mg) of levothyroxine together once weekly on one of her days off work
B. Take levothyroxine with breakfast
C. Continue the current schedule
D. Take levothyroxine at bedtime
E. Take levothyroxine at 6 AM and skip breakfast on workdays

5 A 51-year-old African American man is referred with a diagnosis of hyperthyroidism. The patient was found to have a TSH concentration of 0.29 mIU/L during hospitalization after a motor vehicle crash. A follow-up TSH value obtained by his primary care physician 8 weeks after hospital discharge was 0.27 mIU/L. A repeated value was 0.25 mIU/L. Additional workup performed by the patient's primary care physician before referral included measurement of thyroid hormone, thyroid ultrasonography, and a radioactive iodine uptake and scan. The free T_4 concentration was 1.0 ng/dL (12.9 pmol/L), and the total T_3 concentration was 101 ng/dL (1.6 nmol/L). Thyroid ultrasonography showed 3 subcentimeter thyroid nodules without a suspicious appearance, and the radioactive iodine uptake and scan showed a homogeneous pattern and uptake value of 26% at 24 hours.

At today's appointment, the patient has no concerns other than longstanding anxiety, which has not changed recently. He takes fluoxetine. He has been unsuccessful in quitting cigarette smoking. His physical examination findings are unremarkable with a normal-sized thyroid gland without palpable nodules and normoactive patellar reflexes.

Which of the following is this patient's most likely diagnosis?

A. Recovery from euthyroid sick syndrome
B. Subclinical hyperthyroidism
C. Normal thyroid function
D. Abnormal TSH due to fluoxetine therapy
E. Central hypothyroidism

6 A 33-year-old woman undergoes thyroidectomy following diagnosis of thyroid cancer. Pathology shows multifocal intrathyroidal papillary thyroid cancer. Three foci are identified in total: a 1.5-cm focus in the right lobe and foci of 3 mm and 7 mm in the left lobe. No abnormal lymph nodes are identified at the time of surgery. The patient initiates thyroid hormone replacement and returns to discuss whether radioactive remnant ablation is indicated. Her postoperative thyroglobulin concentration is 0.3 ng/mL (0.3 µg/L) while taking levothyroxine to achieve a TSH concentration of 0.3 mIU/L. A joint decision is made that due to her low risk, disease radioactive administration for remnant ablation is not indicated.

Cervical ultrasonography performed annually does not show any abnormal lymph nodes and the patient is monitored uneventfully, including during a subsequent pregnancy. She is lost to follow-up after her pregnancy. Approximately 2 years later, she has a chest CT for reasons unrelated to thyroid cancer, and innumerable subcentimeter nodules are noted throughout the lungs bilaterally, most prominent in the lower lung fields. A serum thyroglobulin measurement at the time is 14 ng/mL (14 µg/L) with a concurrent TSH value of 0.25 mIU/L.

Which of the following accurately describes the patient's disease burden, risk category, and prognosis at the time of her initial diagnosis?

A. The risk of this patient having distant metastases was approximately 1%
B. The patient likely had cervical lymph node metastases that were unappreciated
C. This patient was classified as being in the American Thyroid Association high-risk category
D. This patient was classified as being in the American Thyroid Association intermediate-risk category
E. The risk of this patient having distant metastases was approximately 15%

7 A 56-year-old man undergoes thyroidectomy following discovery of a 4.5-cm thyroid nodule classified as a follicular neoplasm of undetermined significance. Molecular testing shows positivity for a *PPARG* fusion. Pathology shows a 5-cm focus of Hurthle-cell carcinoma with negative margins and negative lymph nodes. His postoperative thyroglobulin concentration is 150 ng/mL (150 µg/L) while taking levothyroxine. The patient is initially advised against receiving radioactive iodine. His local endocrinologist explains that Hurthle-cell cancer does not concentrate radioactive iodine and therefore would not be effective. The patient seeks a second opinion and is advised to proceed with radioactive iodine therapy. Undecided about the best course of action, the patient seeks a third opinion as to whether it would be beneficial for him to receive radioactive iodine therapy. CT of the chest and abdomen is performed, which reveals lesions in the liver that are consistent with metastatic disease.

Answer	Radioactive iodine uptake may be seen in some lesions	Decreased recurrence after radioactive iodine has been seen	Improved overall survival has been seen after radioactive iodine	Radioactive iodine is recommended for tumors >4 cm	Radioactive iodine is recommended for postoperative basal thyroglobulin levels >10 ng/mL (>10 μg/L)
A.	No	No	Yes	No	Yes
B.	Yes	Yes	No	Yes	Yes
C.	No	Yes	No	No	No
D.	Yes	No	Yes	Yes	Yes
E.	Yes	Yes	Yes	No	No

Which of the above summarizes the published guidelines or literature regarding radioactive iodine use in treating Hurthle-cell cancer and may explain the divergent opinions of the 2 specialists (see table)*?*

8 A 37-year-old woman from Myanmar was traveling by plane to visit her family in the United States. During the plane flight, she felt nauseated and dizzy. Upon arrival in the United States, she vomited and had a syncopal episode. She was taken to the emergency department by her family, where she felt partially recovered after intravenous fluids were administered.

The patient has no notable medical conditions, although she has not felt entirely well for the past 2 years. She was briefly hospitalized 3 years ago after sustaining a snake bite, from which she seemed to recover. On physical examination, she is a slender woman with a small thyroid gland, cool dry skin, and sluggish deep tendon reflexes.

An initial laboratory assessment is undertaken, but the hospital computer system is shut down after a suspected cyber attack and only partial laboratory results are immediately available:

Serum sodium = 128 mEq/L (136-142 mEq/L) (SI: 128 mmol/L [136-142 mmol/L])
Serum TSH = 0.2 mIU/L (0.5-5.0 mIU/L)

The remaining results are promised within 30 minutes, but meanwhile the patient becomes disorientated and confused.

Which of the following is the best therapy for this patient pending the recovery of her remaining laboratory results?

A. Intravenous levothyroxine
B. Oral levothyroxine
C. Oral methimazole
D. Intravenous hydrocortisone
E. Intravenous hydrocortisone followed by intravenous levothyroxine

9 A 27-year-old woman is newly diagnosed with Graves hyperthyroidism and has recently started methimazole, 30 mg daily. She has no evidence of orbitopathy. She and her husband are planning a first pregnancy within the next 1 to 2 years, and she is very concerned about the risks that Graves disease will pose for a potential fetus. Her menses are regular, and she has no other relevant medical history.

Which of the following is the best strategy to reduce the risk of fetal malformations in this scenario?

A. Recommend radioactive iodine treatment at least 6 months before pregnancy with normalization of TSH on levothyroxine before conception
B. Change from methimazole to propylthiouracil before conception
C. Change from methimazole to propylthiouracil as soon as pregnancy is diagnosed
D. Decrease the methimazole dosage to the lowest possible to maintain free T_4 just above the upper normal limit once pregnancy is diagnosed
E. Recommend a block-and-replace therapy with both an antithyroid drug and levothyroxine

10 A 58-year-old man with widely metastatic papillary thyroid carcinoma returns for follow-up. He underwent total thyroidectomy 8 years ago. He has subsequently been treated 3 times with radioactive iodine (cumulative dose 370 mCi). There was no uptake on his posttreatment scans after his second and third treatments. On recent PET-CT imaging, he had diffuse lung metastases throughout both lobes and widespread mediastinal lymphadenopathy. He has no brain lesions.

On physical examination, his blood pressure is 122/74 mm Hg, and pulse rate is 74 beats/min. His weight is 142 lb (64.5 kg). He has been experiencing rapidly worsening exertional dyspnea.

Laboratory test results:

Serum TSH = 0.1 mIU/L (0.5-5.0 mIU/L)
Serum thyroglobulin = 1245 ng/mL (3-42 ng/mL) (SI: 1245 µg/L [3-42 µg/L]) (substantially increased from his last measurement 6 months ago)
Thyroglobulin antibodies, negative

Which of the following is the best next step in his treatment?

A. Cytotoxic chemotherapy with doxorubicin and cisplatin
B. Lenvatinib
C. Ipilimumab
D. Palbociclib
E. Vandetinib

11 A 27-year-old woman presents with nervousness, palpitations, itchy eyes, and weight loss of 20 lb (9.1 kg) over the last 3 months. On physical examination, her pulse rate is 110 beats/min. She has moderate proptosis and a diffuse goiter with bruit and moderate tremor. Her serum free T_4 and T_3 levels are moderately elevated, and baseline liver function and complete blood cell count are normal. Methimazole, 30 mg daily, and atenolol are started and her symptoms improve, but she develops hepatic transaminase enzyme elevations (5 times the upper normal limit). Methimazole is stopped. Radioiodine therapy is recommended, but the patient declines this treatment. Atenolol is changed to propranolol. One week later, her thyroid hormone levels have doubled and her liver enzyme levels continue to rise.

Which of the following is the best approach now?

A. Resume methimazole at a 50% lower dosage
B. Start propylthiouracil and closely follow liver function
C. Give supersaturated potassium iodide (SSKI) for 3 to 4 weeks and refer for thyroidectomy
D. Maximize β-adrenergic blockade and refer for thyroidectomy
E. Start dexamethasone, start SSKI, and optimize β-adrenergic blockade before surgery

12 A 54-year-old woman with surgical hypothyroidism and type 2 diabetes is referred for a progressively increasing levothyroxine dosage requirement over the past 12 months. Other medications include metformin, lisinopril, and aspirin. She acknowledges some recent weight gain, but she reports strict adherence to her therapeutic regimen and takes no over-the-counter preparations.

On physical examination, her blood pressure is 140/88 mm Hg. She has no palpable tissue in the thyroid bed, normal deep-tendon reflexes, and moderate lower-extremity edema.

Laboratory test results:

Serum TSH = 8.7 mIU/L (0.5-5.0 mIU/L)
Free T_4 = 1.0 ng/dL (0.8-1.8 ng/dL) (SI: 12.9 pmol/L [10.30-23.17 pmol/L])
Total cholesterol = 305 mg/dL (<200 mg/dL [optimal]) (SI: 7.90 mmol/L [<5.18 mmol/L])
Triglycerides = 880 mg/dL (<150 mg/dL [optimal]) (SI: 9.94 mmol/L [<1.70 mmol/L])
Serum albumin = 2.6 g/dL (3.5-5.0 g/dL) (SI: 26 g/L [35-50 g/L])
Hemoglobin A_{1c} = 7.1% (4.0%-5.6%) (54 mmol/mol [20-38 mmol/mol])
Urinalysis, positive for protein (2.2 g/g creat)

Which of the following is the most likely cause of this patient's increasing levothyroxine dosage requirement?

A. Metformin therapy
B. Medication nonadherence
C. Celiac disease
D. Euthyroid sick syndrome
E. Nephrotic syndrome

13 A 27-year-old woman with a 10-year history of Hashimoto hypothyroidism has been trying to become pregnant and is now 1 week late for her menses. A home pregnancy kit had a positive result. She takes levothyroxine, 125 mcg daily. Thyroid function tests 1 month ago documented a serum TSH value of 3.2 mIU/L. Her primary care physician requests management advice.

Which of the following recommendations is most appropriate?

A. Decrease levothyroxine to achieve a target TSH concentration of 2.5 mIU/L
B. Continue the current levothyroxine dosage
C. Increase levothyroxine by 30%
D. Increase levothyroxine by 40%
E. Increase levothyroxine by 50%

14 A 37-year-old man was diagnosed with Graves hyperthyroidism 2 months ago, and methimazole, 40 mg daily, was prescribed. He is taking his medication regularly. He has developed a sore throat and fever and now presents to the emergency department.

On physical examination, his temperature is 101.8°F (38.8°C), pulse rate is 90 beats/min, pharynx is without exudate, and there is no cervical adenopathy.

Laboratory test results (2 weeks ago):

Free T_4 = 2.1 ng/dL (0.8-1.8 ng/dL)
(SI: 27.1 pmol/L [10.30-23.17 pmol/L])
TSH = 0.01 mIU/L (0.5-5.0 mIU/L)
Liver-associated enzymes, normal
Complete blood cell count with differential, normal

Which of the following is the best next step in this patient's management?

A. Increase the methimazole dosage
B. Switch methimazole to propylthiouracil
C. Obtain throat culture and start amoxicillin
D. Repeat complete blood cell count with differential
E. Admit to the hospital for impending thyroid storm

15 A 62-year-old woman with weight gain and fatigue is found by her primary care physician to have an elevated serum TSH level. Levothyroxine is prescribed without the patient experiencing any resolution of her symptoms. Based on her primary care physician's concern about her unanticipated biochemical response to treatment, she is then referred for assistance in managing levothyroxine replacement therapy. In addition to levothyroxine, she takes calcium and a multivitamin with iron.

On physical examination, her pulse rate is 80 beats/min, she has no goiter or thyroidectomy scar, and her deep tendon reflexes are normal. Serial thyroid function test results and levothyroxine dosing are shown (*see table*).

Date	TSH (reference range, 0.5-5.0 mIU/L)	Free T_4 (reference range, 0.8-1.8 ng/dL [SI: 10.30-23.17 pmol/L])	Levothyroxine dosage
January	11.9 mIU/L	1.3 ng/dL (SI: 16.7 pmol/L)	None
March	10.2 mIU/L	1.8 ng/dL (SI: 23.2 pmol/L)	75 mcg daily
May	10.7 mIU/L	2.1 ng/dL (SI: 27.0 pmol/L)	112 mcg daily

Which of the following is the most likely explanation for these findings?

A. Poor absorption of levothyroxine
B. Resistance to thyroid hormone
C. TSH-secreting pituitary adenoma
D. Poor adherence to therapy
E. Heterophilic antibody interference with the TSH assay

16 A 64-year-old woman with longstanding hypothyroidism is referred to you because of very high levothyroxine dosage requirements. Previously she had maintained normal TSH values while taking levothyroxine, 112 mcg daily. However, over the past 2 years, the patient's levothyroxine dosage has been as high as 600 mcg daily without good biochemical control of her hypothyroidism. She reports strict adherence to her treatment regimen. On physical examination, there is no goiter, but you note a large abdominal mass that extends into the pelvis.

Laboratory test results:

Serum TSH = 178 mIU/L (0.5-5.0 mIU/L)
Free T_4 = 0.4 ng/dL (0.8-1.8 ng/dL)
(SI: 5.1 pmol/L [10.30-23.17 pmol/L])
Free T_3 = 0.26 pg/mL (2.3-4.2 pg/mL)
(SI: 0.4 pmol/L [3.53-6.45 pmol/L])
Reverse T_3 = 413 ng/dL (10-24 ng/dL)
(SI: 6.4 nmol/L [0.15-0.37 nmol/L])

The tumor is most likely to contain excessive amounts of which of the following?

A. Type 3 deiodinase
B. Monocarboxylase transporter 8
C. Sodium-iodine transporter
D. Thyroid peroxidase
E. Pendrin

17 A 37-year-old woman who is having difficulty losing weight is referred for abnormal thyroid function test results. She is otherwise asymptomatic and takes no medications. Her mother has hypothyroidism. On physical examination, her pulse rate is 86 beats/min. Her thyroid is slightly enlarged without nodules or bruit, there is no tremor, and deep tendon reflexes are normal.

Laboratory test results:

TSH = 0.12 mIU/L (0.5-5.0 mIU/L)
Free T_4 = 1.7 ng/dL (0.8-1.8 ng/mL)
(SI: 21.9 pmol/L [10.30-23.17 pmol/L])
Total T_3 = 154 ng/dL (70-200 ng/dL)
(SI: 2.4 nmol/L [1.08-3.08 nmol/L])
Thyroid-stimulating immunoglobulin = 124%
(normal ≤120%)

Which of the following is the best next step in this patient's management?

A. Start methimazole, 20 mg daily
B. Start atenolol, 50 mg daily
C. Treat with radioiodine therapy
D. Repeat laboratory tests in 3 months
E. Start an iodine-containing multivitamin

18 A 35-year-old man presents with a new palpable 2-cm thyroid nodule. Thyroid ultrasonography demonstrates the following finding in the right thyroid lobe (*see image, arrow*).

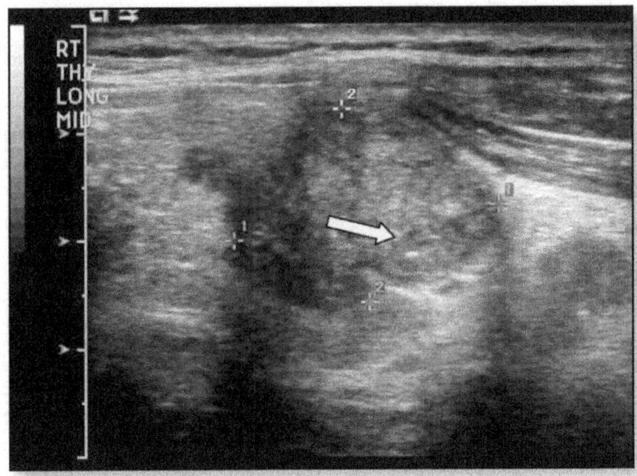

On the basis of the ultrasound pattern observed, what is the likelihood of thyroid cancer?

A. 70%-90%
B. 20%-40%
C. 10%-20%
D. <3%
E. Ultrasonographic patterns do not predict thyroid cancer risk

19 A 38-year-old woman with a history of a 3.0-cm papillary thyroid cancer treated 2 years ago with thyroidectomy and radioiodine ablation is referred for follow-up. Physical examination reveals a 1.5-cm, level 3 lymph node on the left side of the neck. Neck ultrasonography shows bilateral cervical adenopathy. Her serum thyroglobulin concentration is 3.2 ng/mL (3.2 μg/L) at baseline, and it rises to 19.2 ng/mL (19.2 μg/L) after recombinant human TSH. Her whole-body scan, however, is negative. PET-CT shows uptake in the neck corresponding to the palpable lymph node, but FNA biopsy shows only reactive changes.

Which of the following is the best next step in this patient's management?

A. Left lateral radical neck dissection
B. PET-CT after recombinant human TSH
C. MRI of the neck
D. FNA biopsy again and measurement of thyroglobulin in aspirate
E. Surveillance testing again in 1 year

20 A 69-year-old man with tall-cell variant of papillary thyroid cancer invading the strap muscles and extending to the trachea undergoes total thyroidectomy. The surgeon scrapes tumor off the trachea but is unable to remove tumor surrounding the recurrent laryngeal nerve. The surgeon's assessment is that there is gross residual disease remaining in the patient's neck. The patient receives therapeutic radioiodine therapy using an activity of 200 mCi ^{131}I. A whole-body scan performed 7 days after radioiodine therapy shows only faint uptake in the thyroid bed.

Which of the following is the most appropriate next step in this patient's management?

A. External beam radiation therapy to the thyroid bed
B. Tyrosine kinase inhibitor therapy
C. Repeated radioiodine therapy in 3 to 6 months, using dosimetry
D. Chemotherapy with doxorubicin and cisplatin
E. No treatment unless disease progresses

21 A 57-year-old man with Graves disease develops agranulocytosis while taking methimazole. Methimazole is stopped and white blood cell counts recover, but he develops nausea and vomiting and presents to the emergency department.

On physical examination, his temperature is 103°F (39.4°C), pulse rate is 140 beats/min and irregular, and crackles are heard to the mid lung fields. Free T_4 and T_3 levels are 3 times the upper normal limit. He is admitted to the intensive care unit and receives antipyretics, intravenous propranolol, hydrocortisone, and oral potassium iodide therapy. His condition continues to deteriorate and urgent thyroidectomy is planned.

Which additional measure could be considered for this patient before thyroidectomy?

A. Hemodialysis
B. Replacement of propranolol with atenolol
C. Plasmapheresis
D. Intravenous immunoglobulin therapy
E. Cholestyramine therapy

22 An 18-year-old man has a palpable 2-cm neck mass (*see CT images 1 and 2, arrows*). He reports having been treated with antibiotics previously after developing pain and redness in this area. Results from thyroid function tests are normal. Ultrasonography (*image* 3) confirms a cystic mass juxtaposed to the hyoid bone.

Image 1, sagittal view

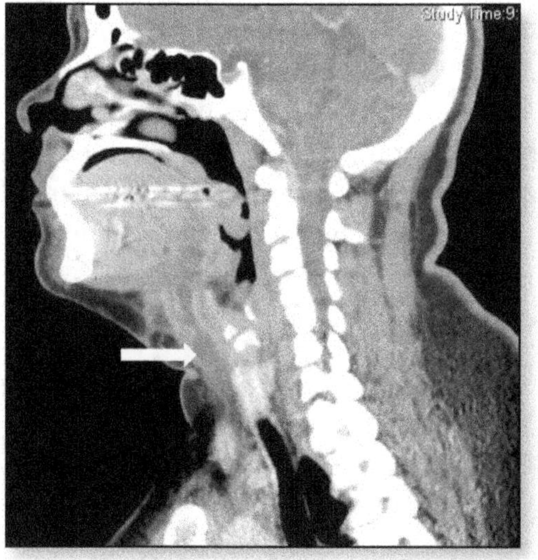

Image 2, coronal view

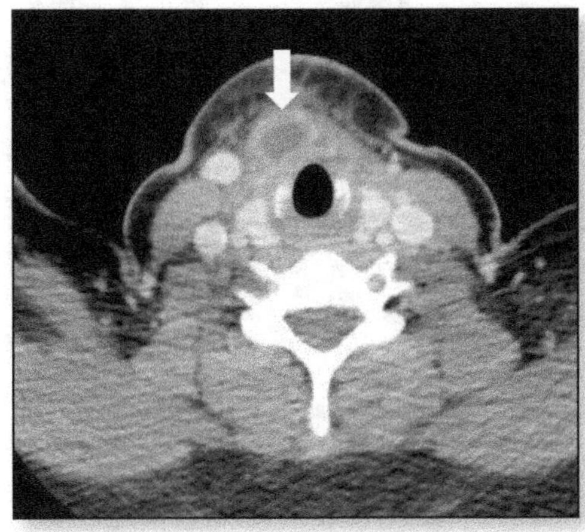

Image 3

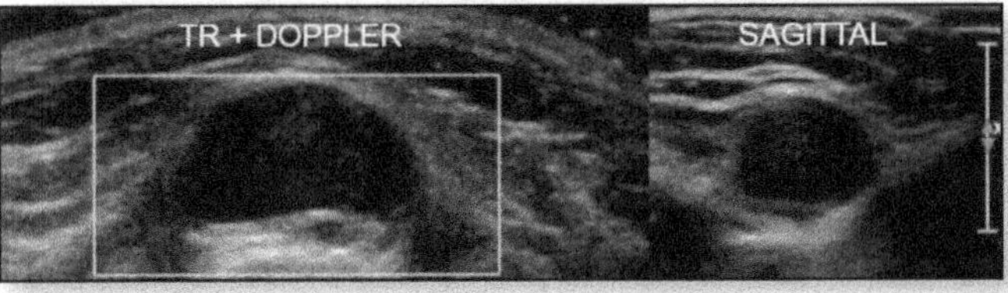

Which of the following is the best management approach for this patient?

A. No treatment now; antibiotics if there is recurrence of infection
B. Surgical resection of the cystic mass, combined with total thyroidectomy
C. Radioactive iodine therapy
D. Surgical resection of the cystic mass
E. Initiation of levothyroxine therapy to achieve TSH suppression

23 A 59-year-old man presents for follow-up of Graves hyperthyroidism that was diagnosed 5 months ago. At presentation he had no signs or symptoms of Graves orbitopathy. He has been treated with methimazole.

Thyroid function test results:

TSH = 0.02 mIU/L (0.5-5.0 mIU/L)
Free T_4 = 1.5 ng/dL (0.8-1.8 ng/dL)
(SI: 19.3 pmol/L [10.30-23.17 pmol/L])
Total T_3 = 140 ng/dL (70-200 ng/dL)
(SI: 2.2 nmol/L [1.08-3.08 nmol/L])

He now reports new bilateral retrobulbar eye aches and occasional tearing starting within the past 3 weeks. On examination, mild eyelid erythema, eyelid swelling, inflammation of the caruncle, and chemosis are present. There is no injection. He has no pain or diplopia with lateral gaze. Vision is normal. There is lid retraction bilaterally that is less than 2 mm. Hertel exophthalmometer measurements are 18 mm on the right eye and 19 mm on the left eye.

Which of the following is the best initial step in this patient's management?

A. Orbital decompression surgery
B. Botulinum toxin therapy to extraocular muscles
C. Rituximab
D. Elevation of the head of the bed
E. Methylprednisolone

24 A 25-year-old man is referred for a 2.5-cm right thyroid nodule. His father had thyroid cancer. The patient has been in good health. Physical examination confirms the right thyroid nodule and reveals no cervical adenopathy. The rest of the examination findings are unremarkable, with the exception of an erythematous patch of skin on the upper back (*see image*) that the patient notes to be highly pruritic and present since childhood. Biopsy of this lesion demonstrates thickened epidermis, increased melanin granules in the basal layer, and accumulation of amyloid in the dermal papillae.

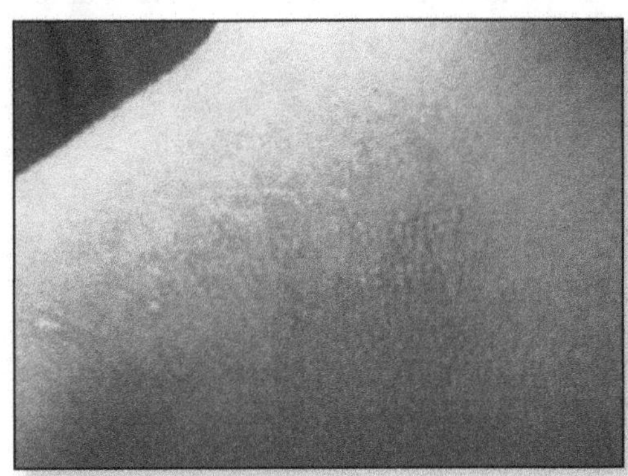

Which of the following is the most likely thyroid diagnosis?

A. Medullary thyroid cancer
B. Papillary thyroid cancer
C. Metastatic disease to the thyroid
D. Thyroid amyloidosis
E. Hashimoto thyroiditis

25 Papillary thyroid cancer is diagnosed in a 40-year-old woman during pregnancy, and thyroidectomy is performed during the second trimester. There is extensive local invasion, and positive lymph nodes are identified in the central and lateral compartments. She initiates breastfeeding after delivery. Treatment with radioactive iodine ^{131}I is planned. The patient is aware that iodine is a component of breast milk and asks for recommendations concerning lactation and radioactive iodine treatment.

Which of the following recommendations is most appropriate?

A. Defer radioactive iodine treatment until the infant is at least 12 months old
B. Continue breastfeeding; pump and discard breast milk for 3 to 4 days after radioactive iodine treatment before resuming breastfeeding
C. Stop breastfeeding 3 weeks before the radioactive iodine treatment
D. Stop breastfeeding 3 months before the radioactive iodine treatment
E. Continue breastfeeding and treat the patient with amifostine before radioactive iodine therapy is delivered

26 A 77-year-old woman with a history of Hashimoto hypothyroidism since age 42 years presents with rapid thyroid enlargement over the course of several weeks. She reports a sensation of discomfort and pressure in her neck. While taking levothyroxine, her serum TSH concentration is 1.34 mIU/L and her TPO antibody level is 462 IU/mL (462 kIU/L). Ultrasonography shows a markedly heterogeneous gland with a 5.4-cm left-sided nodule. FNA biopsy of the nodule is performed (*see image*).

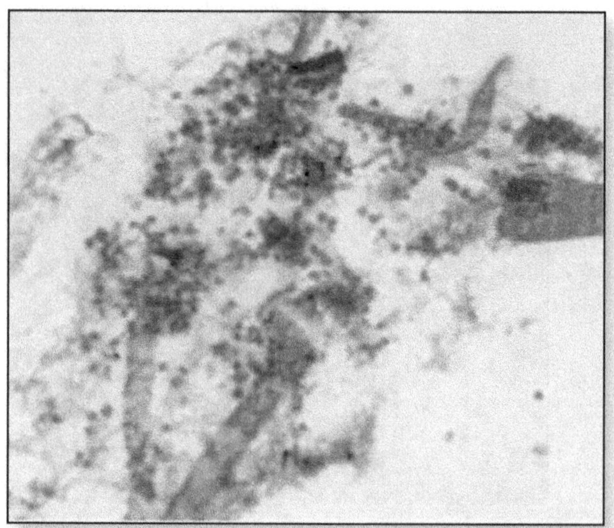

Which of the following is the best next step in this patient's management?

A. ^{123}I scan
B. Total thyroidectomy
C. Repeated FNA biopsy with flow cytometry
D. Repeated FNA biopsy with gene classifier testing
E. Repeated FNA with testing for the pathogenic variants associated with thyroid cancer

27 A 47-year-old woman is found to have a left thyroid nodule. Thyroid ultrasonography shows a 4.8-cm hypoechoic nodule without calcification or hypervascularity and a 0.5-cm right anechoic nodule, with no suspicious lymph nodes. The patient undergoes FNA biopsy of the dominant nodule with cytologic findings of a follicular neoplasm. Repeated FNA biopsy with molecular analysis reveals a *PAX8/PPARG* rearrangement.

Which of the following is the most appropriate next step in this patient's management?

A. Refer for total thyroidectomy
B. Perform thyroid ultrasonography again in 6 months
C. Perform FNA biopsy again in 6 months
D. Perform molecular analysis again in 6 months
E. Refer for diagnostic lobectomy

28 A 52-year-old woman presents with enlargement of her anterior neck over the last 6 months. Her TSH concentration is 0.96 mIU/L (0.5-5.0 mIU/L). Ultrasonography shows a 4.2-cm simple cyst in the left lobe extending into the isthmus. After aspiration of 10 cc of dark brown fluid, the nodule decreases in size to 3.1 cm. Cytopathologic results are interpreted as Bethesda I (nondiagnostic). Three months after her initial visit and cyst aspiration, repeated ultrasonography shows that the cyst fluid has completely reaccumulated. She describes a constant pressure sensation in her anterior neck and discomfort when she lies flat. The patient strongly wishes to avoid surgery.

Which of the following is the best option for control of compressive symptoms?

A. Reaspiration of the cyst
B. Ethanol injection of the cyst
C. Radiofrequency ablation
D. Laser ablation
E. Radioactive iodine treatment

ENDOCRINE BOARD REVIEW

Adrenal Board Review

Tobias Else, MD

1 ANSWER: C) Discuss the diagnosis of pseudopheochromocytoma

This is a classic case of a patient with a diagnosis of pseudopheochromocytoma (Answer C). She has symptoms that could be consistent with a pheochromocytoma or paraganglioma, yet the plasma metanephrines were only minimally elevated. Plasma metanephrines are constantly secreted by chromaffin tumors. In the setting of minimal elevation, a 24-hour urine collection for metanephrines (Answer A) would not be helpful. Although pseudopheochromocytoma is probably more commonly encountered than true pheochromocytoma, there is little research on this entity. Patients with pseudopheochromocytoma experience sudden blood pressure surges not triggered by emotional distress, but are generally very symptomatic, mimicking true pheochromocytoma spells. This patient's biochemical and imaging studies do not support the diagnosis of a true pheochromocytoma. Cardiovascular events in patients with pseudopheochromocytoma appear to be rare. Affected patients are often well-educated individuals and successful in their careers. Exploration of psychosocial factors often reveals a history of abuse or trauma. Therapy is difficult and must be a multipronged approach, including treatment of the acute episodes of hypertension, as well as psychopharmacologic and psychotherapeutic approaches. A first step should be confident reassurance that the patient does not have a pheochromocytoma (Answer C).

This patient's adrenal nodule is rather small and is extremely unlikely to produce symptoms. For a lesion to elicit symptoms, one would expect a mass of at least 2.5 to 3.0 cm accompanied by 2- to 3-fold elevated normetanephrine levels. Normetanephrine values are more often false-positive than are metanephrine values. Elevated metanephrine levels are always concerning when they are above the normal range. In cases where normetanephrine levels are elevated, clonidine-suppression testing is a good option to exclude pheochromocytoma.

Additional cross-sectional imaging with MRI (Answer E) or functional imaging with ^{123}I-MIBG SPECT-CT or ^{68}Ga-DOTATATE PET-CT (Answer B) is unlikely to reveal any results that would confirm a pheochromocytoma in this patient. The fact that the left adrenal gland and the small nodule are positive is not unusual. Even normal adrenal glands, particularly the left adrenal, are often positive on ^{123}I-MIBG SPECT-CT, representing physiologic activity. Moreover, the heart is mildly MIBG-avid on ^{123}I-MIBG SPECT-CT. Absence of physiologic MIBG uptake in the heart is a good surrogate parameter for a hypercatecholaminergic state, such as a pheochromocytoma. Therefore, proceeding with adrenalectomy (Answer D) would be wrong.

EDUCATIONAL OBJECTIVE

Identify pseudopheochromocytoma as a common differential diagnosis of true pheochromocytoma.

REFERENCE(S)

Mann SJ. Severe paroxysmal hypertension (pseudopheochromocytoma). *Curr Hypertens Rep.* 2008;10(1):12-18. PMID: 18367021

Lenders JW, Duh QY, Eisenhofer G, et al; Endocrine Society. Pheochromocytoma and paraganglioma: an Endocrine Society clinical practice guideline. *J Clin Endocrinol Metab.* 2014;99(6):1915-1942. PMID: 24893135

Mamilla D, Gonzales MK, Esler MD, Pacak K. Pseudopheochromocytoma. *Endocrinol Metab Clin North Am.* 2019;48(4):751-764. PMID: 31655774

2 ANSWER: B) Sleep study

This patient is obese and has hypertension, mild hypogonadism, and possibly primary aldosteronism. He also has typical symptoms of obstructive sleep apnea (OSA). A sleep study (Answer B) is the best approach for confirming OSA. OSA can be associated with false-positive elevations of urine metanephrines, with often normal or borderline elevated plasma free metanephrines. Therefore, OSA would most likely explain the increase in this patient's urine normetanephrine. Other conditions that can cause false-positive normetanephrine values are tricyclic antidepressants, norepinephrine uptake inhibitors, and heart failure. Functional imaging (Answers C and D) would not be helpful, as the patient is unlikely to have a chromaffin tumor. Doxazosin does not typically cause false-positive metanephrine levels, so holding this agent and measuring plasma metanephrine again (Answer E) is incorrect.

This patient also has hypogonadism and a borderline-positive screen for primary aldosteronism. Both endocrine disorders can accompany OSA. It is a matter of debate as to whether they are related to obesity (which is also present in this patient) or OSA. In the absence of any classic symptoms or signs of hypercortisolism, screening for hypercortisolism (Answer A) is less important. One could consider screening this patient for subclinical Cushing syndrome, which is generally of adrenal origin, and the 1-mg dexamethasone-suppression test would be the best choice, as 24-hour urine is often within the normal range. However, it should be interpreted in conjunction with other tests for adrenal hypercortisolism, as elevated cortisol-binding globulin in obesity can lead to false-positive results on 1-mg dexamethasone-suppression testing. With low-normal potassium and borderline-positive screening for primary aldosteronism, one could consider rescreening or confirmatory testing for this condition.

He will most likely benefit from multimodal therapy with weight-loss strategies, nocturnal breathing support, and possibly the addition of a mineralocorticoid antagonist.

EDUCATIONAL OBJECTIVE

Evaluate for obstructive sleep apnea as a cause of increased metanephrines.

REFERENCE(S)

Funder JW, Carey RM, Mantero F, et al. The management of primary aldosteronism: case detection, diagnosis, and treatment: an Endocrine Society clinical practice guideline. *J Clin Endocrinol Metab.* 2016;101(5):1889-1916. PMID: 26934393

Bhasin S, Brito JP, Cunningham GR, et al. Testosterone therapy in men with hypogonadism: an Endocrine Society clinical practice guideline. *J Clin Endocrinol Metab.* 2018;103(5):1715-1744. PMID: 29562364

Gilardini L, Lombardi C, Redaelli G, et al. Effect of continuous positive airway pressure in hypertensive patients with obstructive sleep apnea and high urinary metanephrines. *J Hypertens.* 2018;36(1):199-204. PMID: 28800040

3 ANSWER: A) Medication given as prophylaxis for postoperative nausea

This patient with obesity, diabetes, and hypertension has had an episode of mild postsurgical hypotension and tachycardia, responsive to fluid resuscitation. She has hyperglycemia and mild hyponatremia. Clinically, the rapid resolution of symptoms with intravenous fluids, as well as the presence of hyperglycemia are not consistent with adrenal insufficiency. Hyperglycemia and low cortisol are most likely due to the presurgical administration of dexamethasone (Answer A). Dexamethasone, 4 to 8 mg, is routinely given to patients with risk factors for postoperative nausea and vomiting (female sex, nonsmoker, emetogenic surgery).

Inhaled anesthetics (Answer E) are not associated with adrenal insufficiency. Etomidate, sometimes used in anesthetic protocols, can induce a transient adrenally insufficient state due to

11-hydroxylase inhibition. While opioids in the acute and chronic setting can alter the hypothalamic-pituitary-adrenal axis, nonopioid drugs or low-dosage tramadol (Answer B) do not pose this risk. Metastasis from solid tumors (Answer D) almost never cause adrenal insufficiency. Indeed, the adrenal cortex gets pushed to the periphery, but remains present and functional with even large metastasis. Moreover, adrenal metastasis from colon cancer is rare. Adrenal metastases are more typical for lung cancer, breast cancer, kidney cancer, or melanoma. This patient does not have any other risk factors, symptoms, or signs consistent with preexisting adrenal insufficiency (Answer C). When considering adrenal insufficiency in the acute postsurgical setting, it is most important to evaluate for anticoagulation or bleeding disorders, which predispose to adrenal hemorrhage. However, the clinical scenario would be much more serious.

If the patient did not receive any glucocorticoids for postoperative nausea and vomiting, it would be worthwhile to explore prior use of glucocorticoids in inhalers, nasal spray, musculoskeletal injections, or topical application, all of which can suppress the hypothalamic-pituitary-adrenal axis.

EDUCATIONAL OBJECTIVE

List the various conditions treated with glucocorticoids and explain their effect on adrenal function.

REFERENCE(S)

Gan TJ, Diemunsch P, Habib AS, et al; Society for Ambulatory Anesthesia. Consensus guidelines for the management of postoperative nausea and vomiting [published corrections appear in *Anesth Analg.* 2014;118(3):689 and *Anesth Analg.* 2015;120(2):494]. *Anesth Analg.* 2014;118(1): 85-113. PMID: 24356162

Bornstein SR, Allolio B, Arlt W, et al. Diagnosis and treatment of primary adrenal insufficiency: an Endocrine Society clinical practice guideline. *J Clin Endocrinol Metab.* 2016;101(2):364-389. PMID: 26760044

4 ANSWER: B) Lynch syndrome (hereditary nonpolyposis colon cancer)

This patient has adrenocortical cancer and a classic family history of Lynch syndrome (Answer B), which includes colon cancer and uterine cancer, often diagnosed at a young age (<50 years), as core syndromic expression. Individuals with Lynch syndrome are also predisposed to developing pancreatic cancer, ovarian cancer, prostate cancer, and sebaceous gland cancers. Lynch syndrome is caused by germline pathogenic variants in the *MSH2, MSH6, PMS2,* or *MLH1* genes, and immunohistochemical staining for the gene products can be used to screen the pathologic specimen. Adrenal cancer occurs in a minority of patients with Lynch syndrome, but the prevalence of Lynch syndrome among patients with adrenocortical cancer is the same as in patients with colon or uterine cancer (3%-5%), making evaluation for this familial cancer syndrome worthwhile in patients with adrenal cancer.

Li-Fraumeni syndrome (Answer A) is a cancer syndrome predisposing to young-onset breast cancer, lung cancer, sarcomas, brain cancer, and adrenal cancer. Up to 80% of all children with adrenal cancer have a germline pathogenic variant in the *TP53* gene, and *TP53* pathogenic variants can be found in adult patients with adrenal cancer (up to 2%-3%). However, the family history in this case is not typical of Li-Fraumeni syndrome. In a significant number of cases, the family history will be entirely negative, as up to 20% of all pathogenic *TP53* variants are de novo.

Familial adenomatous polyposis (Answer C) predisposes to colon polyps and colon cancer (usually age 20-40 years), as well as to some other tumors. Adrenal adenomas are more common in patients with familial adenomatous polyposis, but adrenal cancer is rare.

The adrenal phenotype in Carney complex (Answer D), with the main manifestations of GH hypersecretion, cardiac myxomas, and testicular large-cell calcifying Sertoli-cell tumors, is primary pigmented nodular adrenal disease, with hypercortisolism and normal-sized adrenal glands. Adrenal cancer has been described, but it is rare among patients with Carney complex/primary pigmented nodular adrenal disease due to germline pathogenic *PRKAR1A* variants.

Multiple endocrine neoplasia type 1 (Answer E) predisposes to primary hyperparathyroidism (usually before age 40 years), pituitary adenomas, and foregut neuroendocrine tumors. Cushing syndrome can be due to adrenal tumors, pituitary tumors, or ectopic ACTH or corticotropin-releasing hormone production by neuroendocrine tumors. There is an increased incidence of adrenal tumors in multiple endocrine neoplasia type 1. Up to 40% of affected patients have at least 1 adrenal nodule, but they are usually benign. Although the relative risk for adrenal cancer is increased in patients with multiple endocrine neoplasia, the personal and family history in this patient is not suggestive of this syndrome.

EDUCATIONAL OBJECTIVE

Describe the hereditary predisposition to adrenocortical carcinoma.

REFERENCE(S)

Fassnacht M, Dekkers OM, Else T, et al. European Society of Endocrinology clinical practice guidelines on the management of adrenocortical carcinoma in adults, in collaboration with the European Network for the Study of Adrenal Tumors. *Eur J Endocrinol.* 2018;179(4):G1-G46. PMID: 30299884

Raymond VM, Everett JN, Furtado LV, et al. Adrenocortical carcinoma is a lynch syndrome-associated cancer [*J Clin Oncol.* 2013;31(28):3612]. *J Clin Oncol.* 2013;31(24):3012-3018. PMID: 23752102

5 ANSWER: D) Adrenal lymphoma

This patient has bilateral adrenal masses and findings suggestive of primary adrenal insufficiency (tiredness, fatigue, nausea, weight loss, orthostatic hypertension, hyponatremia, hyperkalemia, low cortisol, and elevated ACTH). The most common causes of adrenal insufficiency are congenital adrenal hyperplasia (usually 21-hydroxylase deficiency [Answer A]), autoimmune adrenalitis (Answer B), and, in young men, adrenoleukodystrophy. However, this patient does not have a classic history of any of these conditions, and with the latter 2 conditions the adrenal glands appear small or normal on imaging. When considering the differential diagnosis of adrenal insufficiency with bilateral adrenal enlargement in an adult patient, the main considerations are infectious or granulomatous disease, adrenal hemorrhage, or infiltrative disease such as lymphoma (Answer D). Common infections that lead to adrenal enlargement and adrenal insufficiency are tuberculosis and histoplasmosis (Answer E). However, this patient has no risk factors for either of these 2 diseases, he does not live in an area where histoplasmosis is endemic, and his chest CT shows no abnormalities. In the setting of tuberculosis, the adrenal glands can also show significant areas of calcification. Another rare differential diagnosis would be adrenal involvement with sarcoidosis. Adrenal hemorrhage, not an answer option, is a possibility, but in that setting, the patient's history would usually reveal anticoagulation therapy or a bleeding disorder. While adrenal metastasis from melanoma (Answer C) is common, adrenal insufficiency almost never occurs in this setting. Metastases usually do not destroy adrenocortical tissue—the tissue simply remains functionally intact in the periphery of even large adrenal metastases.

After exclusion of pheochromocytoma by documenting normal plasma free metanephrines, an adrenal biopsy would reveal the correct diagnosis in this patient. Particularly with diffuse large B-cell lymphoma, adrenal involvement is quite common and is part of the clinical risk score to predict central nervous system involvement.

EDUCATIONAL OBJECTIVE

Describe the causes of bilateral adrenal enlargement with adrenal insufficiency.

REFERENCE(S)

Bornstein SR, Allolio B, Arlt W, et al. Diagnosis and treatment of primary adrenal insufficiency: an Endocrine Society clinical practice guideline. *J Clin Endocrinol Metab.* 2016;101(2):364-389. PMID: 26760044

Rashidi A, Fisher SI. Primary adrenal lymphoma: a systematic review. *Ann Hematol.* 2013;92(12): 1583-1593. PMID: 23771429

6 **ANSWER: A) Cholestyramine**

This patient has longstanding adrenal insufficiency without a dosage change in hydrocortisone. She has symptoms and signs of adrenal insufficiency despite taking the same hydrocortisone dosage. When considering causes of insidious worsening of symptoms and signs of adrenal insufficiency, one should consider additional endocrinopathies, medication changes, or other systemic diseases. Autoimmune adrenalitis occurs as part of other autoimmune disorders and endocrinopathies.

Cholestyramine (Answer A) is commonly used to treat chronic diarrhea due to its bile acid–sequestering properties. Cholestyramine also binds hydrocortisone and prevents its absorption. The patient should be advised to take hydrocortisone at least 1 hour before the cholestyramine, which usually resolves the issue.

While Hashimoto disease (Answer C) might explain some of her symptoms, she does not have typical hypothyroid symptoms and her free T_4 concentration is normal and TSH concentration is only slightly elevated. Hydrocortisone requirements are not typically affected by low thyroid hormone levels. An increased requirement would rather be expected with hyperthyroidism (eg, Graves disease), which leads to increased metabolism of hydrocortisone. Several medications can increase hydrocortisone requirements. Usually, inducers of *CYP3A4* increase cortisol metabolism. While physiologically only a small fraction of cortisol is metabolized through 6β-hydroxylation by CYP3A4, induction of this enzyme can significantly increase this fraction. Common inducers of CYP3A4 are mitotane, carbamazepine, phenytoin, and St. John's Wort.

Proton-pump inhibitors (Answer B) are not known to influence hydrocortisone metabolism or absorption. Estrogen-containing oral contraceptives (Answer D) do increase cortisol-binding globulin and can pose a challenge when measuring total serum cortisol (eg, 1-mg dexamethasone-suppression test), but there is no effect on the total daily hydrocortisone requirement. While biotin can interfere with several immunoassays, there is no biologic effect that would require adjustment of the hydrocortisone dosage. Atrophic gastritis (Answer E) is commonly observed in patients with polyglandular autoimmune syndrome, but it does not alter hydrocortisone requirements.

EDUCATIONAL OBJECTIVE

Identify medications that can alter hydrocortisone metabolism and absorption.

REFERENCE(S)

Bornstein SR, Allolio B, Arlt W, et al. Diagnosis and treatment of primary adrenal insufficiency: an Endocrine Society clinical practice guideline. *J Clin Endocrinol Metab.* 2016;101(2):364-389. PMID: 26760044

Johansson C, Adamsson U, Stierner U, Lindsten T. Interaction by cholestyramine on the uptake of hydrocortisone in the gastrointestinal tract. *Acta Med Scand.* 1978;204(6):509-512. PMID: 735882

7 **ANSWER: E) Plasma ACTH measurement**

The biochemical diagnosis of hypercortisolemia relies on 3 screening tests: 24-hour urinary free cortisol excretion, late-night salivary cortisol measurement, and overnight 1-mg dexamethasone-suppression test. None of these studies is perfect and they all have limitations. The value of any of these tests depends greatly on the pretest probability of Cushing syndrome. This patient has a high pretest probability of Cushing syndrome on the basis of her history and physical examination findings. In addition, she has a known adrenal mass. Although the referral was to evaluate the adrenal mass, most adenomas that produce clinically significant hypercortisolemia are larger than 2.5 cm in diameter, so it is unlikely that this tumor is causing cortisol excess.

Biopsy of the mass (Answer D) would only reveal cortical cells or other tissue, and it would not address the functional state of the adrenal mass. In general, adrenal biopsy should only be considered in the setting of metastatic cancer and after exclusion of a pheochromocytoma. Similarly, adrenal MRI (Answer B) might confirm that the tumor is a lipid-rich cortical adenoma, but this will not aid in the evaluation. She has 2 very abnormal salivary cortisol values and a very abnormal result following an overnight dexamethasone-suppression test, so hypercortisolemia is established. Therefore, another type of screening such as urinary free cortisol measurement is not necessary. Instead, subtyping of the different etiologies of Cushing syndrome is the next step to determine whether the cortisol excess is ACTH-dependent or ACTH-independent. This is accomplished with a plasma ACTH measurement (Answer E). In this case, the plasma ACTH value was 60 pg/mL (13.2 pmol/L), and the patient had pituitary Cushing disease. The adrenal tumor was a red herring.

The purpose of the dexamethasone corticotropin-releasing hormone test (Answer C) is to distinguish pseudocushing state (defined as physiologic or pathologic elevation of cortisol levels not caused by hypothalamic-pituitary-adrenal axis pathologies) from pathologic hypercortisolism when other testing and physical examination findings are equivocal. This patient has significant biochemical abnormalities and suggestive physical exam findings, so this distinction is not necessary. Plasma renin activity (Answer A) would be relevant if one were screening for primary aldosteronism but not for the evaluation of hypercortisolemia.

EDUCATIONAL OBJECTIVE

Recommend measurement of plasma ACTH as the initial differential diagnostic test in the subtyping of Cushing syndrome.

REFERENCE(S)

Findling JW, Raff H. Cushing's syndrome: important issues in diagnosis and treatment. *J Clin Endocrinol Metab.* 2006;91(10):3746-3753. PMID: 16868050

Kidambi S, Raff H, Findling JW. Limitations of nocturnal salivary cortisol and urine free cortisol in the diagnosis of mild Cushing's syndrome. *Eur J Endocrinol.* 2007;157(6):725-731. PMID: 18057379

Alexandraki KI, Grossman AB. Is urinary free cortisol of value in the diagnosis of Cushing syndrome? *Curr Opin Endocrinol Diabetes Obes.* 2011;18(4): 259-263. PMID: 21681089

Pecori Giraldi F, Saccani A, Cavagnini F; Study Group on the Hypothalamo-Pituitary-Adrenal Axis of the Italian Society of Endocrinology. Assessment of ACTH assay variability: a multicenter study. *Eur J Endocrinol.* 2011;164(4):505-512. PMID: 21252174

8 ANSWER: E) Make no changes in his corticosteroid dosages

The treatment of primary adrenal insufficiency with glucocorticoid and mineralocorticoid replacement has evolved over the past 30 years. Hydrocortisone dosages as high as 30 to 40 mg daily (Answer C) were routinely administered years ago. These dosages were often associated with signs and symptoms of excessive glucocorticoid exposure, such as decreased bone mineral density. In healthy individuals, the daily secretion of cortisol is only 6 to 7 mg/m^2 (or approximately 8 to 12 mg daily). Most patients with primary adrenal insufficiency need only 15 to 25 mg of hydrocortisone in divided daily doses (even less in many patients with secondary adrenal insufficiency). Almost all patients with primary adrenal insufficiency require mineralocorticoid replacement. Fludrocortisone is the treatment of choice. The fludrocortisone dosage is usually titrated on the basis of electrolyte composition, blood pressure, and plasma renin activity. A plasma renin activity less than 5 ng/mL per h is a reasonable treatment target.

This patient has evidence of adequate mineralocorticoid replacement, and a dosage increase in fludrocortisone (Answer D) is not indicated. However, monitoring the adequacy of glucocorticoid replacement is more difficult. It is currently impossible to mimic the diurnal rhythm of cortisol. It is well known that the early-morning increase in cortisol begins at approximately 3:00 AM in patients with normal sleep–wake cycles. Glucocorticoid negative feedback on ACTH is complex, and ACTH levels usually remain elevated in patients with primary adrenal insufficiency despite adequate glucocorticoid replacement. Measurement of plasma ACTH in patients with adrenal insufficiency may be helpful if low-normal or subnormal levels are found. This suggests excessive glucocorticoid exposure and the need for a dosage reduction.

Because this patient is doing very well on his current replacement therapy, the modest increase in ACTH is of no concern and no change in treatment is warranted (Answer E). Some clinicians prescribe prednisone therapy (Answer A). However, there is no acceptable physiologic replacement dosage of prednisone. Because its active metabolite, prednisolone, has a very high affinity for the glucocorticoid receptor and a long plasma half-life, it is often associated with clinical features of excessive glucocorticoid exposure. The addition of 0.75 mg of dexamethasone at bedtime (Answer B) may suppress ACTH to near the reference range, but it would most likely cause iatrogenic Cushing syndrome. Reviewing the stress dosing of glucocorticoid replacement in patients with adrenal insufficiency is always indicated and should be done at nearly every visit.

EDUCATIONAL OBJECTIVE

Assess the adequacy of glucocorticoid and mineralocorticoid support in patients with primary adrenal insufficiency and recognize that plasma ACTH is usually elevated in this setting.

REFERENCE(S)

Bleicken B, Hahner S, Loeffler M, Ventz M, Allolio B, Quinkler M. Impaired subjective health status in chronic adrenal insufficiency: impact of different glucocorticoid replacement regimens. *Eur J Endocrinol.* 2008;159(6):811-817. PMID: 18819943

Hahner S, Loeffler M, Bleicken B, et al. Epidemiology of adrenal crisis in chronic adrenal insufficiency: the need for new prevention strategies. *Eur J Endocrinol.* 2010;162(3):597-602. PMID: 19955259

Bornstein SR, Allolio B, Arlt W, et al. Diagnosis and treatment of primary adrenal insufficiency: an Endocrine Society clinical practice guideline. *J Clin Endocrinol Metab.* 2016;101(2):364-389. PMID: 26760044

9 ANSWER: A) Unable to localize

For adrenal venous sampling, the cortisol concentrations in the adrenal vein samples are used to determine whether the adrenal veins were accessed and to correct for the fractional dilution of the adrenal vein blood with mixed venous blood. This ratio of cortisol in the adrenal vein blood to the cortisol in the mixed venous blood is often called the selectivity index. The selectivity index on both sides should be greater than 2 if adrenal venous sampling is performed without cosyntropin and greater than 3 if performed with cosyntropin infusion. Otherwise, the sample does not contain sufficient adrenal vein blood to interpret the results, and the study should not be interpreted unless both selectivity indices are greater than these minimum values. Usually, the right side, which is more difficult to access, fails the selectivity index test. If the aldosterone-to-cortisol ratio in the left adrenal vein is much lower than in the mixed venous blood, also called "contralateral suppression," aldosterone production can sometimes be confidently localized to the right adrenal, but conclusive cut-off values are not known. Note that contralateral suppression is not always observed in studies with convincing lateralization, so lack of contralateral suppression does not equate to bilateral aldosterone production.

Because the selectivity index on the right side is only 1.1 times higher than that of the mixed venous blood, the study was not successful (thus, Answer A is correct and Answer D is incorrect). Although it is possible that both adrenal glands are the source (Answer C), this conclusion cannot be drawn because of the low selectivity index on the right side. For the reasons stated above, the adrenal venous sampling study did not yield enough information to localize the aldosterone production (thus, Answers B and E are incorrect), even though all the information required for interpretation (aldosterone and cortisol from the adrenal veins and mixed venous blood) was available. Plasma metanephrines can also be used to confirm successful access of the adrenal veins, but the values cannot be used mathematically to correct for dilution with mixed venous blood.

EDUCATIONAL OBJECTIVE
Interpret results of adrenal venous sampling.

REFERENCE(S)

Rossi GP, Auchus RJ, Brown M, et al. An expert consensus statement on the use of adrenal vein sampling for the subtyping of primary aldosteronism. *Hypertension.* 2014;63(1):151-160. PMID: 24218436

Dekkers T, Deinum J, Schultzekool LJ, et al. Plasma metanephrine for assessing the selectivity of adrenal venous sampling. *Hypertension.* 2013;62(6): 1152-1157. PMID: 24082051

Funder JW, Carey RM, Mantero F, et al. The management of primary aldosteronism: case detection, diagnosis, and treatment: an Endocrine Society Clinical Practice Guideline. *J Clin Endocrinol Metab.* 2016;101(5):1889-1916. PMID: 26934393

10 ANSWER: A) No changes

The treatment of 21-hydroxylase deficiency requires glucocorticoid to replace the cortisol deficiency and to limit the rise in ACTH, thus controlling the adrenal-derived androgen excess. Relatively tight control of androgen (and thus estrogen) excess is necessary in childhood to prevent premature development of secondary sexual characteristics and bone maturation. Serum 17-hydroxyprogesterone, which accumulates immediately before the enzymatic block, is used for diagnosis and is also measured to titrate therapy in children. 17-Hydroxyprogesterone is a very sensitive measure of disease control when small amounts of androgens and estrogens are detrimental. In adults, disease control is relaxed somewhat as tolerated, because small amounts of adrenal-derived sex steroid compared to gonadal synthesis are not damaging. Overtreatment can cause iatrogenic Cushing syndrome with long-term complications. Scenarios requiring intensified therapy in adults include when women are attempting pregnancy and when men have testicular adrenal rest tumors.

This woman, who has no androgen excess symptoms, regular menses, and absence of cushingoid features, has disease control that is clinically at goal. Not surprisingly, her androstenedione and testosterone are in the normal female reference range, and her plasma renin activity is normal. 17-Hydroxyprogesterone tends to rise before the next dose of hydrocortisone, but a high 17-hydroxyprogesterone level alone—especially just before a hydrocortisone dose—is not an indication for intensified therapy. Hence, no change in therapy is indicated (Answer A).

Increasing in the hydrocortisone dosage (Answer B) or further dividing her dose (Answer D) is not necessary. In fact, her hydrocortisone dosage could be reduced slightly, but that is not a listed option. Note that DHEA-S is typically low and rarely elevated in the setting of classic 21-hydroxylase deficiency. Dexamethasone given at bedtime is the most effective way to prevent the early-morning ACTH rise and thus control the androgen excess. However, dexamethasone is difficult to titrate and easily causes iatrogenic Cushing syndrome, particularly when given at bedtime (Answer C). A dosage of 1 mg daily is far too high for a small adult such as this patient. Stopping fludrocortisone (Answer E) would cause volume depletion, so it should not be discontinued.

EDUCATIONAL OBJECTIVE
Guide the treatment of congenital adrenal hyperplasia on the basis of clinical and laboratory information.

REFERENCE(S)

Auchus RJ, Arlt W. Approach to the patient: the adult with congenital adrenal hyperplasia. *J Clin Endocrinol Metab.* 2013;98(7):2645-2655. PMID: 23837188

Arlt W, Willis DS, Wild SH, et al; United Kingdom Congenital Adrenal Hyperplasia Adult Study Executive (CaHASE). Health status of adults with congenital adrenal hyperplasia: a cohort study of 203 patients. *J Clin Endocrinol Metab.* 2010;95(11): 5110-5121. PMID: 20719839

Casteràs A, De Silva P, Rumsby G, Conway GS. Reassessing fecundity in women with classical congenital adrenal hyperplasia (CAH): normal pregnancy rate but reduced fertility rate. *Clin Endocrinol (Oxf).* 2009;70(6):833-837. PMID: 19250265

11 ANSWER: E) Measure serum aldosterone and plasma renin activity

The recommended functional evaluation of an incidentally discovered adrenal mass includes:

- Measurement of plasma or urinary metanephrines to exclude pheochromocytoma
- Overnight dexamethasone-suppression test to exclude hypercortisolemia
- Measurement of plasma renin and serum aldosterone (Answer E) to exclude primary aldosteronism (only in hypertensive patients)

This patient had normal results for the first 2 tests. While plasma metanephrine measurement has many false-positive results, the test has high negative predictive value, and further testing for pheochromocytoma (Answer A) is not necessary. If the dexamethasone-suppression test result were equivocal, serum DHEA-S and plasma ACTH (Answer C) could be used to further assess for autonomous cortisol excess, but these tests are not necessary if the dexamethasone-suppression test result is normal. Furthermore, clinically significant hypercortisolemia is uncommon if an adrenal adenoma is smaller than 2.4 cm in diameter. Because this patient has hypertension, he should be screened for primary aldosteronism, even with a normal serum potassium level. Of normokalemic hypertensive patients with an incidental adrenal tumor, 5% to 10% have primary aldosteronism. In fact, this patient did have primary aldosteronism, and after evaluation, he underwent left adrenalectomy with subsequent improvement in his blood pressure.

Characterization of adrenal nodules by imaging is the mainstay to diagnose potential malignancy. As a first step, the density of this mass should be measured. If the density on this noncontrast CT is less than 10 Hounsfield units, then this is a lipid-rich adenoma and no further imaging follow-up is required. If the density of the mass is indeterminate (>10 Hounsfield units), there are 3 options: (1) immediate further imaging characterization (eg, MRI [Answer B]); (2) repeated imaging in 6 to 12 months (Answer D); or (3) surgery. However, in the absence of a clear classification as an indeterminate mass, the evaluation for primary aldosteronism should be conducted first. In addition, this is a small homogeneous mass, which is unlikely to represent a malignant tumor. Even if not definitively a benign lipid-rich adenoma, the options of repeated imaging or further imaging evaluation are more reasonable than surgery.

EDUCATIONAL OBJECTIVE

Evaluate an incidentally discovered adrenal tumor for hormone production.

REFERENCE(S)

Zeiger MA, Siegelman SS, Hamrahian AH. Medical and surgical evaluation and treatment of adrenal incidentalomas. *J Clin Endocrinol Metab.* 2011;96(7): 2004-2015. PMID: 21632813

Bernini G, Moretti A, Argenio G, Salvetti A. Primary aldosteronism in normokalemic patients with adrenal incidentalomas. *Eur J Endocrinol.* 2002;146(4):523-529. PMID: 11916621

Fassnacht M, Arlt W, Bancos I, et al. Management of adrenal incidentalomas: European Society of Endocrinology Clinical Practice Guideline in collaboration with the European Network for the Study of Adrenal Tumors. *Eur J Endocrinol.* 2016;175(2):G1-G34. PMID: 27390021

12 ANSWER: C) Etomidate

Drugs that inhibit cortisol synthesis include aminoglutethimide, ketoconazole, metyrapone, and etomidate (Answer C), as well as new drugs under development such as the 11β-hydroxylase inhibitor osilodrostat. Etomidate is frequently administered intravenously in preparation for rapid intubation in the emergency department. Etomidate inhibits 11β-hydroxylase, the last step in cortisol synthesis and an enzyme unique to the cortisol pathway. Etomidate is very effective for control of hypercortisolemia in acutely ill patients with Cushing syndrome. Etomidate is best used in intubated patients, as in this vignette, in whom any sedative effects are less of a concern. However, even in the awake patient, etomidate can often be safely used, as dosages resulting in inhibition of cortisol production are about 10-fold lower than levels needed to achieve sedation. Etomidate has the advantages of intravenous

2 A 33-year-old woman presents to her primary care physician for an annual visit. She feels well and has no concerns. She has a history of gestational diabetes during a pregnancy 5 years ago. She has no history of hypertension, dyslipidemia, or cardiovascular disease. Her only medication is a daily multivitamin. She has no known family history of diabetes and does not smoke cigarettes or drink alcohol. She exercises regularly.

On physical examination, her blood pressure is 120/70 mm Hg and BMI is 23.0 kg/m^2. The rest of her examination findings are unremarkable.

Her current hemoglobin A_{1c} level is 5.4% (36 mmol/mol).

Regarding lifelong screening with respect to her prediabetes/diabetes risk, how often should she be screened?

A. No screening needed
B. At least every year
C. At least every 3 years
D. At least every 5 years
E. At least every 10 years

3 A 58-year-old man with a 14-year history of diabetes is referred for a second opinion regarding high-dosage insulin therapy. He currently takes insulin glargine, 75 units twice daily; insulin aspart, 50 units with each meal; and metformin, 2000 mg daily. His preprandial and postprandial fingerstick blood glucose levels range between 100 and 250 mg/dL (5.6-13.9 mmol/L). He does not report any hypoglycemic events.

On physical examination, his BMI is 46 kg/m^2 and blood pressure is 130/79 mm Hg.

Laboratory test results:

Hemoglobin A_{1c} = 7.6% (4.0%-5.6%) (60 mmol/mol [20-38 mmol/mol])
Estimated glomerular filtration rate = 68 mL/min per 1.73 m^2 (>60 mL/min per 1.73 m^2)

You decide to convert his insulin to regular U500.

Which of the following is the best next step in this patient's regimen?

A. 100 units 3 times daily before meals
B. 120 units 3 times daily before meals
C. 140 units before breakfast and 100 units before dinner
D. 180 units before breakfast and 120 units before dinner
E. 220 units before breakfast and 140 units before dinner

4 An emergency department physician requests an endocrine consult regarding diabetes management for a 62-year-old woman. She presented with chest pain, which started few hours ago. In the emergency department, her initial blood glucose fingerstick concentration was 340 mg/dL (18.9 mmol/L); she was given 10 units of regular insulin based on a sliding scale. She has a 20-year history of type 1 diabetes, hypertension, dyslipidemia, and coronary artery disease. Her outpatient regimen includes insulin detemir, mealtime insulin lispro, metformin, metoprolol, lisinopril, rosuvastatin, and aspirin. Her blood glucose fingerstick values at home range from 60 to 250 mg/dL (3.3-13.9 mmol/L) without a real pattern.

On physical examination, her BMI is 29 kg/m^2 and blood pressure is 140/90 mm Hg. She has a soft systolic murmur. Examination findings are otherwise unremarkable.

Her most recent hemoglobin A_{1c} measurement a few months ago was 7.6% (60 mmol/mol). During a discussion with the patient about her medical history, her speech becomes slurred and she suddenly loses consciousness. A blood glucose fingerstick value is 38 mg/dL (2.1 mmol/L).

Which of the following is the best treatment to administer?

A. Subcutaneous glucagon, 3 mg
B. Intravenous 50% dextrose, 100 mL
C. Intranasal glucagon, 3 mg
D. Intraoral glucose gel, 24 g
E. Glucose tablets, 15 g

administration and rapid onset. Ultimately, the patient will need cytotoxic chemotherapy to control ACTH excess from a likely small cell lung cancer.

Mitotane (Answer A) is adrenolytic, but it takes weeks to have an effect. Pasireotide (Answer B) is only effective in treating Cushing disease. Ketoconazole (Answer D) is relatively contraindicated due to elevated transaminases and must be administered orally. Mifepristone (Answer E) can be used to treat any form of hypercortisolemia and it might be effective in this patient, but it is orally administered, and hypokalemia should be corrected before dosing.

EDUCATIONAL OBJECTIVE

Differentiate among drugs that lower cortisol production.

REFERENCE(S)

Alexandraki KI, Grossman AB. Therapeutic strategies for the treatment of severe Cushing's syndrome. *Drugs.* 2016;76(4):447-458. PMID: 26833215

Preda VA, Sen J, Karavitaki N, Grossman AB. Etomidate in the management of hypercortisolaemia in Cushing's syndrome: a review. *Eur J Endocrinol.* 2012;167(2):137-143. PMID: 22577107

Fleseriu M, Petersenn S. Medical therapy for Cushing's disease: adrenal steroidogenesis inhibitors and glucocorticoid receptor blockers. *Pituitary.* 2015;18(2):245-252. PMID: 25560275

13 ANSWER: D) Increase the hydrocortisone dosage to 40 mg on arising and 20 mg in the early afternoon

This woman had severe Cushing disease for a prolonged period. Her pituitary surgery was successful with histologic confirmation of adenoma resection plus undetectable cortisol and ACTH. Further she had a low DHEA-S, which is often elevated in Cushing disease before surgery, but it significantly drops as a result of the absent ACTH stimulation of the adrenal cortex. Her hypothalamic-pituitary-adrenal axis will remain suppressed for many months, and she requires cortisol replacement therapy. Not surprisingly, she is suffering from cortisol withdrawal syndrome. Laboratory testing confirms central adrenal insufficiency, so no further testing for recurrent disease (Answers A and C) is required. Instead, she needs to have her hydrocortisone dosage increased (Answer D). While the current dosage might seem supraphysiologic, it is still very low relative to her cortisol exposure when she had Cushing disease. Patients even experience cortisol withdrawal syndrome when their Cushing disease is not cured but ACTH and cortisol production is significantly lowered.

Because her cortisol deficiency is central, her renin-angiotensin-aldosterone axis is functional, and both standing blood pressure and serum potassium are normal. Fludrocortisone (Answer B) is therefore unnecessary. DHEA-S decreases following cure of Cushing disease and can remain low for years despite recovery of cortisol production. Some literature suggests that DHEA replacement (Answer E) is beneficial for women with permanent adrenal insufficiency in the chronic setting, but the benefits are mostly for sexuality and do not address cortisol withdrawal. In several months, it might be appropriate to consider DHEA supplementation.

Ancillary medications to aid symptoms include selective serotonin reuptake inhibitors for mood problems and nonsteroidal anti-inflammatory drugs for myalgias. The hydrocortisone dosage is gradually tapered as symptoms abate to allow axis recovery. For those with severe glucocorticoid-induced myopathy, physical therapy is very important from the midpoint of the recovery phase.

EDUCATIONAL OBJECTIVE

Manage cortisol withdrawal syndrome following cure of Cushing disease.

REFERENCE(S)

Bhattacharyya A, Kaushal K, Tymms DJ, Davis JR. Steroid withdrawal syndrome after successful treatment of Cushing's syndrome: a reminder. *Eur J Endocrinol.* 2005;153(2):207-210. PMID: 16061825

Kleiber H, Rey F, Temler E, Gomez F. Dissociated recovery of cortisol and dehydroepiandrosterone sulphate after treatment for Cushing's syndrome. *J Endocrinol Invest.* 1991;14(6):489-492. PMID: 1663528

El Asmar N, Rajpal A, Selman WR, Arafah BM. The value of perioperative levels of ACTH, DHEA, and DHEA-S and tumor size in predicting recurrence of Cushing disease. *J Clin Endocrinol Metab.* 2018;103(2):477-445. PMID: 29244084

Nieman LK, Biller BM, Findling JW, et al; Endocrine Society. Treatment of Cushing's syndrome: an Endocrine Society Clinical Practice Guideline. *J Clin Endocrinol Metab.* 2015;100(8):2807-2831. PMID: 26222757

14 ANSWER: E) Fasting serum glucose level

Mifepristone is a competitive antagonist for both the glucocorticoid receptor and the progesterone receptor. It is used for the treatment of Cushing syndrome in patients with glucose intolerance or diabetes mellitus. Because mifepristone also antagonizes the feedback inhibition of cortisol on the adenoma, ACTH and cortisol production often rises in Cushing disease when patients are on treatment but not enough to offset the beneficial effects of glucocorticoid receptor blockade in peripheral tissues. Consequently, serum cortisol, urinary free cortisol (Answer A), or plasma ACTH (Answer C) cannot be used to titrate therapy.

Because of potent progesterone receptor antagonism, menses cease during mifepristone therapy. Furthermore, endometrial hypertrophy and vaginal bleeding can occur weeks to months after starting therapy. Thus, return of regular monthly menses (Answer B) cannot be used as a guide.

Blood pressure (Answer D) can decrease after several weeks of treatment, but blood pressure can also rise if the cortisol increases sufficiently. A rise in cortisol increases mineralocorticoid receptor activation, yet mifepristone does not antagonize the mineralocorticoid receptor. Thus, hypertension and hypokalemia can also occur or worsen on treatment. Hence, blood pressure is not a reliable measure of therapeutic adequacy.

If elevated, serum glucose (Answer E) decreases rapidly with mifepristone treatment, and the improved glycemic control is a reliable indicator of therapeutic effect. Additional parameters include weight loss, decrease in waist circumference and regression of cushingoid features, but these changes take much longer than the immediate reduction in glucose.

EDUCATIONAL OBJECTIVE

Titrate mifepristone therapy for Cushing disease on the basis of clinical and biochemical data.

REFERENCE(S)

Castinetti F, Fassnacht M, Johanssen S, et al. Merits and pitfalls of mifepristone in Cushing's syndrome. *Eur J Endocrinol.* 2009;160(6):1003-1010. PMID: 19289534

Fleseriu M, Biller BM, Findling JW, Molitch ME, Schteingart DE, Gross C; SEISMIC Study Investigators. Mifepristone, a glucocorticoid receptor antagonist, produces clinical and metabolic benefits in patients with Cushing's syndrome. *J Clin Endocrinol Metab.* 2012;97(6):2039-2049. PMID: 22466348

15 ANSWER: E) No further testing

During critical illness, cortisol rises and remains elevated without circadian rhythm for days to weeks until recovery occurs. Furthermore, cortisol production is resistant to suppression from exogenous glucocorticoids such as dexamethasone. The more gravely ill the patient, the greater the stimulus for cortisol production and the less the cortisol rises with cosyntropin. Viewed this way, cortisol and its attenuated rise with cosyntropin are prognostic factors in critical illness. In addition, many critically ill patients are hypoproteinemic, with low albumin and low plasma cortisol-binding capacity as in this patient, such that the total serum cortisol underestimates the concentration of free and biologically active cortisol. For patients with serum albumin concentrations less than 2.5 g/dL (<25 g/L), the serum free cortisol is uniformly normal even when the serum total cortisol concentration is 12 to 18 µg/dL (331.1-496.6 nmol/L), which is below the conventional cutoff for a normal response. In addition, newer cortisol immunoassays and mass spectrometry assays yield values about 30% lower than older immunoassays. For these reasons, this patient does not have adrenal insufficiency and requires no further testing or therapy (Answer E).

Serum DHEA-S (Answer B) is a useful measure of adrenal function in combination with cortisol, as DHEA-S production is also ACTH-dependent. However, in critical illness, DHEA-S falls and DHEA rises. Thus, serum DHEA-S cannot be used to adjudicate adrenal function in critical illness. Plasma ACTH (Answer C) will not influence the interpretation of the cosyntropin-stimulation test and can be low or low-normal after several days of critical illness. Critical illness is a contraindication to an insulin tolerance test (Answer A), and cortisol values from a low-dose cosyntropin-stimulation test (Answer D) would have to be corrected for hypoproteinemia as well.

EDUCATIONAL OBJECTIVE
Interpret cortisol dynamics in critical illness.

REFERENCE(S)

Sprung CL, Annane D, Keh D, et al; CORTICUS Study Group. Hydrocortisone therapy for patients with septic shock. *N Engl J Med.* 2008;358(2):111-124. PMID: 18184957

Arafah BM. Hypothalamic pituitary adrenal function during critical illness: limitations of current assessment methods. *J Clin Endocrinol Metab.* 2006;91(10):3725-3745. PMID: 16882746

Sam S, Corbridge TC, Mokhlesi B, Comellas AP, Molitch ME. Cortisol levels and mortality in severe sepsis. *Clin Endocrinol (Oxf).* 2004;60(1):29-35. PMID: 14678284

Hamrahian AH, Oseni TS, Arafah BM. Measurements of serum free cortisol in critically ill patients. *N Engl J Med.* 2004;350(16):1629-1638. PMID: 15084695

Annane D, Sebille V, Troche G, Raphael JC, Gajdos P, Bellissant E. A 3-level prognostic classification in septic shock based on cortisol levels and cortisol response to corticotropin. *JAMA.* 2000;283(8):1038-1045. PMID: 10697064

Al-Aridi R, Abdelmannan D, Arafah BM. Biochemical diagnosis of adrenal insufficiency: the added value of dehydroepiandrosterone sulfate measurements. *Endocr Pract.* 2011;17(2):261-270. PMID: 21134877

Arlt W, Hammer F, Sanning P, et al. Dissociation of serum dehydroepiandrosterone and dehydroepiandrosterone sulfate in septic shock. *J Clin Endocrinol Metab.* 2006;91(7):2548-2554. PMID: 16608898

Raverot V, Richet C, Morel Y, Raverot G, Borson-Chazot F. Establishment of revised diagnostic cut-offs for adrenal laboratory investigation using the new Roche Diagnostics Elecsys® Cortisol II assay. *Ann Endocrinol (Paris).* 2016;77(5):620-622. PMID: 27449530

16 ANSWER: E) Refer for inferior petrosal sinus sampling

This woman has convincing biochemical and clinical evidence of ACTH-dependent Cushing syndrome. In most young women with this clinical picture, the etiology is Cushing disease due to an ACTH-producing pituitary adenoma, but ectopic ACTH syndrome cannot be excluded. In addition, this patient's ACTH level is quite high for pituitary Cushing disease, and the MRI does not clearly identify a tumor. Thus, before referring for surgery (Answer B), the source of ACTH should be identified with inferior petrosal sinus sampling (Answer E).

Although oral contraceptives can cause false-positive results on dexamethasone-suppression testing due to increased corticosteroid-binding globulin, the magnitude of post-dexamethasone cortisol is typically less than 5.0 µg/dL (<138 nmol/L), and the test is unnecessary given the salivary cortisol values, which are readily interpretable (thus, Answer A is incorrect). Likewise, additional demonstration of hypercortisolemia such as urinary free cortisol excretion (Answer C) is not necessary and will not identify the source of ACTH. Mifepristone therapy is indicated for patients with Cushing syndrome that is not curable with surgery or in patients who are not surgical candidates and in whom diabetes or glucose intolerance is present. This patient is a surgical candidate and is not hyperglycemic; furthermore, the starting dosage of mifepristone is 300 mg daily (thus, Answer D is incorrect).

EDUCATIONAL OBJECTIVE
Evaluate ACTH-dependent hypercortisolism.

REFERENCE(S)

Nieman LK, Biller BM, Findling JW, et al. The diagnosis of Cushing's syndrome: an Endocrine Society clinical practice guideline. *J Clin Endocrinol Metab.* 2008;93(5):1526-1540. PMID: 18334580

Ilias I, Torpy DJ, Pacak K, et al. Cushing's syndrome due to ectopic corticotropin secretion: twenty years' experience at the National Institutes of Health. *J Clin Endocrinol Metab.* 2005;90(8): 4955-4962. PMID: 15914534

Lacroix A, Feelders RA, Stratakis CA, Nieman LK. Cushing's syndrome. *Lancet.* 2015;386(9996): 913-927. PMID: 26004339

17 ANSWER: C) Adrenocortical carcinoma

Functional benign adrenal adenomas nearly always produce a single active hormone as their final product. Large cortisol-producing adenomas sometimes co-secrete aldosterone, but usually one hormone excess is dominant, while the second is mild. In contrast, overt, clinically manifested excess of more than one active steroid, such as glucocorticoid and androgen excess, is characteristic of adrenal cancer. Furthermore, the rapid progression of androgen excess alone, with very high testosterone and virilization (voice deepening), is worrisome for an adrenal or ovarian tumor. The mineralocorticoid excess in this patient, which is disproportionate to the cortisol and aldosterone concentrations, suggests elevation of cortisol precursors, primarily corticosterone and 11-deoxycorticosterone. Adrenal carcinomas tend to be relatively deficient in 11β-hydroxylase activity, leading to elevation of 11-deoxycortisol and further upstream intermediates, which can account for the robust androgen and mineralocorticoid excess with normal or modestly elevated cortisol. In particular, the elevation of DHEA-S in parallel to testosterone and the 11-deoxycortisol elevation is almost pathognomonic for adrenocortical carcinoma. Hypokalemia in patients with adrenal cancer can arise from severe hypercortisolism overwhelming 11β-hydroxysteroid dehydrogenase type 2 in the kidney, mineralocorticoid production, or compression of the kidney and renal vasculature causing hyperreninemic hyperaldosteronism.

Macronodular adrenocortical hyperplasia (Answer A) typically manifests with pure cortisol excess, and the mineralocorticoid excess is due to cortisol and parallels cortisol production. DHEA-S is typically normal in hypercortisolemic patients with macronodular hyperplasia rather than suppressed as is often the case in hypercortisolemic patients with unilateral adrenal cortical adenomas, but this preservation of DHEA-S does not account for the profound androgen excess in this patient. While mild or nonclassic 11β-hydroxylase deficiency (Answer B) has been described, these patients have mild androgen excess and rarely have hypertension; the abrupt onset in this vignette is also inconsistent with a genetic etiology. Anabolic steroid abuse (Answer E) could account for the androgen excess but not the mineralocorticoid excess. Ovarian hyperthecosis (Answer D) is another cause of hirsutism and hyperandrogenemia. However, onset is usually more insidious and testosterone levels are not as elevated as they are in this patient. Most importantly, DHEA-S is usually not significantly elevated in the setting of ovarian hyperthecosis.

EDUCATIONAL OBJECTIVE

Suspect adrenocortical carcinoma on the basis of clinical features.

REFERENCE(S)

Arlt W, Biehl M, Taylor AE, et al. Urine steroid metabolomics as a biomarker tool for detecting malignancy in adrenal tumors. *J Clin Endocrinol Metab.* 2011;96(12):3775-3784. PMID: 21917861

Messer CK, Kirschenbaum A, New MI, Unger P, Gabrilove JL, Levine AC. Concomitant secretion of glucocorticoid, androgens, and mineralocorticoid by an adrenocortical carcinoma: case report and review of literature. *Endocr Pract.* 2007;13(4): 408-412. PMID: 17669719

Fassnacht M, Dekkers OM, Else T, et al. European Society of Endocrinology clinical practice guidelines on the management of adrenocortical carcinoma in adults, in collaboration with the European Network for the Study of Adrenal Tumors M. *Eur J Endocrinol.* 2018;179(4):G1-G46. PMID: 30299884

18 ANSWER: C) *VHL*

The susceptibility genes for pheochromocytoma and paraganglioma are listed (*see table*).

Classic von Hippel–Lindau syndrome involves retinal and cerebellar hemangioblastomas, pancreatic islet-cell tumors, and renal cell cancer, but pheochromocytoma can also be part of the syndrome and is sometimes the only manifestation. In contrast to the biochemical profile of pheochromocytomas associated with multiple endocrine neoplasia 2A and 2B, pheochromocytomas in von Hippel–Lindau syndrome almost invariably produce norepinephrine and normetanephrine. Thus, given this patient's laboratory test results, the gene most likely responsible for pheochromocytoma in this kindred is *VHL* (Answer C).

Establishing a genetic diagnosis is important, as it will further inform future surveillance for other associated tumors. In this case, the patient should be monitored for renal cell cancer and pancreatic neuroendocrine tumors. Confirming a genetic diagnosis also serves as the basis for further family cascade screening (first-degree relatives are at 50% risk of carrying the same pathogenic variant). Evaluation would be indicated even in the absence of a positive family history, as roughly one-third of all patients with von Hippel–Lindau syndrome do not have a positive family history.

Syndrome	**Gene(s)**	**Tumor locations**	**Hormone products**	**Other features**
Familial paraganglioma type 1	*SDHD*	Head and neck paraganglioma, multiple; mediastinal paraganglioma; rarely adrenal medulla	NE, DA, or none	Clear cell renal cell carcinoma, gastrointestinal stromal tumor, pituitary adenoma, pulmonary chondroma
Familial paraganglioma type 2	*SDHAF2*	Head and neck paraganglioma, multiple; rarely adrenal medulla	Unknown	Unknown
Familial paraganglioma type 3	*SDHC*	Head and neck paraganglioma; mediastinal paraganglioma	NE or none	Unknown
Familial paraganglioma type 4	*SDHB*	Abdominal and pelvic paraganglioma; mediastinal paraganglioma; rarely adrenal medulla	NE, DA, or none	Often malignant paraganglioma; clear cell renal cell carcinoma, gastrointestinal stromal tumor, pituitary adenoma, pulmonary chondroma
Familial paraganglioma	*SDHA*	Head and neck or other paraganglioma; adrenal medulla	Unknown	Unknown
Multiple endocrine neoplasia type 2A and 2B	*RET*	Adrenal medulla, bilateral	E>>NE	Medullary thyroid carcinoma, hyperparathyroidism; marfanoid habitus and mucosal ganglioneuromas (2B only)
Neurofibromatosis type 1	*NF1*	Adrenal medulla	E or E and NE	Café-au-lait spots, neurofibromas, carcinoid tumors, peripheral nerve sheath tumors
von Hippel–Lindau syndrome	*VHL*	Adrenal medulla, bilateral; rarely paraganglioma	NE>>DA	Retinal and central nervous system hemangioblastomas, clear cell renal cell carcinoma, pancreatic islet-cell tumors, other
Familial pheochromocytoma	*TMEM127*	Adrenal medulla	NE and E	Renal cell carcinoma
Familial pheochromocytoma	*MAX*	Adrenal medulla, bilateral	NE and E	Unknown
Fumarate hydratase deficiency	*FH*	Head and neck paraganglioma; adrenal medulla	NE	Papillary renal cell carcinoma, uterine fibroids, cutaneous leiomyoma

Abbreviations: DA, dopamine; E, epinephrine; NE, norepinephrine.

Pathogenic variants in the *SDH* genes (Answer D) predispose to the development of paragangliomas, and pathogenic variants in *TMEM127* (Answer E) and *MAX* are rare causes of pheochromocytoma. *RET* pathogenic variants (Answer A), which cause multiple endocrine neoplasia type 2A and 2B, are a more common cause of bilateral pheochromocytoma. However, tumors associated with these syndromes almost invariably produce epinephrine and metanephrine. Pheochromocytoma is not a characteristic tumor of multiple endocrine neoplasia type 1, which is caused by pathogenic variants in the *MEN1* gene (Answer B). Patients with neurofibromatosis type 1 can have bilateral pheochromocytomas. Neurofibromatosis type 1 remains a clinical diagnosis with the presence of other features, such as neurofibromas, Lisch nodules, and axillary freckling.

EDUCATIONAL OBJECTIVE

Compare the genetics and hormonal function of different familial pheochromocytoma syndromes.

REFERENCE(S)

Pacak K, Wimalawansa SJ. Pheochromocytoma and paraganglioma. *Endocr Pract.* 2015;21(4):406-412. PMID: 25716634

Fishbein L, Merrill S, Fraker DL, Cohen DL, Nathanson KL. Inherited mutations in pheochromocytoma and paraganglioma: why all patients should be offered genetic testing. *Ann Surg Oncol.* 2013;20(5):1444-1450. PMID: 23512077

19 ANSWER: D) Refer for laparoscopic right adrenalectomy

The evaluation of ACTH-independent hypercortisolism prompted by the incidental discovery of an adrenocortical adenoma is slightly different than screening for Cushing disease based on clinical suspicion. For an adrenal adenoma, the dexamethasone-suppression test evaluates the autonomous cortisol production when ACTH is completely suppressed, and its sensitivity is the highest among the conventional tests. Additional tests that assess the chronic state of the hypothalamic-pituitary-adrenal axis in these patients use a first-morning plasma ACTH measurement and a random DHEA-S measurement, which is an ACTH-dependent product of the adrenal cortex. Urinary free cortisol excretion is elevated in a minority of patients and is not a very sensitive test for detecting subtle hypercortisolism of any type.

A substantial body of literature now documents the long-term health consequences of mild autonomous cortisol excess, most commonly derived from adrenal adenomas. These tumors are typically larger than 2.4 cm in diameter, as in this patient, and although exact minimal criteria for mild autonomous cortisol excess are debated, the 3 main tests (ACTH, DHEA-S, and dexamethasone-suppressed cortisol) are all consistently abnormal in this patient. This patient was initially clinically observed because she had only osteoporosis and borderline hypertension as possible manifestations of hypercortisolism. However, hypertension has now worsened, she has become obese, and she has developed diabetes. The DHEA-S concentration has further decreased because of persistent hypercortisolism of adrenal origin (suppression of pituitary ACTH drive). The major morbidity that improves with adrenalectomy is hypertension. However, autonomous cortisol excess from adrenal adenomas is associated with a host of other conditions, such as osteoporosis, glucose intolerance, cardiovascular events, and death, thus justifying the recommendation for surgical right adrenalectomy (Answer D).

Retrospective and prospective studies have shown that patients without elevated urinary free cortisol excretion might benefit from surgery. Thus, delaying medical or surgical therapy until urinary free cortisol is clearly elevated (Answer A) is incorrect. Also, this degree of cortisol excess can cause morbidities. The patient does not have ACTH-dependent Cushing syndrome and therefore petrosal sinus sampling (Answer B) is not indicated. There is also no concern for adrenocortical carcinoma, as there is only an insidious worsening of symptoms and the mass was initially clearly benign with a density of less than –5 Hounsfield units. Therefore, imaging for malignant transformation (Answer E) is incorrect. Surgery as a final therapy is preferred over any medical treatment, including mifepristone (Answer C), which is indicated for patients with failed surgery or those who are not surgical candidates.

Indeed, this patient needed postsurgical hydrocortisone replacement due to suppression of the contralateral adrenal gland—post hoc evidence for presurgical hypercortisolism.

EDUCATIONAL OBJECTIVE

Guide the management of patients with subclinical Cushing syndrome and mild autonomous cortisol excess.

REFERENCE(S)

Morelli V, Reimondo G, Giordano R, et al. Long-term follow-up in adrenal incidentalomas: an Italian multicenter study. *J Clin Endocrinol Metab.* 2014;99(3):827-834. PMID: 24423350

Chiodini I, Morelli V, Salcuni AS, et al. Beneficial metabolic effects of prompt surgical treatment in patients with an adrenal incidentaloma causing biochemical hypercortisolism. *J Clin Endocrinol Metab.* 2010;95(6):2736-2745. PMID: 20375210

Di Dalmazi G, Vicennati V, Garelli S, et al. Cardiovascular events and mortality in patients with adrenal incidentalomas that are either non-secreting or associated with intermediate phenotype or subclinical Cushing's syndrome: a 15-year retrospective study. *Lancet Diabet Endocrinol.* 2014;2(5):396-405. PMID: 24795253

20 ANSWER: B) Induces hepatic CYP3A4 activity

Mitotane therapy for adrenal cancer lowers cortisol production by several mechanisms besides direct adrenal toxicity. Among the more important effects, mitotane is one of the most potent inducers of CYP3A4 and drug metabolism (thus, Answer B is correct). CYP3A4 also metabolizes hydrocortisone, primarily by 6β-hydroxylation, and 6β-hydroxycortisol production increases 10-fold with mitotane therapy. While mitotane actually increases (not decreases) corticosteroid-binding globulin (thus, Answer A is incorrect), this effect would, if anything, slows cortisol metabolism. Mitotane has no significant effect on cortisol (hydrocortisone) absorption (Answer C) or urinary excretion (Answer D). Mitotane inhibits rather than induces 5α-reductase activity (thus, Answer E is incorrect), and because 5α-reduction is one means of cortisol catabolism, this action would also slow cortisol elimination.

EDUCATIONAL OBJECTIVE

Explain mitotane's effect on hepatic CYP3A4 activity and drug metabolism.

REFERENCE(S)

Chortis V, Taylor AE, Schneider P, et al. Mitotane therapy in adrenocortical cancer induces CYP3A4 and inhibits 5α-reductase, explaining the need for personalized glucocorticoid and androgen replacement. *J Clin Endocrinol Metab.* 2013;98(1):161-171. PMID: 23162091

Kroiss M, Quinkler M, Lutz WK, Allolio B, Fassnacht M. Drug interactions with mitotane by induction of CYP3A4 metabolism in the clinical management of adrenocortical carcinoma. *Clin Endocrinol (Oxf).* 2011;75(5):585-591. PMID: 21883349

Sbiera S, Leich E, Liebisch G, et al. Mitotane inhibits sterol-o-acyl transferase 1 triggering lipid- mediated endoplasmic reticulum stress and apoptosis in adrenocortical carcinoma cells. *Endocrinology.* 2015;156(11):3895-3908. PMID: 26305886

21 ANSWER: E) Serum 11-deoxycortisol measurement

The elevated ACTH and low cortisol values indicate a primary adrenal problem, which manifests as hypertension and hypokalemia. The differential diagnosis for ACTH-dependent mineralocorticoid excess is best approached considering the pathologic mineralocorticoid in each case:

- Aldosterone
  - Glucocorticoid-remediable aldosteronism (familial hyperaldosteronism type 1)
- Cortisol
  - Cushing syndrome; apparent mineralocorticoid excess (genetic or licorice)
- 11-Deoxycorticosterone
  - 17α-hydroxylase deficiency, 11β-hydroxylase deficiency

In this case, the cortisol and aldosterone are both suppressed, which excludes apparent mineralocorticoid excess and glucocorticoid-remediable aldosteronism (thus, Answers B and D are incorrect). Although 17-hydroxyprogesterone is elevated, 21-hydroxylase deficiency causes hypotension rather than hypertension. Thus, genotyping the *CYP21A2* gene (Answer C) is incorrect. Measurement of serum 17-hydroxypregnenolone (Answer A) assesses for 3β-hydroxysteroid dehydrogenase deficiency, which also causes hypotension. Given the patient's normal virilization and Middle Eastern ancestry, he has 11β-hydroxylase deficiency, which is diagnosed by documenting an elevated 11-deoxycortisol concentration (Answer E). Note that 17-hydroxyprogesterone also accumulates behind the block at 11-hydroxylase, but it is not as high as it is in 21-hydroxylase deficiency. The remaining etiology is 17α-hydroxylase deficiency, but this defect also causes androgen deficiency, which is inconsistent with the clinical picture. Serum 11-deoxycorticosterone is elevated in both 11β- and 17α-hydroxylase deficiency, but 11-deoxycortisol is elevated in only 11β-hydroxylase deficiency. In 17α-hydroxylase deficiency, corticosterone is also elevated. In both conditions, the mineralocorticoids defend against adrenal crises, despite cortisol deficiency.

EDUCATIONAL OBJECTIVE

Construct the differential diagnosis of ACTH-dependent mineralocorticoid excess and diagnose 11β-hydroxylase deficiency.

REFERENCE(S)

Parajes S, Loidi L, Reisch N, et al. Functional consequences of seven novel mutations in the CYP11B1 gene: four mutations associated with nonclassic and three mutations causing classic 11β-hydroxylase deficiency. *J Clin Endocrinol Metab.* 2010;95(2): 779-788. PMID: 20089618

Zachmann M, Tassinari D, Prader A. Clinical and biochemical variability of congenital adrenal hyperplasia due to 11 beta-hydroxylase deficiency. A study of 25 patients. *J Clin Endocrinol Metab.* 1983;56(2):222-229. PMID: 6296182

Miller WL, Auchus RJ. The molecular biology, biochemistry, and physiology of human steroidogenesis and its disorders [published correction appears in *Endocr Rev.* 2011;32(4):579]. *Endocr Rev.* 2011;32(1):81-151. PMID: 21051590

22 ANSWER: A) Overnight dexamethasone-suppression test (1 mg)

The evaluation of ACTH-independent hypercortisolism prompted by the incidental discovery of an adrenocortical adenoma is slightly different than screening for Cushing disease based on clinical suspicion. For the adrenal adenoma, the dexamethasone-suppression test evaluates the autonomous cortisol production when ACTH is completely suppressed, and its sensitivity is the highest among the conventional tests (thus, Answer A is correct).

Assessing 24-hour urinary free cortisol excretion (Answer B) is not a very sensitive test for detecting subtle hypercortisolism of any type. Although late-night serum or salivary cortisol measurement is better than urinary cortisol measurement, none of these tests is very sensitive for early ACTH-independent disease (thus, Answer C is incorrect). Serum DHEA-S reflects chronic ACTH stimulation of the adrenal (with some caveats), but the option to measure DHEA-S is not listed, and serum DHEA measurement (Answer D) has no role in the evaluation of hypercortisolism. Similarly, plasma ACTH measurement (Answer E) in the early morning is a useful adjunctive test, but it is associated with false-positive and false-negative results.

EDUCATIONAL OBJECTIVE

Select the appropriate first test in the evaluation of early ACTH-independent hypercortisolism from an adrenocortical adenoma.

REFERENCE(S)

Morelli V, Reimondo G, Giordano R, et al. Long-term follow-up in adrenal incidentalomas: an Italian multicenter study. *J Clin Endocrinol Metab.* 2014;99(3):827-834. PMID: 24423350

Eller-Vainicher C, Morelli V, Salcuni AS, et al. Post-surgical hypocortisolism after removal of an adrenal incidentaloma: is it predictable by an accurate endocrinological work-up before surgery? *Eur J Endocrinol.* 2010;162(1):91-99. PMID: 19797503

Fassnacht M, Arlt W, Bancos I, et al. Management of adrenal incidentalomas: European Society of Endocrinology Clinical Practice Guideline in collaboration with the European Network for the Study of Adrenal Tumors. *Eur J Endocrinol.* 2016;175(2):G1-G34. PMID: 27390021

Calcium & Bone Board Review

Natalie Cusano, MD, MS

1 ANSWER: E) Romosozumab

Romosozumab (Answer E) is a monoclonal antibody against sclerostin that has been approved for treatment of postmenopausal women with osteoporosis at high risk for fracture. It results in both an increase in bone formation markers and a decrease in bone resorption markers. Romosozumab is given as a subcutaneous injection once monthly for 12 months, with subsequent need for antiresorptive therapy. Development of romosozumab began after identification of sclerostin as the genetic basis for high bone density in patients with sclerosteosis and van Buchem disease. Romosozumab was found to be highly effective in decreasing risk of vertebral fractures vs placebo in the FRAME trial (relative risk, 0.27 in the romosozumab arm at 12 months; $P < .001$), as well as vs alendronate therapy in the ARCH trial (relative risk, 0.63 in the romosozumab arm at 12 months; $P = .003$). In the ARCH trial, there was an imbalance in the number of adjudicated serious cardiovascular events in the romosozumab vs alendronate arms (2.5% vs 1.9%, respectively). The cause of this imbalance is unclear, as there was no imbalance in cardiovascular events in the FRAME trial, and no excess cardiovascular risk noted in patients with sclerosteosis or van Buchem disease with a congenital absence of sclerostin. Romosozumab has been approved by the FDA with a boxed warning that therapy should not be initiated in patients who have had a myocardial infarction or stroke within the preceding year. Therefore, romosozumab is contraindicated for this patient.

Abaloparatide (Answer D) should be strongly considered in this patient with multiple vertebral fractures at high risk for future fracture; however, therapy with alendronate (Answer A), zoledronic acid (Answer B), and denosumab (Answer C) would not be incorrect.

EDUCATIONAL OBJECTIVE

Identify cardiovascular contraindications for romosozumab therapy.

REFERENCE(S)

Cosman F, Crittenden DB, Adachi JD, et al. Romosozumab treatment in postmenopausal women with osteoporosis. *N Engl J Med.* 2016;375(16):1532-1543. PMID: 27641143

Evenity (romosozumab-aqqg) [prescribing information]. Thousand Oaks, CA: Amgen. 2019. www.accessdata.fda.gov/drugsatfda_docs/label/2019/761062s000lbl.pdf

Rosen CJ. Romosozumab - promising or practice changing? *N Engl J Med.* 2017;377(15):1479-1480. PMID: 28892459

Saag KG, Petersen J, Brandi ML, et al. Romosozumab or alendronate for fracture prevention in women with osteoporosis. *N Engl J Med.* 2017;377(15):1417-1427. PMID: 28892457

2 ANSWER: D) Genetic testing for *GNA11* and *AP2S1* pathogenic variants

Familial hypocalciuric hypercalcemia (FHH) is a rare disease resulting in a rightward shift of a patient's calcium-sensing curve. Patients with FHH do not shut off production of PTH in response to a serum calcium value that for the general population would be considered hypercalcemic. There are 3 variants of the disease: type 1 due to pathogenic variants in the calcium-sensing receptor gene (*CASR*), type 2 caused by pathogenic variants in the guanine nucleotide–binding protein (G-protein) subunit α_{11} gene (*GNA11*), and type 3 due to pathogenic variants in the adaptor-related protein complex 2, sigma 1 subunit gene (*AP2S1*). Patients with FHH have low urinary calcium excretion, calculated with the following formula:

[urine calcium (mg/24 h) × serum creatinine (mg/dL)] / [urine creatinine (mg/24 h) × serum calcium (mg/dL)]

A urinary calcium-to-creatinine ratio less than 0.01 is consistent with a diagnosis of FHH, although patients must be vitamin D replete (>20 ng/mL [>49.9 mmol/L]) with good renal function for the collection to be interpretable. A patient with no identifiable *CASR* pathogenic variants and clinical concern for FHH should have *GNA11* and *AP2S1* genetic testing (Answer D). This patient was documented to have a pathogenic variant in *AP2S1*.

While FHH is a benign disease that does not carry an increased risk of nephrolithiasis or osteoporosis as does primary hyperparathyroidism, patients with FHH type 3 may have significant hypercalcemia and clinical symptoms related to high serum calcium. A case series demonstrated successful cinacalcet therapy for 3 patients with FHH type 3.

It is important to distinguish between FHH and primary hyperparathyroidism, as surgical treatment is not indicated in patients with FHH. Thus, preoperative localization studies (Answers A and B) or referral to a parathyroid surgeon (Answer C) is incorrect. Pathogenic variants in the *PHEX* gene (Answer E) result in X-linked hypophosphatasia, a genetic disorder causing rickets and phosphate wasting.

EDUCATIONAL OBJECTIVE

Distinguish familial hypocalciuric hypercalcemia from primary hyperparathyroidism.

REFERENCE(S)

Eastell R, Brandi ML, Costa AG, D'Amour P, Shoback DM, Thakker RV. Diagnosis of asymptomatic primary hyperparathyroidism: proceedings of the Fourth International Workshop. *J Clin Endocrinol Metab.* 2014;99(10):3570-3579. PMID: 25162666

Howles SA, Hannan FM, Babinsky VN, et al. Cinacalcet for symptomatic hypercalcemia caused by AP2S1 mutations. *N Engl J Med.* 2016;374(14): 1396-1398. PMID: 27050234

3 ANSWER: B) Alendronate, 70 mg weekly for 1 year

This patient has been treated with denosumab therapy for 10 years with significant improvements in bone density. Her most recent bone density values are within the osteopenic range at all sites. It is reasonable to plan for an upcoming "drug holiday" due to the rare adverse effects of osteonecrosis of the jaw and atypical femoral fracture associated with antiresorptive therapy. However, cessation of denosumab results in an increase in bone resorption markers above pretreatment values for approximately 24 months after the last dose. Bone mineral density returns to pretreatment values within 18 months of the last denosumab injection. Abrupt discontinuation of denosumab therapy has been associated with increased risk of multiple vertebral fractures, as early as 7 months from the last dose. Prior vertebral fracture, as in this patient, is a predictor of multiple vertebral fractures after discontinuation of denosumab. Thus, a drug holiday from antiresorptive therapy (Answer A) is not the best option at this time. The FDA insert for denosumab recommends considering transition to another antiresorptive agent if denosumab is discontinued. Therapy with alendronate for 1 year (Answer B) before a drug holiday is reasonable.

A drug holiday should be considered for this patient, and therapy with ibandronate indefinitely (Answer C) is incorrect. Teriparatide (PTH [1-34]) (Answer D) is contraindicated in this patient with a history of skeletal radiation. Romosozumab (Answer E) acts as both an osteoanabolic and antiresorptive treatment, resulting in an increase in bone formation markers and a decrease in bone resorption markers. Since osteonecrosis of the jaw and atypical femoral fracture have been reported with romosozumab therapy, treatment with an oral bisphosphonate for 1 year followed by a drug holiday is a better choice.

EDUCATIONAL OBJECTIVE

Explain the vertebral fracture risk involved in cessation of denosumab.

REFERENCE(S)

Cummings SR, Ferrari S, Eastell R, et al. Vertebral fractures after discontinuation of denosumab: a post hoc analysis of the randomized placebo-controlled FREEDOM trial and its extension. *J Bone Miner Res.* 2018;33(2):190-198. PMID: 29105841

Prololia (denosumab) [prescribing information]. Thousand Oaks, CA: Amgen. 2018. www.accessdata.fda.gov/drugsatfda_docs/label/2018/125320s186lbl.pdf

Lewiecki EM. New and emerging concepts in the use of denosumab for the treatment of osteoporosis. *Ther Adv Musculoskelet Dis.* 2018;10(11):209-223. PMID: 30386439

4 ANSWER: B) Calcium citrate, 600 mg 4 times daily

Absorption of calcium carbonate is pH-dependent. In one experiment, only 1% of 500 mg of calcium carbonate was dissolved in 500 mL of water after 1 hour at 98.6°F (37°C) at a neutral pH, with 100% dissolving at a pH of 2.5, similar to that observed in the stomach. Proton-pump inhibitors inhibit the parietal cell H+ K+ATPase pump, leading to suppressed acid secretion and increased stomach pH. There have been multiple case reports of acute hypocalcemia in patients with hypoparathyroidism on calcium carbonate subsequently treated with a proton-pump inhibitor. Absorption of calcium citrate is not pH-dependent, and patients with hypoparathyroidism who will be starting a proton-pump inhibitor should be transitioned to a regimen of calcium citrate (Answer B) since calcium carbonate (Answers A and E) is not well absorbed in this setting. rhPTH (1-84) (Answer C) has not been studied in patients with acute hypocalcemia. While there are case reports of use of PTH (1-34) (Answer D) in acute hypocalcemia, it is not standard treatment. Hydrochlorothiazide (Answer E) can be used to treat hypercalciuria, but it is not used for acute hypocalcemia.

Of note, there are also multiple cases of euparathyroid individuals developing functional hypoparathyroidism caused by hypomagnesemia related to proton-pump inhibitor use, since the secretion of PTH is magnesium-dependent.

EDUCATIONAL OBJECTIVE

Recognize problems with calcium absorption in the setting of proton-pump inhibitor use.

REFERENCE(S)

Bilezikian JP, Brandi ML, Cusano NE, et al. Management of hypoparathyroidism: present and future. *J Clin Endocrinol Metab.* 2016;101(6): 2313-2324. PMID: 26938200

Epstein M, McGrath S, Law F. Proton-pump inhibitors and hypomagnesemic hypoparathyroidism. *N Engl J Med.* 2006;355(17):1834-1836. PMID: 17065651

Milman S, Epstein EJ. Proton pump inhibitor-induced hypocalcemic seizure in a patient with hypoparathyroidism. *Endocr Pract.* 2011;17(1): 104-107. PMID: 21041166

Vallejo F, Sum M. Acute hypocalcemia from proton pump inhibitor use. In: *Hypoparathyroidism: A Clinical Casebook*. Cusano NE, ed. Switzerland: Springer; 2020:9-15.

5 ANSWER: D) Hydrochlorothiazide, 25 mg daily, and calcium carbonate, 500 mg only with exercise

Genetic testing should be considered for patients with nonsurgical hypoparathyroidism. This patient was found to have autosomal dominant hypocalcemia type 1 due to an activating pathogenic variant in the *CASR* gene, causing a leftward shift of the calcium-sensing curve. Autosomal dominant hypocalcemia type 1 is the mirror disorder of familial hypocalciuric hypercalcemia type 1. The activating defect in the *CASR* gene that causes hypoparathyroidism, despite the relatively low PTH concentrations, results in increased renal calcium excretion. Autosomal dominant hypocalcemia should be considered in a patient with high urinary calcium excretion in the absence of treatment with calcium or calcitriol. Patients with autosomal dominant hypocalcemia are at high risk for renal complications, including kidney stones and kidney failure.

Asymptomatic patients can be monitored without calcium or calcitriol therapy (Answers A, B, and C) unless serum calcium is very low, since treatment will worsen hypercalciuria. Hydrochlorothiazide (Answer D) and a low-sodium diet should be started in patients with hypercalciuria to reduce risk. Patients with hypoparathyroidism often need higher dosages of hydrochlorothiazide to reduce renal calcium excretion. This patient has symptoms of hypocalcemia with exercise, and a calcium supplement can be considered, as needed, when she exercises. She does not have difficult-to-control disease with conventional therapy, and treatment with rhPTH (1-84) (Answer E) is not necessary. Of note, patients with known *CASR* pathogenic variants were excluded from the pivotal REPLACE trial of rhPTH (1-84) therapy, although PTH (1-34) was shown to reduce the need for calcium supplementation.

EDUCATIONAL OBJECTIVE

Manage the increased renal risk in patients with autosomal dominant hypocalcemia.

REFERENCE(S)

Bilezikian JP, Brandi ML, Cusano NE, et al. Management of hypoparathyroidism: present and future. *J Clin Endocrinol Metab.* 2016;101(6):2313-2324. PMID: 26938200

Winer KK, Kelly A, Johns A, et al. Long-term parathyroid hormone 1-34 replacement therapy in children with hypoparathyroidism. *J Pediatr.* 2018;203:391-399. PMID: 30470382

6 ANSWER: E) Measure PTH again in 5 months (before her next denosumab injection)

Denosumab is a known cause of hyperparathyroidism. PTH concentrations can rise within the first 1 to 3 months after an injection, typically decreasing towards normal before the next injection. Measurement of PTH in 5 months (before her next injection) (Answer E) is thus the correct answer. This transient PTH elevation in healthy individuals following inhibition of bone resorption with bisphosphonates or denosumab may be a compensatory mechanism in order to maintain normal serum calcium. There is no indication to stop denosumab therapy (Answer C) if PTH levels are elevated. The patient's 25-hydroxyvitamin D level is sufficient, and there is no benefit to further increase vitamin D supplementation (Answer D).

The diagnosis of normocalcemic primary hyperparathyroidism requires elevated PTH concentrations in the absence of secondary causes for hyperparathyroidism. The expert panel from the Fourth International Workshop on the Management of Asymptomatic Primary Hyperparathyroidism recommended that the PTH level remain above the normal range on at least 2 subsequent measurements during a 3- to 6-month period to confirm hyperparathyroidism. Ordering parathyroid imaging (Answer A) or referring to a parathyroid surgeon (Answer B) is incorrect since she has had only a single elevated PTH measurement that may be ascribed to a medication causing hyperparathyroidism.

EDUCATIONAL OBJECTIVE

Identify medications that cause hyperparathyroidism.

REFERENCE(S)

Eastell R, Brandi ML, Costa AG, D'Amour P, Shoback DM, Thakker RV. Diagnosis of asymptomatic primary hyperparathyroidism: proceedings of the Fourth International Workshop. *J Clin Endocrinol Metab.* 2014;99(10):3570-3579. PMID: 25162666

Pawlowska M, Cusano NE. An overview of normocalcemic primary hyperparathyroidism. *Curr Opin Endocrinol Diabetes Obes.* 2015;22(6):413-421. PMID: 26512768

7 ANSWER: E) Working with a dietician to resolve energy deficiency

Relative energy deficiency in sport (RED-S) is a syndrome consisting of disordered eating (or low energy availability), oligomenorrhea/amenorrhea, and decreased bone mineral density. RED-S is a more inclusive and comprehensive term for what was formally referred to as the "female athletic triad."

While this patient's BMI is normal, she has evidence of functional amenorrhea and relative energy deficiency. The Endocrine Society guidelines for functional hypothalamic amenorrhea recommend correcting the energy imbalance (Answer E) to improve function of her hypothalamic-pituitary-ovarian axis, which should also improve bone mineral density.

The guidelines recommend against use of oral contraceptive pills (Answer A) for the sole purpose of regaining menses or improving bone mineral density. There has been lack of clear benefit in studies evaluating bone density effects of oral contraceptive pills vs placebo in women with functional amenorrhea. There are some data that transdermal estrogen with progesterone may be of benefit in women who have not had return of menses after a trial of nutritional, psychological, and/or modified exercise intervention. Transdermal estrogen may improve bone density more than oral contraceptive pills because it does not affect IGF-1 secretion, a bone-trophic hormone that oral contraceptive pills down-regulate. The guidelines recommend against using bisphosphonates (Answer B), denosumab (Answer C), testosterone, or leptin to improve bone mineral density in women with functional amenorrhea. Short-term teriparatide therapy (Answer D) can be considered in rare cases of women with functional amenorrhea in the setting of delayed fracture healing and very low bone mineral density. This patient has had good fracture healing, and treatment with teriparatide is not indicated.

EDUCATIONAL OBJECTIVE

Treat low bone density in a patient with functional hypothalamic amenorrhea/ relative energy deficiency in sport.

REFERENCE(S)

Ackerman KE, Singhal V, Slattery M, et al. Effects of estrogen replacement on bone geometry and microarchitecture in adolescent and young adult oligoamenorrheic athletes: a randomized trial. *J Bone Miner Res.* 2020;35(2):248-260. PMID: 31603998

Gordon CM, Ackerman KE, Berga SL, et al. Functional hypothalamic amenorrhea: an Endocrine Society clinical practice guideline. *J Clin Endocrinol Metab.* 2017;102(5):1413-1439. PMID: 28368518

8 ANSWER: B) Primary hyperparathyroidism

Primary hyperparathyroidism (Answer B) is one of the most common endocrine disorders and is diagnosed in the setting of hypercalcemia with an elevated or inappropriately normal PTH. This patient's PTH concentration, although technically within normal limits, is inappropriate in the setting of hypercalcemia. In primary hyperparathyroidism, PTH facilitates the conversion of 25-hydroxyvitamin D to 1,25-dihydroxyvitamin D, and up to 25% of patients have frankly elevated 1,25-dihydroxyvitamin D levels.

Familial hypocalciuric hypercalcemia (FHH) (Answer A) is a rare, benign disorder caused by loss-of-function pathogenic variants in the gene encoding the calcium-sensing receptor. Patients with FHH usually have a positive family history, although a given patient could represent an index case. The extremely high penetrance of FHH ensures that virtually all patients develop hypercalcemia by their third decade. In FHH, 24-hour urinary calcium excretion is typically less than 100 mg with a calcium-to-creatinine clearance ratio less than 0.01, while typically the ratio is greater than 0.02 in patients with primary hyperparathyroidism. It can be difficult to distinguish between FHH and primary hyperparathyroidism when the ratio is between 0.01 and 0.02; however, patients must be vitamin D replete (>20 ng/mL [>49.9 mmol/L]) with good renal function for the collection to be interpretable. In younger patients, genetic testing may assist with making the diagnosis.

In granulomatous disease (Answer C), while 1,25-dihydroxyvitamin D is typically elevated because macrophages in the granulomas synthesize the active metabolite of vitamin D, PTH levels are also suppressed. PTH levels would also be suppressed in the case of calcitriol toxicity (Answer D). In humoral hypercalcemia of malignancy (Answer E), PTH levels are classically undetectable because endogenous PTH is suppressed and PTHrP, a major cause of humoral hypercalcemia of malignancy, is not detected by immunoassays for PTH.

EDUCATIONAL OBJECTIVE
Diagnose primary hyperparathyroidism.

REFERENCE(S)

Cusano NE, Bilezikian JP. Parathyroid hormone in the evaluation of hypercalcemia. *JAMA.* 2014;312(24):2680-2681. PMID: 25536261

Eastell R, Brandi ML, Costa AG, D'Amour P, Shoback DM, Thakker RV. Diagnosis of asymptomatic primary hyperparathyroidism: proceedings of the Fourth International Workshop. *J Clin Endocrinol Metab.* 2014;99(10):3570-3579. PMID: 25162666

9 ANSWER: A) Zoledronic acid

A number of clinical trials have demonstrated that women with breast cancer treated with aromatase inhibitors experience higher rates of bone loss and fragility fractures, particularly in the first 1 to 2 years of therapy, compared with rates in women treated with tamoxifen. Thus, recommending no intervention (Answer E) is incorrect. Current recommendations are to optimize calcium and vitamin D supplementation and perform DXA screening. International guidelines recommend antiresorptive treatment for patients initiating aromatase inhibitor therapy with a T-score of 2.0 or less regardless of additional risk factors, for the duration of aromatase inhibitor treatment. In addition, patients with any 2 of the following risk factors should receive antiresorptive therapy: T-score of 1.5 or less, age greater than 65 years, low BMI (<20 kg/m^2), family history of hip fracture, personal history of fragility fracture after age 50 years, oral corticosteroid use of greater than 6 months, and current cigarette smoking (or history of).

Several large clinical trials in postmenopausal women with early-stage breast cancer have shown that aromatase inhibitor–induced bone loss can be prevented by treatment with antiresorptive agents at the onset of aromatase inhibitor therapy. The drug regimen that has been studied most extensively is intravenous zoledronic acid (4 mg every 6 months) (Answer A). Oral bisphosphonates can also be used in this setting, although clinical trial data are not nearly as extensive. Denosumab, 60 mg subcutaneously every 6 months, has also been shown to reduce both fractures and cancer recurrence in postmenopausal women with early-stage breast cancer. Calcitonin (Answer B) is a weak antiresorptive agent that would not be appropriate in this patient. Teriparatide (Answer C) is contraindicated in patients with a history of radiation therapy due to increased risk of osteosarcoma. Raloxifene (Answer D), a selective estrogen receptor modulator, significantly reduces estrogen receptor–positive breast cancer in women with osteoporosis, but it is not approved for use in women with a diagnosis of breast cancer.

EDUCATIONAL OBJECTIVE
Manage low bone mass in the setting of breast cancer and aromatase inhibitor therapy.

REFERENCE(S)

Hadji P, Aapro MS, Body JJ, et al. Management of aromatase inhibitor-associated bone loss (AIBL) in postmenopausal women with hormone sensitive breast cancer: joint position statement of the IOF, CABS, ECTS, IEG, ESCEO IMS, and SIOG. *J Bone Oncol.* 2017;7:1-12. PMID: 28413771

Wagner-Johnston ND, Sloan JA, Liu H, et al. 5-year follow-up of a randomized controlled trial of immediate versus delayed zoledronic acid for the prevention of bone loss in postmenopausal women with breast cancer starting letrozole after tamoxifen: N03CC (Alliance) trial. *Cancer.* 2015;121(15):2537-2543. PMID: 25930719

Brufsky AM, Harker WG, Beck JT, et al. Final 5-year results of Z-FAST trial: adjuvant zoledronic acid maintains bone mass in postmenopausal breast cancer patients receiving letrozole. *Cancer.* 2012;118(5):1192-1201. PMID: 21987386

Gnant M, Pfeiler G, Steger GG, et al; Austrian Breast and Colorectal Cancer Study Group. Adjuvant denosumab in postmenopausal patients with hormone receptor-positive breast cancer (ABCSG-18): disease-free survival results from a randomised, double-blind, placebo-controlled, phase 3 trial. *Lancet Oncol.* 2019;20(3):339-351. PMID: 30795951

10 ANSWER: E) Her spine bone mineral density was measured incorrectly

It is always important to look at the images and numbers of a DXA study, particularly when the results do not make sense. Although gains in bone mineral density at one site and loss at another are possible, this situation is very uncommon. In this patient's images, the placement of the spine analysis bars is incorrect, one level higher up than in the previous study (ie, L4 on the current study is actually L3) (Answer E). After correct reanalysis, she had a significant 2.1% improvement in spine bone mineral density.

Her hip images are correct (thus, Answer D is incorrect). She appears to be responding to risedronate (thus, Answer B is incorrect) and therefore she is most likely taking it correctly (thus, Answer A is incorrect). The gains seen in the hip are higher than the least significant change, assumed to be 2.8% for the total hip and 5% for the femoral neck in clinical DXA studies. There is no reason to suspect that she has an undiagnosed secondary cause of osteoporosis (Answer C).

EDUCATIONAL OBJECTIVE

Carefully review DXA images and identify common technical errors.

REFERENCE(S)

Watts NB. Fundamentals and pitfalls of bone densitometry using dual-energy X-ray absorptiometry (DXA). *Osteoporos Int.* 2004;15(11):847-854. PMID: 15322740

Schousboe JT, Shepherd JA, Bilezikian JP, Baim S. Executive summary of the 2013 international society for clinical densitometry position development conference on bone densitometry. *J Clin Densitom.* 2013;16(4):455-466. PMID: 24183638

11 ANSWER: A) 25-Hydroxyvitamin D

Shown on the radiograph is a Looser zone, characteristic of osteomalacia. Mechanical stress of blood vessels overlying the uncalcified cortical bone affected by osteomalacia is thought to cause "pseudofractures" that appear as transverse zones of rarefaction, sometimes as wide as 1 cm, often multiple, and generally symmetric. Typical locations are the ischium, ilium, pubis, femur, tibia, radius, fibula, lower ribs, and scapula.

This patient had malabsorption of both vitamin D and calcium after bariatric surgery, and she did not adhere to calcium and vitamin D supplementation. Her serum 25-hydroxyvitamin D level (Answer A) was undetectable (<7 ng/mL [<17.5 nmol/L]). High-dosage vitamin D_3, 50,000 IU daily, did not correct the vitamin D deficiency, but ultraviolet light (increased sun exposure) was successful. Chemical clues to osteomalacia include hypocalcemia, hypophosphatemia, and elevated alkaline phosphatase. Measuring FGF-23 (Answer C), 1,25-dihydroxyvitamin D (Answer B), intact PTH (Answer D), and C-telopeptide (Answer E) would not clarify the diagnosis.

EDUCATIONAL OBJECTIVE

Identify clinical and radiographic findings in osteomalacia after gastric bypass (severe vitamin D deficiency).

REFERENCE(S)

Karefylakis C, Näslund I, Edholm D, Sundbom M, Karlsson FA, Rask E. Vitamin D status 10 years after primary gastric bypass: gravely high prevalence of hypovitaminosis D and raised PTH levels. *Obes Surg.* 2014;24(3):343-348. PMID: 24163201

Bal BS, Finelli FC, Shope TR, Koch TR. Nutritional deficiencies after bariatric surgery. *Nat Rev Endocrinol.* 2012;8(9):544-556. PMID: 22525731

Reginato AJ, Falasca GF, Pappu R, McKnight B, Agha A. Musculoskeletal manifestations of osteomalacia: report of 26 cases and literature review. *Semin Arthritis Rheum.* 1999;28(5):287-304. PMID: 10342386

Thacher TD, Clarke BL. Vitamin D insufficiency. *Mayo Clin Proc.* 2011;86(1):50-60. PMID: 21193656

Bhan A, Rao AD, Rao DS. Osteomalacia as a result of vitamin D deficiency. *Endocrinol Metab Clin North Am.* 2010;39(2):321-331. PMID: 20511054

12 ANSWER: A) Begin alendronate

This man has an acute vertebral compression fracture at L1 that is symptomatic. This warrants intervention with antiresorptive therapy regardless of the DXA results because vertebral fractures are strong independent predictors of both future vertebral and nonvertebral fractures. Repeating the DXA now (Answer E) is unlikely to be helpful given his degenerative arthritis at the spine, and the results will not change recommended therapy. The correct answer is to begin alendronate (Answer A) because it is an approved and effective therapy in this setting.

Teriparatide (Answer C) is contraindicated in a man who has received pelvic irradiation. Invasive procedures, such as bone biopsy and kyphoplasty (Answer D), are not indicated in the acute setting given the absence of clinical or biochemical evidence (ie, his alkaline phosphatase level is normal) of recurrent bladder cancer or other malignancy. Patients with acute vertebral fractures from osteoporosis should generally not be referred for vertebral augmentation (kyphoplasty or vertebroplasty) unless severe pain has not responded to medical therapies.

Because there are no large randomized controlled trials showing antifracture efficacy for testosterone in men with osteoporosis, testosterone therapy (Answer B) should be considered only for hypogonadal men who are symptomatic, have an organic cause for the hypogonadism, have testosterone levels less than 200 ng/dL (<6.9 nmol/L), and/or are not candidates for other therapies. Due to reports of cardiovascular complications, testosterone is not an ideal therapy for a 72-year-old man. In hypogonadal men with benign prostatic hypertrophy, testosterone therapy, along with a 5α-reductase inhibitor such as finasteride, has been given without exacerbating benign prostatic hypertrophy. However, even men with marked hypogonadism have good skeletal responses to bisphosphonate therapy without correction of hypogonadism.

EDUCATIONAL OBJECTIVE

Manage an acute vertebral fracture in an elderly man.

REFERENCE(S)

Watts NB, Adler RA, Bilezikian JP, et al; Endocrine Society. Osteoporosis in men: an Endocrine Society clinical practice guideline. *J Clin Endocrinol Metab.* 2012;97(6):1802-1822. PMID: 22675062

Cosman F, de Beur SJ, LeBoff MS, et al; National Osteoporosis Foundation. Clinician's guide to prevention and treatment of osteoporosis. *Osteoporos Int.* 2014;25(10):2359-2381. PMID: 25182228

McConnell CT Jr, Wippold FJ 2nd, Ray CE Jr, et al. ACR appropriateness criteria for management of vertebral compression fractures. *J Am Coll Radiol.* 2014;11(8):757-763. PMID: 24935074

13 ANSWER: E) Decrease the cinacalcet dosage

This patient's PTH level is lower than the goal in patients undergoing dialysis and may indicate underlying adynamic bone disease. Because of the low PTH and hypocalcemia, the cinacalcet dosage should be decreased (Answer E). Adynamic bone disease, a type of renal osteodystrophy (now called chronic kidney disease–mineral bone disorder [CKD-MBD]), is present in at least one-third of patients receiving dialysis. Adynamic bone disease is characterized by markedly low bone turnover, no accumulation of osteoid, and high fracture risk. Serum PTH levels in adynamic bone disease are relatively low (usually <100 pg/mL [<100 ng/L]) compared with levels in patients undergoing dialysis who have other forms of CKD-MBD.

In patients with end-stage kidney disease, there is resistance to PTH due at least in part to increased N-terminal truncated PTH (7-84), which counteracts the effect of the 1-84 whole molecule on bone. This can be exacerbated by the use of cinacalcet, as well as overly aggressive treatment with calcitriol, both of which reduce PTH secretion. This patient's low alkaline phosphatase level is also consistent with a low bone turnover state.

Increasing the calcitriol dosage (Answer A) would further suppress PTH, which is not a desired outcome. Decreasing the calcitriol dosage (Answer B) may worsen the hypocalcemia. Teriparatide (Answer C) has been used anecdotally in some patients with end-stage renal disease, low bone turnover, and fractures, but it is not an approved therapy in this context. Although denosumab (Answer D) can be used in patients receiving dialysis, it would be inappropriate to administer it now in the face of hypocalcemia, vitamin D deficiency, and probable adynamic bone disease. A potent antiresorptive agent would theoretically worsen the adynamic bone disease and increase fracture risk.

Impaired mineralization, osteitis fibrosa cystica, and mixed renal osteodystrophy are other forms of CKD-MBD, but these diagnoses are unlikely given the laboratory findings. Osteitis fibrosa cystica and high bone turnover are associated with elevated PTH, osteomalacia is associated with very low 25-hydroxyvitamin D, and mixed renal osteodystrophy is associated with both findings.

EDUCATIONAL OBJECTIVE

Diagnose and manage adynamic bone disease in a patient undergoing dialysis.

REFERENCE(S)

Cannata-Andía JB, Rodriguez García M, Gómez Alonso C. Osteoporosis and adynamic bone in chronic kidney disease. *J Nephrol.* 2013;26(1): 73-80. PMID: 23023723

Hruska KA, Mathew S. Chronic kidney disease mineral bone disorder (CKD-MBD). In: Rosen CJ, Compston JE, Lian JB, eds. Primer on the Metabolic Bone Diseases and Disorders of Mineral Metabolism. Washington, DC: The American Society for Bone and Mineral Research; 2008:343-349.

Brandenburg VM, Floege J. Adynamic bone disease: bone and beyond. *NDT Plus.* 2008;1(3):135-147. PMID: 25983860

Kidney Disease: Improving Global Outcomes (KDIGO) CKD-MBD Work Group. KDIGO clinical practice guideline for the diagnosis, evaluation, prevention, and treatment of chronic kidney disease-mineral and bone disorder (CKD-MBD). *Kidney Int Suppl.* 2009;(Suppl 113):S1-S130. PMID: 19644521

14 ANSWER: B) Zoledronic acid

The 2017 guidelines from the American College of Rheumatology recommend some type of pharmacologic treatment for adults 40 years and older with a moderate fracture risk, defined as a glucocorticoid-adjusted FRAX risk of 10% to 19% for major osteoporotic fracture or 1.1% to 2.9% for hip fracture.

Alendronate, risedronate, zoledronic acid (Answer B), teriparatide (Answer C), and denosumab (Answer D) (but not ibandronate [Answer A]) are all FDA approved for management of glucocorticoid-induced osteoporosis. Because there is still controversy about the link between esophageal cancer and oral bisphosphonate use, it may be preferable to start with intravenous zoledronic acid (Answer B) rather than an oral bisphosphonate in a patient with Barrett esophagus.

Teriparatide (Answer C) is usually reserved for patients with prevalent vertebral fractures or much lower vertebral T-scores—in the frankly osteoporotic range. Given limited safety data, denosumab (Answer D) is generally not recommended as first-line therapy in patients taking multiple immunosuppressive drugs or biologic drugs.

Finally, the low FRAX scores underestimate the fracture risk in patients on long-term glucocorticoid therapy. FRAX does not account for the disproportionate negative effects of glucocorticoids on spinal trabecular bone and does not include spinal bone mineral density in the calculation. Therefore, recommending no therapeutic intervention (Answer E) is incorrect despite the patient's low FRAX scores.

EDUCATIONAL OBJECTIVE

Determine whether pharmacologic treatment to reduce fracture risk is necessary in a patient taking glucocorticoids.

REFERENCE(S)

Buckley L, Guyatt G, Fink HA, et al. 2017 American College of Rheumatology guideline for the prevention and treatment of glucocorticoid-induced osteoporosis. *Arthritis Rheumatol.* 2017;69(8): 1521-1537. PMID: 28585373

Venuturupalli SR, Sacks W. Review of new guidelines for the management of glucocorticoid induced osteoporosis. *Curr Osteoporos Rep.* 2013;11(4):357-364. PMID: 24114241

Leib ES, Saag KG, Adachi JD, et al; FRAX(®) Position Development Conference Members. Official Positions for FRAX(®) clinical regarding glucocorticoids: the impact of the use of glucocorticoids on the estimate by FRAX(®) of the 10 year risk of fracture from Joint Official Positions Development Conference of the International Society for Clinical Densitometry and International Osteoporosis Foundation on FRAX(®). *J Clin Densitom.* 2011;14(3):212-219. PMID: 21810527

15 ANSWER: D) Obtain lateral spine radiographs

A frequent clinical question is when or if to give a "bisphosphonate holiday" to patients with osteoporosis who have been on either oral or intravenous bisphosphonates for several years. Because bisphosphonates have a long retention in the skeleton, they may continue to exhibit antifracture efficacy even after therapy is stopped. The decision to stop bisphosphonate therapy must be individualized. Studies have shown that after 3 years of annual intravenous zoledronic acid or 5 years of oral bisphosphonate therapy, it is reasonable to reassess each patient and determine whether a bisphosphonate holiday may be considered. Patients and physicians worry about the risk of rare but devastating adverse effects (such as osteonecrosis of the jaw and atypical femur fractures) that seem to be correlated with duration of bisphosphonate therapy.

Data from the FLEX and HORIZON extension trials show that many patients can stop bisphosphonate therapy temporarily after 3 to 5 years without loss of bone mineral density or increased fracture risk. However, some subgroups of patients appear to be at higher risk for bone loss or fractures after stopping therapy. For these patients, the options include either continuing the bisphosphonate for up to 10 years with periodic reassessment or stopping the bisphosphonate and switching to a different agent. Patients at higher risk include those with a history of hip or vertebral fractures, multiple fractures, T-score of −2.5 or lower at the hip, or other factors placing them "at high risk" for fractures.

The correct answer in this case is to obtain lateral spine radiographs (Answer D). This patient no longer has osteoporosis by DXA criteria and has not sustained a known clinical fracture. Thus, he might qualify for a "bisphosphonate holiday" (Answer B). However, the loss of height over the past 4 years and moderate kyphosis suggest that he is likely to have 1 or more vertebral fracture that would move him into a very high-risk category. Presence of a prevalent vertebral fracture would prompt either continued antiresorptive therapy with a bisphosphonate for up to 10 years (such as alendronate [Answer A]) or a switch to denosumab or teriparatide. Radiographs of asymptomatic patients with loss of height and/or kyphosis are recommended because up to 70% of vertebral fractures are clinically silent. While many clinicians use measurement of fasting serum C-telopeptide (Answer C) to determine whether or when patients should discontinue bisphosphonates and whether or when they should resume therapy, there are no data to support this approach. Routine radiographs of the proximal femurs (Answer E) are not recommended as part of the evaluation of asymptomatic patients on bisphosphonate therapy.

Finally, it is important to note that not all bisphosphonates are the same. Alendronate and zoledronic acid have much longer retention in bone than do ibandronate or risedronate. With the latter 2 bisphosphonates, decreases in bone density can occur within 6 to 12 months—thus, drug holidays, if given at all, must be short.

EDUCATIONAL OBJECTIVE

Assess the appropriateness of "bisphosphonate holidays" in osteoporosis management.

REFERENCE(S)

Black DM, Schwartz AV, Ensrud KE, et al; FLEX Research Group. Effects of continuing or stopping alendronate after 5 years of treatment: the Fracture Intervention Trial Long-term Extension (FLEX): a randomized trial. *JAMA.* 2006;296(24): 2927-2938. PMID: 17190893

Black DM, Reid IR, Boonen S, et al. The effect of 3 versus 6 years of zoledronic acid treatment of osteoporosis: a randomized extension to the HORIZON-Pivotal Fracture Trial (PFT). [published correction appears in *J Bone Miner Res.* 2012;27(12):2612]. *J Bone Miner Res.* 2012;27(2): 243-254. PMID: 22161728

Adler RA, Fuleihan GE, Bauer DC, et al. Managing osteoporosis in patients on long-term bisphosphonate treatment: report of a Task force of the American Society for Bone and Mineral Research. *J Bone Miner Res.* 2016;31(1):16-35. PMID: 26350171

16 ANSWER: D) Risedronate

This patient has no symptoms of testosterone deficiency and no indication that his mildly low testosterone is "organic." Because there are no large randomized controlled trials showing antifracture effectiveness for testosterone in men with osteoporosis, testosterone therapy (Answers A and B) should only be considered for hypogonadal men who are symptomatic, have an organic cause for the hypogonadism, have testosterone levels less than 200 ng/dL (<6.9 nmol/L), and/or are not candidates for other therapies. If he were symptomatic or had lower testosterone levels, testosterone therapy with a 5a-reductase inhibitor such as finasteride could be given without exacerbating his benign prostatic hypertrophy. However, even men with marked hypogonadism respond well to antiosteoporosis therapy without correction of the hypogonadism. He should be offered treatment with an agent approved to treat osteoporosis in men and one that reduces fracture risk, such as risedronate (Answer D). Teriparatide (Answer E) is generally not a first-line agent for osteoporosis and is best reserved for those with vertebral fractures or very low bone mineral density. Hydrochlorothiazide (Answer C) can be used for management of hypercalciuria, but this patient has a urine calcium excretion within the reference range for men.

EDUCATIONAL OBJECTIVE

Recommend appropriate management of male osteoporosis in the setting of borderline-low testosterone.

REFERENCE(S)

Watts NB, Adler RA, Bilezikian JP, et al; Endocrine Society. Osteoporosis in men: an Endocrine Society clinical practice guideline. *J Clin Endocrinol Metab.* 2012;97(6):1802-1822. PMID: 22675062

Boonen S, Lorenc RS, Wenderoth D, Stoner KJ, Eusebio R, Orwoll ES. Evidence for safety and efficacy of risedronate in men with osteoporosis over 4 years of treatment: results from the 2-year, open-label, extension study of a 2-year, randomized, double-blind, placebo-controlled study. *Bone.* 2012;51(3):383-388. PMID: 22750403

17 ANSWER: C) Cholecalciferol, 4000 IU daily

The average serum 25-hydroxyvitamin D response to 1000 IU of vitamin D daily for 8 to 12 weeks is an increase of about 12 ng/mL (30.0 nmol/L). In this vignette, the patient's level would be expected to increase from 8 to 20 ng/mL (20.0 to 49.9 nmol/L) over a period of 2 to 3 months. Instead, due to class 3 obesity, his 25-hydroxyvitamin D level may only increase by a few nanograms per deciliter, a very blunted response. Therefore, recommending cholecalciferol, 400 or 1000 IU daily (Answers A and B), will not normalize his 25-hydroxyvitamin D level.

A number of studies have shown that patients who are overweight or obese require much higher dosages of vitamin D than normal-weight participants to achieve adequate levels. Obese patients are estimated to require 2 to 3 times the usual daily dose of cholecalciferol to achieve adequate levels. The mechanism is not well understood. The closest dosage to what would be needed to correct the vitamin D deficiency in this patient is cholecalciferol, 4000 IU daily (Answer C). The dosage could be adjusted in 8 to 12 weeks after rechecking the 25-hydroxyvitamin D level. Giving 10,000 IU cholecalciferol weekly (Answer D) would only provide about 1700 IU daily and thus would not be adequate. Finally, there is no role for treating with activated vitamin D or calcitriol (Answer E) in this setting.

EDUCATIONAL OBJECTIVE

Recommend appropriate vitamin D supplementation for obese patients.

REFERENCE(S)

Heaney RP, Davies KM, Chen TC, Holick MF, Barger-Lux MJ. Human serum 25-hydroxycholecalciferol response to extended oral dosing with cholecalciferol [published correction appears in *Am J Clin Nutr.* 2003;78(5):1047]. *Am J Clin Nutr.* 2003;77(1):204-210. PMID: 12499343

Ekwaru JP, Zwicker JD, Holick MF, Giovannucci E, Veugelers PJ. The importance of body weight for the dose response relationship of oral vitamin D supplementation and 25-hydroxyvitamin D in healthy volunteers. *PLoS One.* 2014;9(11):e111265. PMID: 25372709

Holick MF, Binkley NC, Bischoff-Ferrari HA, et al; Endocrine Society. Evaluation, treatment, and prevention of vitamin D deficiency: an Endocrine Society clinical practice guideline. *J Clin Endocrinol Metab.* 2011;96(7):1911-1930. PMID: 21646368

18 ANSWER: E) Severe hypocalcemia

Denosumab, a human monoclonal antibody against RANK ligand, is approved for treatment of osteoporosis, as well as metastatic solid tumors such as breast cancer. It is a very potent inhibitor of osteoclastic bone resorption. Unlike bisphosphonates, denosumab is not cleared via the kidneys and has no effect on renal function (thus, Answer A is incorrect). Although cases of osteonecrosis of the jaw (Answer B) have been reported with both bisphosphonates and denosumab, this is very unlikely after only 1 dose of the drug. Severe flulike syndromes (Answer C) (also known as "acute phase reactions") are much more common with intravenous bisphosphonates than with denosumab. Potent antiresorptive agents such as denosumab have not been shown to impair fracture healing (Answer D).

The major adverse effect to be expected in this setting is profound, symptomatic hypocalcemia (Answer E) within 7 to 10 days following denosumab administration. Patients at greatest risk for this complication are those with significantly impaired renal function and high bone turnover with elevated alkaline phosphatase, as demonstrated in this patient. The potent inhibition of osteoclastic bone resorption by denosumab stops the efflux of calcium from bone and can lower serum calcium dramatically. The usual physiologic responses to hypocalcemia, such as a rise in PTH and calcitriol production, that would normally lead to increased renal tubular reabsorption of calcium and increased gut absorption of calcium, will not work in the setting of renal failure. This woman also has a very low vitamin D level. Therefore, even if renal function were better, she would still be at risk for an inadequate homeostatic response due to very low vitamin D substrate.

EDUCATIONAL OBJECTIVE

Anticipate the risk of symptomatic hypocalcemia following denosumab in the setting of renal failure.

REFERENCE(S)

Dave V, Chiang CY, Booth J, Mount PF. Hypocalcemia post denosumab in patients with chronic kidney disease stage 4-5. *Am J Nephrol.* 2015;41(2):129-137. PMID: 25790847

Body JJ, Bone HG, de Boer RH, et al. Hypocalcaemia in patients with metastatic bone disease treated with denosumab. *Eur J Cancer.* 2015;51(13): 1812-1821. PMID: 26093811

Kinoshita Y, Arai M, Ito N, et al. High serum ALP level is associated with increased risk of denosumab-related hypocalcemia in patients with bone metastases from solid tumors. *Endocr J.* 2016;63(5):479-484. PMID: 26860123

Stopeck AT, Lipton A, Body JJ, et al. Denosumab compared with zoledronic acid for the treatment of bone metastases in patients with advanced breast cancer: a randomized, double-blind study. *J Clin Oncol.* 2010;28(35):5132-5139. PMID: 21060033

19 ANSWER: B) Decrease calcium supplementation

Patients with hypoparathyroidism cannot stimulate renal tubular reabsorption of filtered calcium due to lack of PTH effect on the kidneys. Therefore, calcium and calcitriol supplementation in the management of chronic hypoparathyroidism can lead to hypercalciuria, nephrolithiasis, nephrocalcinosis, and renal insufficiency. Epidemiologic studies have shown markedly increased relative risks (3- to 6-fold) of renal dysfunction among those with both surgical and nonsurgical hypoparathyroidism. Because of this, it is important to encourage patients to minimize excessive calcium intake, to take the lowest possible calcitriol dosage, and to try to maintain serum calcium in the low-normal or even slightly low range, typically between 8 and 9 mg/dL (2.0-2.3 mmol/L). It is also important to monitor urinary calcium excretion and avoid hypercalciuria. Because this patient has hypercalciuria, continuing the current regimen (Answer A) is not optimal. Sevelamer (Answer C), a phosphate binder, is not indicated for this mild hyperphosphatemia and would not address his hypercalciuria. His calcium × phosphate product is less than 55 mg^2/dL^2, so there is no urgency for a phosphate binder.

The best option is to recommend that he gradually decrease his excessive intake of calcium supplements (Answer B). Patients with hypoparathyroidism can experience unpleasant symptoms of muscle cramps, spasms, and paresthesias, particularly during or after exercise. Therefore, it is important to gradually try to achieve a lower calcium intake that is both safe and tolerable.

The approval of recombinant human PTH (1-84) (Answer D) for management of permanent hypoparathyroidism offers another option, but it is extremely expensive. Moreover, this should be reserved for patients who cannot be managed well on conventional therapy. Guidelines for its use are discussed in the provided references. Thiazide diuretics (Answer E) may be useful adjunctive therapy for some patients with persistent hypercalciuria who are unable to lower calcium intake due to hypocalcemic symptoms. It is reasonable to try a thiazide diuretic in these cases, particularly if serum calcium is on the lower end of normal with persistent hypercalciuria. Often, high dosages (such as 50 mg daily of hydrochlorothiazide or more) are needed to normalize urinary calcium excretion, but some patients respond well to lower dosages. Concomitant potassium-sparing diuretics such as amiloride and low-salt diets may be useful adjunctive therapies. When starting thiazides, serum calcium may rise, allowing reduction in the calcitriol dosage.

Other risks for patients with permanent surgical hypoparathyroidism include neuropsychiatric disease, infections, and seizures. Among those with nonsurgical hypoparathyroidism, there is a higher occurrence of ischemic cardiovascular disease, cataracts, and fractures.

EDUCATIONAL OBJECTIVE
Manage chronic surgical hypoparathyroidism.

REFERENCE(S)

Bilezikian JP, Khan A, Potts JT Jr, et al. Hypoparathyroidism in the adult: epidemiology, diagnosis, pathophysiology, target-organ involvement, treatment, and challenges for future research. *J Bone Miner Res.* 2011;26(10):2317-2337. PMID: 21812031

Clarke BL, Brown EM, Collins MT, et al. Epidemiology and diagnosis of hypoparathyroidism. *J Clin Endocrinol Metab.* 2016;101(6): 2284-2299. PMID: 26943720

Bilezikian JP, Brandi ML, Cusano NE, et al. Management of hypoparathyroidism: present and future. *J Clin Endocrinol Metab.* 2016;101(6): 2313-2324. PMID: 26938200

20 ANSWER: D) Serum cortisol and ACTH

This patient has autoimmune polyendocrine syndrome type 1 (APS type 1) due to a pathogenic variant in the autoimmune regulator gene (*AIRE*) and presents with symptoms and signs of Addison disease. APS type 1 is also known by the acronym APECED (autoimmune polyendocrinopathy-candidiasis-ectodermal dystrophy). The classic presentation includes at least 2 of the following 3 major clinical components: chronic mucocutaneous candidiasis, primary hypoparathyroidism, and autoimmune adrenal insufficiency. The physical examination notes ectodermal dystrophy of the fingernails. Hyperpigmentation from adrenal insufficiency would also be expected on exam. Primary adrenal insufficiency may be diagnosed before clinical symptoms by checking for antibodies against the 21-hydroxylase enzyme, but in this case, serum cortisol and ACTH (Answer D) must be measured immediately. Given the physical examination findings, one would expect to find hyponatremia, hyperkalemia, and elevated ACTH, along with a low or "normal" serum cortisol (which is being maximally stimulated). Pending the results, a formal cosyntropin-stimulation test should be done.

Serum ceruloplasmin measurement (Answer A) is used to diagnose Wilson disease, a genetic syndrome in which copper accumulates in tissues, including the parathyroid glands. Classic findings include Kayser-Fleischer rings, liver damage, and neuropsychiatric symptoms. Serum ferritin, iron, and total iron-binding capacity (Answer B) can be used to screen for hemochromatosis ("bronze diabetes"), but that would not fit the clinical picture. Transglutaminase antibodies (Answer C) can be used to diagnose celiac disease. While up to 80% of patients with APECED have malabsorption or other gastrointestinal illness, celiac disease is not typical. Hypothyroidism can occur with APECED, although this patient's symptoms are more consistent with adrenal insufficiency and prompt diagnosis of adrenal insufficiency is critical. Therefore, TSH measurement (Answer E) is not the best next step.

EDUCATIONAL OBJECTIVE
Diagnose Addison disease as part of autoimmune polyendocrine syndrome type 1.

REFERENCE(S)

Weiler FG, Dias-da-Silva MR, Lazaretti-Castro M. Autoimmune polyendocrine syndrome type 1: case report and review of literature. *Arq Bras Endocrinol Metabol.* 2012;56(1):54-66. PMID: 22460196

Akirav EM, Ruddle NH, Herold KC. The role of AIRE in human autoimmune disease. *Nat Rev Endocrinol.* 2011;7(1):25-33. PMID: 21102544

Eisenbarth GS, Gottlieb PA. Autoimmune polyendocrine syndromes. *N Engl J Med.* 2004;350(20): 2068-2079. PMID: 15141045

Ferre EM, Rose SR, Rosenzweig SD, et al. Redefined clinical features and diagnostic criteria in autoimmune polyendocrinopathy-candidiasis-ectodermal dystrophy. *JCI Insight.* 2016;1(13). pii: e88782. PMID: 27588307

21 ANSWER: A) FGF-23 measurement

This patient has tumor-induced osteomalacia caused by a benign mesenchymal tumor that is secreting FGF-23 (Answer A). This causes renal tubular loss of phosphate and inhibits 1α-hydroxylase, resulting in low 1,25-dihydroxyvitamin D levels. These tumors are typically located in the skin, bones, or connective tissue (eg, sinuses) and may be difficult to localize. Imaging to localize the tumor includes nuclear medicine techniques such as bone scan, octreotide scan, or PET. In difficult cases, serum FGF-23 measurement in selective venous sampling may be used to localize the extremity from which FGF-23 is being secreted. Tumor removal (if it can be located and removed) normalizes renal phosphate handling within hours to days.

Hypophosphatemia induced by tenofovir (and adefovir) is part of a more generalized syndrome known as Fanconi syndrome in which multiple substances such as bicarbonate, glucose, uric acid, potassium, and phosphate are "wasted" in the urine (Answer C). This patient has no evidence of this syndrome. Low levels of 24,25-dihydroxyvitamin D (Answer B) can be useful to diagnose patients with hypercalcemia and kidney stones who have pathogenic variants in the *CYP24A1* gene. While the severity of X-linked hypophosphatasia caused by pathogenic variants in *PHEX* (Answer D) varies widely, even among members of the same family, the disease is completely penetrant and not expected to first cause symptoms later in life. A sestamibi scan (Answer E) is not helpful in diagnosing tumor-induced osteomalacia.

EDUCATIONAL OBJECTIVE

Diagnose tumor-induced osteomalacia by measuring FGF-23.

REFERENCE(S)

Ruppe MD, Jan de Beur SM. Disorders of phosphate homeostasis. In: Rosen CJ, Compston JE, Lian JB, eds. *Primer on the Metabolic Bone Diseases and Disorders of Mineral Metabolism.* Washington, DC: The American Society for Bone and Mineral Research; 2008:601-612.

Jan de Beur SM. Tumor-induced osteomalacia. *JAMA.* 2005;294(10):1260-1267. PMID: 16160135

Andreopoulou P, Dumitrescu CE, Kelly MH, et al. Selective venous catheterization for the localization of phosphaturic mesenchymal tumors. *J Bone Miner Res.* 2011;26(6):1295-1302. PMID: 21611969

22 ANSWER: C) 25-Hydroxyvitamin D measurement

Although this patient may have Paget disease, other causes of elevated alkaline phosphatase must be considered before proceeding to bone scan, including vitamin D deficiency and/or secondary hyperparathyroidism, particularly given his age and chronic kidney disease. This patient was indeed found to have vitamin D deficiency with secondary hyperparathyroidism. Thus, measurement of 25-hydroxyvitamin D (Answer C) is the correct next step. Although he has been taking 2000 IU of vitamin D daily, this is not enough to maintain a normal 25-hydroxyitamin D level in some patients after bariatric surgery. Serum levels of 1,25-dihyroxyvitamin D are regulated primarily by PTH levels, which in turn are regulated by calcium and/or vitamin D. 1,25-Dihydroxyvitamin D levels do not reflect vitamin D stores, and in vitamin D deficiency, 1,25-dihydroxyvitamin D levels are normal or even elevated due to secondary hyperparathyroidism. Thus, measuring 1,25-dihydroxyvitamin D (Answer D) is incorrect. In this patient, a whole-body bone scan (Answer A) may be spuriously abnormal, showing multiple areas of uptake due to increased bone turnover. Serum C-telopeptide (Answer E) may be elevated, but its measurement will not help to determine the cause of his elevated alkaline phosphatase.

A skeletal survey (Answer B) would be helpful if multiple myeloma were the suspected diagnosis, which is not the case.

EDUCATIONAL OBJECTIVE

Rule out vitamin D deficiency and secondary hyperparathyroidism before evaluating for Paget disease.

REFERENCE(S)

Karefylakis C, Näslund I, Edholm D, Sundbom M, Karlsson FA, Rask E. Vitamin D status 10 years after primary gastric bypass: gravely high prevalence of hypovitaminosis D and raised PTH levels. *Obes Surg.* 2014;24(3):343-348. PMID: 24163201

23 ANSWER: B) Type 1 collagen α 1 and 2 genes (*COL1A1/COL1A2*)

This patient has the mildest form of osteogenesis imperfecta, known as type 1. Inheritance is autosomal dominant, but many pathogenic variants can occur de novo, so the family history may be negative. Patients with osteogenesis imperfecta type 1 have normal stature and little or no skeletal deformity. Fractures occur in childhood or adolescence and decrease markedly after puberty. As is the case in this vignette, affected patients may then present in middle age with "osteoporosis." In 50% of patients, there is early-onset hearing loss before age 40 years. On physical examination, there may be blue sclerae and easy bruising. Joint laxity may be present, but dentinogenesis imperfecta is usually absent. Diagnosis is made by sequencing the genes that encode type 1 collagen (α1 and α2) (*COL1A1/COL1A2*) (Answer B). Pathogenic variants in *COL1A1* or *COL1A2* that cause decreased amounts of normal collagen lead to the mild phenotype seen in patients with osteogenesis imperfecta type 1. Pathogenic variants that disrupt the formation of the normal type I collagen triple helix cause the lethal phenotype seen in type IIA. Posttranslational defects in the interferon-induced transmembrane protein 5 gene (*IFITM5*), FK506-binding protein 10 gene (*FKBP10* [*FKBP65*]), and cartilage-associated protein gene (*CRTAP*) are among the causes of osteogenesis imperfecta in the 10% patients without pathogenic variants in *COL1A1* or *COL1A2*.

The main therapy for osteogenesis imperfecta remains bisphosphonates (intravenous pamidronate and zoledronic acid and oral bisphosphonates). Denosumab has been used in rare case reports. Teriparatide does not dramatically change clinical outcomes. It is hoped that the sclerostin inhibitor romosozumab may have some effectiveness in decreasing fractures in osteogenesis imperfecta, but this awaits clinical trials.

Osteoprotegerin (Answer A) is a cytokine and decoy receptor for the receptor activator of nuclear factor kappa B ligand (RANKL). By binding to RANKL, it reduces differentiation of precursors to osteoclasts and blocks osteoclast production and proliferation, thus reducing bone resorption. Pathogenic variants in this gene have been associated with osteoarthritis but not with the phenotype illustrated in this vignette. Pathogenic variants in the gene encoding the LDL receptor-related protein 5 (Answer C) are involved with the canonical Wnt pathway. Loss-of-function variants can cause osteoporosis-pseudoglioma syndrome, while gain-of-function variants result in a high bone mass phenotype. Pathogenic variants in the vitamin D receptor gene (Answer D) can be found in vitamin D–resistant rickets, but this would be accompanied by a high 1,25-dihydroxyvitamin D level, as well as hypophosphatemia, hypocalcemia, and osteomalacia. Sclerostin, produced by the *SOST* gene (Answer E), is produced by osteocytes and has antianabolic effects on bone formation by suppressing Wnt signaling. Inactivating variants in the *SOST* gene cause syndromes of high bone mass (sclerosteosis and van Buchem disease).

EDUCATIONAL OBJECTIVE

Diagnose osteogenesis imperfecta type 1 (the mildest form).

REFERENCE(S)

Van Dijk FS, Sillence DO. Osteogenesis imperfecta: clinical diagnosis, nomenclature and severity assessment [published correction appears in *Am J Med Genet A.* 2015;167A(5):1178]. *Am J Med Genet A.* 2014;164A(6):1470-1481. PMID: 24715559

Thomas IH, DiMeglio LA. Advances in the classification and treatment of osteogenesis imperfecta. *Curr Osteoporos Rep.* 2016;14(1):1-9. PMID: 26861807

Shapiro JR, Thompson CB, Wu Y, Nunes M, Gillen C. Bone mineral density and fracture rate in response to intravenous and oral bisphosphonates in adult osteogenesis imperfecta. *Calcif Tissue Int.* 2010;87(2):120-129. PMID: 20544187

24 ANSWER: A) Begin hydrochlorothiazide

In patients with multiple stone episodes—most of whom have already increased their fluid intake—thiazide diuretics (Answer A) and citrate supplements are similarly effective in patients with hypercalciuria, as well as in unselected patients. Hydrochlorothiazide acts to enhance renal calcium reabsorption to reduce urinary calcium excretion. Citrate acts as a stone inhibitor. Reducing dietary calcium (Answer D) is counterproductive since dietary calcium binds with dietary oxalate and helps reduce intestinal oxalate absorption.

Hypercalciuria may be caused by increased sodium intake, which leads to increased sodium excretion and an obligatory loss of calcium in the urine; however, this patient's urinary sodium excretion is normal as is his urinary uric acid level. Thus, prescribing allopurinol (Answer B) is incorrect. His urinary oxalate level is normal, so there would be no benefit in reducing dietary oxalate (Answer C). Finally, the urine volume of 2.6 L suggests that increased fluid intake (Answer E) would not be helpful. The goal is to aim for urine volume greater than 2.5 L per day.

Other risk factors for recurrent kidney stones include excessive intake of salt and proteins and high dietary acid load. The intake of vegetables and a vegetarian-type diet is encouraged in stone-forming patients. Consumption of sugar-sweetened soda is associated with a higher risk of stone formation, whereas consumption of coffee, tea, beer, wine, and orange juice is associated with a lower risk.

EDUCATIONAL OBJECTIVE

Recommend a thiazide diuretic as a means to reduce the risk of recurrent kidney stones.

REFERENCE(S)

Fink HA, Wilt TJ, Eldman KE, et al. Medical management to prevent recurrent nephrolithiasis in adults: a systematic review for an American College of Physicians Clinical Guideline [published correction appears in *Ann Intern Med.* 2013;159(3): 230-232]. *Ann Intern Med.* 2013;158(7):535-543. PMID: 23546565

Vigen R, Weideman RA, Reilly RF. Thiazides diuretics in the treatment of nephrolithiasis: are we using them in an evidence-based fashion? *Int Urol Nephrol.* 2011;43(3):813-819. PMID: 20737209

Borghi L, Schianchi T, Meschi T, et al. Comparison of two diets for the prevention of recurrent stones in idiopathic hypercalciuria. *N Engl J Med.* 2002;346(2):77-84. PMID: 11784873

25 ANSWER: C) Intravenous bolus of 150 mg calcium gluconate followed by a continuous calcium gluconate infusion of 1 mg/kg per h

Intravenous calcium should be considered for patients presenting with clinical features of hypocalcemia, including symptoms of paresthesias, carpopedal spasm, bronchospasm or laryngospasm, tetany, seizures, mental status changes, positive Chvostek or Trousseau signs, bradycardia, impaired cardiac contractility, and prolonged QT interval. While some patients with marked hypocalcemia (ie, corrected calcium <7.0 mg/dL [<1.8 mmol/L]) may not be symptomatic, intravenous therapy may be indicated because at those levels, life-threatening features such as laryngeal spasm and seizures can appear acutely. This patient needs rapid correction of hypocalcemia. Calcium gluconate is preferred over calcium chloride because the latter is more likely to cause vein sclerosis and tissue necrosis if extravasated (thus, Answers A and B are incorrect). Dosing at 1 mg/kg per h would be a total dose of 1680 mg daily for a 70-kg patient (thus, Answer C is correct); a higher rate might be required for patients with a profound calcium deficiency. The dose of intravenous calcium is dangerously high in Answer E. rhPTH (1-84) (Answer D) has not been studied in acute hypocalcemia.

Ordering intravenous calcium can be potentially confusing. For intravenous use, a 10-mL ampule of calcium gluconate contains 93 mg of calcium; a 10-mL ampule of 10% calcium chloride contains 272 mg of calcium. In some situations, adding a calcium salt to an intravenous liter bag of 0.9% saline or 5% dextrose requires removing some of the fluid to allow space for the added calcium salt.

EDUCATIONAL OBJECTIVE

Manage acute, severe hypocalcemia.

REFERENCE(S)

Zalonga GP, Chernow B. Hypocalcemia in critical illness. *JAMA.* 1986;256(14):1924-1929. PMID: 3531557

Vetter T, Lohse MJ. Magnesium and the parathyroid. *Curr Opin Nephrol Hypertens.* 2002;11(4):403-410. PMID: 12105390

al-Ghamdi SM, Cameron EC, Sutton RA. Magnesium deficiency: pathophysiologic and clinical overview. *Am J Kidney Dis.* 1994;24(5):737-752. PMID: 7977315

26 ANSWER: B) Genetic testing for pathogenic variants in the multiple endocrine neoplasia type 1 gene (*MEN1*)

It is critical to think about and screen for *MEN1* pathogenic variants (Answer B) in all young patients (<30 years) who present with primary hyperparathyroidism. Up to 10% of patients with primary hyperparathyroidism have a familial (germline) pathogenic variant. Hereditary syndromes should be suspected in anyone with a personal history of other endocrine tumors (especially pancreatic or pituitary) or a family history of parathyroid disease, renal stones, or pancreatic/pituitary tumors in first-degree relatives. These syndromes should also be suspected and screened for in patients presenting with atypical or multigland parathyroid adenomas at any age. Only 2% to 4% of all patients with primary hyperparathyroidism present with multigland adenomas.

In addition to multiple endocrine neoplasia type 1, other more rare causes of multiorgan syndromic primary hyperparathyroidism include multiple endocrine neoplasia type 2, multiple endocrine neoplasia type 4, and hyperparathyroidism–jaw tumor syndrome. Familial idiopathic primary hyperparathyroidism may be a subtype of hyperparathyroidism–jaw tumor syndrome.

The presence of renal stones and high urinary calcium excretion excludes familial hypocalciuric hypercalcemia caused by an inactivating variant in the gene encoding the calcium sensing receptor (*CASR*) (Answer A). Although a 4D CT of the neck (Answer C) would be reasonable in an older patient with persistent primary hyperparathyroidism, in this young man it is mandatory to screen for multiple endocrine neoplasia first because that diagnosis would alter the surgical management and medical follow-up. Another sestamibi scan (Answer D) looking for a second adenoma would not be indicated when all 4 glands may be involved. Calcium supplementation would not be responsible for these laboratory findings, so cessation of this treatment (Answer E) is not necessary.

EDUCATIONAL OBJECTIVE

Pursue the diagnosis of multiple endocrine neoplasia type 1 in young patients presenting with primary hyperparathyroidism.

REFERENCE(S)

Thakker RV, Newey PJ, Walls GV, et al; Endocrine Society. Clinical practice guidelines for multiple endocrine neoplasia 1 (MEN1). *J Clin Endocrinol Metab.* 2012;97(9):2990-3011. PMID: 22723327

Eastell R, Brandi ML, Costa AG, D'Amour P, Shoback DM, Thakker RV. Diagnosis of asymptomatic primary hyperparathyroidism: proceedings of the Fourth International Workshop. *J Clin Endocrinol Metab.* 2014;99(10):3570-3579. PMID: 25162666

Lassen T, Friis-Hansen L, Rasmussen AK, Knigge U, Feldt-Rasmussen U. Primary hyperparathyroidism in young people. When should we perform genetic testing for multiple endocrine neoplasia 1 (MEN-1)? *J Clin Endocrinol Metab.* 2014;99(11): 3983-3987. PMID: 24731012

27 ANSWER: B) Decreases rapidly in the spine and hip (3%-5% in the first year)

When estrogen levels decrease with menopause, bone mineral density decreases at a rate of about 1% to 2% per year. Age-related bone loss is about 0.5% to 1% per year. When estrogen is stopped after at least 5 years of treatment, spine and hip bone mineral density falls by approximately 5% in the first year (Answer B). Similar rapid decreases in bone mineral density are seen after initiation of aromatase inhibitors, androgen-deprivation therapy, and pharmacologic dosages of glucocorticoids.

If her bone mineral density drops by 5% in the next year, her T-score will decrease from −2.2 to around −2.5. There are differing opinions about using osteoporosis drugs for "prevention of osteoporosis," but in a case like this, one might consider offering a few years of alendronate or a dose or two of zoledronic acid—drugs that might have some lingering benefit after treatment is stopped. Other scenarios in which rapid bone loss would be expected and "prevention" should be considered include initiation of aromatase inhibitors, androgen-deprivation therapy, and pharmacologic dosages of glucocorticoids.

EDUCATIONAL OBJECTIVE

Anticipate the rapid bone loss that occurs when estrogen therapy is stopped.

REFERENCE(S)

Neele SJ, Evertz R, de Valk-de Roo GC, Netelenbos JC. Effect of 1 year of discontinuation of raloxifene or estrogen therapy on bone mineral density after 5 years of treatment in healthy postmenopausal women. *Bone.* 2002;30(4):599-603. PMID: 11934652

Gallagher JC, Rapuri PB, Haynatzki G, Detter JR. Effect of discontinuation of estrogen, calcitriol, and the combination of both on bone density and bone markers. *J Clin Endocrinol Metab.* 2002;87(11): 4914-4923. PMID: 12414850

Grey A, Bolland MJ, Horne A, et al. Five years of anti-resorptive activity after a single dose of zoledronate--results from a randomized double-blind placebo-controlled trial. *Bone.* 2012;50(6): 1389-1393. PMID: 22465268

28 ANSWER: C) Worsening arthritis in the hip

Zoledronic acid should improve the component of pain arising from the pagetic involvement of his left hip, but it is not expected to help the pain due to degenerative arthritis and may not prevent arthritis progression (thus, Answer C is correct and Answer D is incorrect). Paget disease does not extend across joint spaces and has never been reported to develop in new bones not involved at diagnosis (thus, Answer A is incorrect). Since he does not have Paget disease in his skull, it will not cause hearing loss (Answer B). Osteonecrosis of the femoral neck (Answer E) is not more likely after treatment with zoledronic acid or in patients with Paget disease of the hip.

Whether all patients with Paget disease should be treated is controversial. Indications for treatment in asymptomatic patients include the following:

- Involvement of a weight-bearing bone (eg, spine or leg)
- Involvement near a joint
- Involvement of the skull
- Serum alkaline phosphatase level greater than 3 times the upper normal limit

Zoledronic acid is clearly the most effective treatment. It normalizes bone turnover markers and maintains normal values for the longest duration of any medication. Normal turnover markers are associated with the normalization of pagetic woven bone to lamellar bone and can eliminate pain arising from pagetic bone. A single dose of zoledronic acid results in many years of disease inactivity in most patients.

EDUCATIONAL OBJECTIVE

Counsel patients that treating Paget disease should effectively eliminate pain attributable to the pagetic bone, but it is not expected to resolve pain due to degenerative arthritis.

REFERENCE(S)

Reid IR, Lyles K, Su G, et al. A single infusion of zoledronic acid produces sustained remissions in Paget disease: data to 6.5 years. *J Bone Miner Res.* 2011;26(9):2261-2270. PMID: 21638319

Langston AL, Campbell MK, Fraser WD, et al; PRISM Trial Group. Randomized trial of intensive bisphosphonate treatment versus symptomatic management in Paget's disease of bone. *J Bone Miner Res.* 2010;25(1):20-31. PMID: 19580457

Ralston SH. Clinical practice. Paget's disease of bone. *N Engl J Med.* 2013;368(7):644-650. PMID: 23406029

Diabetes Mellitus Section 1 Board Review

Serge A. Jabbour, MD

1 **ANSWER: C) Leptin measurement**
This patient has acquired generalized lipodystrophy. The lipodystrophy syndromes are a heterogeneous group of rare disorders that have in common selective deficiency of adipose tissue in the absence of nutritional deprivation or catabolic state.

Lipodystrophies are categorized based on etiology (genetic or acquired) and distribution of lost adipose tissue, affecting the entire body (generalized) or only regions (partial). This yields 4 major categories:

- Congenital generalized lipodystrophy
- Familial partial lipodystrophy
- Acquired generalized lipodystrophy
- Acquired partial lipodystrophy

Acquired generalized lipodystrophy, also known as Lawrence syndrome, is very rare. Generalized fat loss is not present at birth but develops later in life. It occurs over a variable period, ranging from a few weeks to years. Although the pathogenesis of acquired generalized lipodystrophy is unknown, it is hypothesized to be linked to autoimmune destruction of adipocytes. Some patients with acquired generalized lipodystrophy present initially with an autoimmune disease that includes dermatomyositis, Sjogren syndrome, rheumatoid arthritis, systemic sclerosis, and systemic lupus erythematosus. Fat loss occurs within few weeks to years after the onset of the autoimmune condition. Acquired generalized lipodystrophy may coexist with other autoimmune diseases, such as Hashimoto thyroiditis, hemolytic anemia, and chronic active hepatitis.

In patients with acquired generalized lipodystrophy, as a result of generalized fat loss, metabolic abnormalities associated with severe insulin resistance (eg, hypertriglyceridemia, diabetes mellitus, hepatic steatosis, acanthosis nigricans, menstrual irregularities, and polycystic ovary syndrome) may develop soon after the recognition of fat loss. Affected patients have suppressed leptin levels and adiponectin. Thus, leptin measurement (Answer C) is the best next step.

Currently, metreleptin (recombinant human methionyl leptin) is the only drug approved specifically for lipodystrophy. It is approved in the United States as an adjunct to diet for treatment of metabolic complications in patients with generalized lipodystrophy.

Patients with generalized lipodystrophy may need high insulin doses (>200 units daily). Because of the lack of subcutaneous fat, insulin might need to be administered by the intramuscular route. In patients with severe insulin resistance, U500 regular insulin can be used. GLP-1 receptor agonists may not work because of the lack of subcutaneous fat.

Glutamic acid decarboxylase antibodies (Answer A) would be assessed to evaluate for type 1 diabetes, which this patient cannot have as she has severe insulin resistance. *HNF1A* gene testing (Answer D) is done to diagnose maturity-onset diabetes of the young (MODY), which is not the diagnosis in this patient because such individuals typically do well on a secretagogue, although they can end up needing insulin (but at dosages similar to those used in type 1 diabetes). Pathogenic variants in the insulin receptor gene (Answer E) cause type A insulin resistance; affected patients do not have loss of subcutaneous fat as is observed in acquired generalized lipodystrophy.

EDUCATIONAL OBJECTIVE

Diagnose lipodystrophic syndromes.

REFERENCE(S)

Araújo-Vilar D, Santini F. Diagnosis and treatment of lipodystrophy: a step-by-step approach. *J Endocrinol Invest.* 2019;42(1):61-73. PMID: 29704234

Hussain I, Garg A. Lipodystrophy syndromes. *Endocrinol Metab Clin North Am.* 2016;45(4): 783-797. PMID: 27823605

Brown RJ, Araujo-Vilar D, Cheung PT, et al. The diagnosis and management of lipodystrophy syndromes: a multi-society practice guideline. *J Clin Endocrinol Metab.* 2016;101(12):4500-4511. PMID: 27710244

2 ANSWER: C) At least every 3 years

In asymptomatic adults, diabetes screening should be considered in patients who are overweight or obese who have 1 or more of the following risk factors: first-degree relative with diabetes, high-risk race/ethnicity, history of cardiovascular disease, hypertension, HDL-cholesterol level less than 35 mg/dL (<0.91 mmol/L), and/or triglyceride level greater than 250 mg/dL (>2.83 mmol/L), polycystic ovary syndrome (in women), and physical inactivity.

Patients with prediabetes should have annual testing, and women diagnosed with gestational diabetes should have lifelong testing at least every 3 years (Answer C).

According to the American Diabetes Association guidelines, screening for diabetes should begin at age 45 years regardless of other factors such as ethnicity, family history, BMI, blood pressure, and dyslipidemia.

EDUCATIONAL OBJECTIVE

Select the appropriate screening frequency for type 2 diabetes/prediabetes in a woman with a history of gestational diabetes mellitus.

REFERENCE(S)

American Diabetes Association. 2. Classification and diagnosis of diabetes: standards of medical care in diabetes-2020. *Diabetes Care.* 2020;42(Suppl 1): S14-S31. PMID: 31862745

US Preventive Services Task Force. Final Recommendation Statement. Abnormal Blood Glucose and Type 2 Diabetes Mellitus: Screening. April 2018. https://www.uspreventiveservices-taskforce.org/Page/Document/RecommendationStatementFinal/screening-for-abnormal-blood-glucose-and-type-2-diabetes

Pottie K, Jaramillo A, Lewin G, et al; Canadian Task Force on Preventive Health Care. Recommendations on screening for type 2 diabetes in adults [published correction appears in *CMAJ.* 2012;184(16):1815]. *CMAJ.* 2012;184(15): 1687-1696. PMID: 23073674

3 ANSWER: C) 140 units before breakfast and 100 units before dinner

In patients requiring more than 200 units of insulin daily, the volume of insulin given becomes a problem, both in terms of patient comfort and pharmacokinetics. Large-volume insulin injections are poorly absorbed. In these cases, U500 insulin should be considered. There is increasing evidence of more reliable delivery of insulin and successful outcomes with the use of U500 insulin in patients such as the one presented. Although the formulation of U500 is similar to that of regular insulin, the duration of action is up to 13 to 24 hours, permitting adequate delivery with 2 or 3 injections per day. Fortunately, U500 pens are now available and patients with severe insulin resistance are good candidates for U500 insulin.

Recommendations for the conversion from U100 to U500 generally incorporate the baseline U100 insulin doses, as well as the hemoglobin A_{1c} level, to determine appropriate doses of the concentrated insulin. One randomized titration-to-target trial provided a clear and specific recommendation on how to convert from U100 to U500:

- If hemoglobin A_{1c} is >8.0% (>64 mmol/mol) at the time of conversion, use 100% of the U100 insulin total dose
- If hemoglobin A_{1c} is ≤8.0% (≤64 mmol/mol) at the time of conversion, use 80% of the U100 insulin total dose

This patient is on a regimen of 300 units daily (total dose of U100 insulin) with a hemoglobin A_{1c} level of 7.6% (60 mmol/mol); therefore, his U500 dose should be 300 × 0.8 = 240 units daily.

Split of U500 can be done either as twice daily (60% 30 minutes before breakfast and 40% 30 minutes before dinner) or 3 times daily (40% 30 minutes before breakfast, 30% 30 minutes before lunch, and 30% 30 minutes before dinner). In this case, the split based on 240 units daily would be either 140/100 (Answer C) or 100/70/70. The other answers (Answers A, B, D, and E) are incorrect. In Answers A and D, the total daily dose is kept at 300 units, which could lead to more hypoglycemic events if the hemoglobin A_{1c} level is less than 8.0% (<64 mmol/mol). In Answers B and E, it is even worse, as the total daily dose of U500 is increased by 20%.

In the described trial, both twice-daily and thrice-daily regimens led to similar hemoglobin A_{1c} reductions. The only difference was the incidence and rate of documented symptomatic, nonsevere hypoglycemia (glucose ≤70 mg/dL [≤3.9 mmol/L]), which was lower in the thrice-daily group than in the twice-daily group.

EDUCATIONAL OBJECTIVE

Convert a patient's diabetes treatment regimen from U100 insulin to regular U500 insulin.

REFERENCE(S)

Bergen PM, Kruger DF, Taylor AD, Eid WE, Bhan A, Jackson JA. Translating U-500R randomized clinical trial evidence to the practice setting: a diabetes educator/expert prescriber team approach. *Diabetes Educ.* 2017;43(3):311-323. PMID: 28427304

Shaw KF, Valdez CA. Development and implementation of a U-500 regular insulin program in a federally qualified health center. *Clin Diabetes.* 2017;35(3):162-167. PMID: 28761218

Wysham C, Hood RC, Warren ML, Wang T, Morwick TM, Jackson JA. Effect of total daily dose on efficacy, dosing, and safety of 2 dose titration regimens of human regular U500 insulin in severely insulin-resistant patients with type 2 diabetes. *Endocr Pract.* 2016;22(6):653-665. PMID: 26789342

Hood RC, Arakaki RF, Wysham C, Li YG, Settles JA, Jackson JA. Two treatment approaches for human regular U-500 insulin in patients with type 2 diabetes not achieving adequate glycemic control on high-dose U-100 insulin therapy with or without oral agents: a randomized, titration-to-target clinical trial. *Endocr Pract.* 2015;21(7):782-793. PMID: 25813411

4 ANSWER: C) Intranasal glucagon, 3 mg

The American Diabetes Association workgroups recommend that a plasma glucose concentration of 70 mg/dL or less (≤3.9 mmol/L) should serve as an alert to the patient of the possibility of developing clinically important hypoglycemia and should prompt appropriate actions such as ingestion of carbohydrates or, at the very least, repeated measurements of glucose and temporary avoidance of critical tasks such as driving. In 2017, the International Hypoglycaemia Study Group (a joint working group of the American Diabetes Association and the European Association for the Study of Diabetes) proposed a glucose concentration less than 54 mg/dL (<3.0 mmol/L) as sufficiently low to indicate serious, clinically important biochemical hypoglycemia. Severe hypoglycemia was defined as an event requiring the assistance of another person to actively administer carbohydrate, glucagon, or other resuscitative actions.

Various options are available to treat severe hypoglycemia, such as in this patient who lost consciousness, including intravenous dextrose, glucagon (subcutaneous, intramuscular, or intranasal), or intraoral glucose gel. Patients with intravenous access (already in the hospital), can usually be treated quickly by administering

25 to 50 mL (12.5-25 g) of 50% dextrose intravenously. The amount of 100 mL (Answer B) is equivalent to 50 g of dextrose, which could lead to severe rebound hyperglycemia. Patients without intravenous access can be administered glucagon (subcutaneous, intramuscular, or nasal), which usually leads to recovery of consciousness within approximately 15 minutes, although it may be followed by marked nausea or even vomiting. Glucagon is given as 1 mg subcutaneously or intramuscularly (thus, Answer A is incorrect) or as 3 mg intranasally (Answer C). Most experts do no recommend oral gel (Answer D) in patients with severe hypoglycemia, given the lack of supporting evidence showing that buccal absorption of glucose occurs in humans, as well as concerns about aspiration. Administering glucose tablets (Answer E) is incorrect because the patient is unconscious.

EDUCATIONAL OBJECTIVE

Manage severe hypoglycemia in a patient with diabetes mellitus.

REFERENCE(S)

Rickels MR, Ruedy KJ, Foster NC, et al; T1D Exchange Intranasal Glucagon Investigators. Intranasal glucagon for treatment of insulin-induced hypoglycemia in adults with type 1 diabetes: a randomized crossover noninferiority study. *Diabetes Care.* 2016;39(2):264-270. PMID: 26681725

Umpierrez GE, Hellman R, Korytkowski MT, et al; Endocrine Society. Management of hyperglycemia in hospitalized patients in non-critical care setting: an Endocrine Society clinical practice guideline. *J Clin Endocrinol Metab.* 2012;97(1):16-38. PMID: 22223765

Thome J, Byon D. Addressing hypoglycemic emergencies. *US Pharm.* 2018;43(10):HS2-HS6.

5 ANSWER: C) Fasting glucose

A higher risk of insulin resistance and diabetes has been described in patients with HIV infection on antiretroviral therapy compared with risk in uninfected patients. Thus, patients with HIV infection should be screened for diabetes at baseline and after initiation of antiretroviral therapy.

According to the American Diabetes Association guidelines, patients with HIV should be screened for diabetes and prediabetes with a fasting glucose measurement (Answer C) before starting antiretroviral therapy, at the time of switching antiretroviral therapy, and 3 to 6 months after starting or switching antiretroviral therapy. If initial screening results are normal, measuring fasting glucose every year is advised.

In several studies, hemoglobin A_{1c} measurement (Answer B) has been found to underestimate glycemic levels in HIV-infected patients when compared with other diagnostic methods. Explanations for the lower-than-expected hemoglobin A_{1c} values in these patients have been hypothesized. For example, higher mean cell volume and hemolysis are more prevalent in HIV-infected patients. High mean cell volume, as a marker of a greater proportion of younger erythrocytes that have a shorter time to become glycated, suggests greater red blood cell turnover in HIV-infected patients.

Fructosamine (Answer A) and C-peptide (Answer E) are not used to diagnose diabetes. Glutamic acid decarboxylase 65 antibodies (Answer D) can distinguish type 1 from type 2 diabetes once diabetes has been diagnosed.

EDUCATIONAL OBJECTIVE

Appropriately screen for diabetes mellitus in HIV-infected patients.

REFERENCE(S)

American Diabetes Association. 4. Comprehensive medical evaluation and assessment of comorbidities: standards of medical care in diabetes-2020. *Diabetes Care.* 2020;43(Suppl 1):S37-S47. PMID: 31862747

Coelho AR, Moreira FA, Santos AC, et al. Diabetes mellitus in HIV-infected patients: fasting glucose, A1c, or oral glucose tolerance test – which method to choose for the diagnosis? *BMC Infect Dis.* 2018;18(309):1-13. PMID: 29980190

Kim PS, Woods C, Georgoff P, et al. A1C underestimates glycemia in HIV infection. *Diabetes Care.* 2009;32(9):1591-1593. PMID: 19502538

6 ANSWER: E) Serum vitamin B_{12}

This patient has recent onset of peripheral neuropathy and ataxia. She has been on high-dosage metformin for a long time, making vitamin B_{12} deficiency the most likely diagnosis. Metformin reduces intestinal absorption of vitamin B_{12} in up to 30% of patients and lowers serum vitamin B_{12} concentrations in 5% to 10% (Answer E). The dosage and duration of metformin use correlate with the risk of vitamin B_{12} deficiency. While the mechanism is not entirely clear, most evidence points to interference with food-derived B_{12} absorption, primarily in the ileum. The most common neurologic findings in vitamin B_{12} deficiency are symmetric paresthesias or numbness and gait problems. Neuropsychiatric symptoms can be present even in the absence of anemia or macrocytosis, and the lack of these hematologic changes cannot be used to exclude vitamin B_{12} deficiency as a cause of neuropsychiatric symptoms. The current American Diabetes Association standards of care recommend periodic measurement of vitamin B_{12} levels in metformin-treated patients, especially in those with anemia or peripheral neuropathy.

Cortisol measurement (Answer A) is incorrect because there is no evidence for adrenal insufficiency: the patient has no weight loss, hypotension, or electrolytes abnormalities. Taking proton-pump inhibitors can lead to magnesium deficiency (Answer B), which would present as hypocalcemia, hypokalemia, and neuromuscular hyperexcitability, none of which are present in this patient. Biotin can affect TSH levels (Answer C) in certain assays, mimicking hyperthyroidism, unlike in this patient who has a high TSH. In addition, abnormalities in TSH would not explain this patient's presentation with ataxia and peripheral neuropathy. There are no reports of adverse effects of dietary chromium (Answer D). Animal studies suggest that high dosages of chromium are nontoxic because of poor oral bioavailability.

EDUCATIONAL OBJECTIVE

Identify vitamin B_{12} deficiency as an adverse effect of metformin therapy.

REFERENCE(S)

American Diabetes Association. 9. Pharmacologic approaches to glycemic treatment: standards of medical care in diabetes-2020. *Diabetes Care.* 2020;43(Suppl 1):S98-S110. PMID: 31862752

Yang W, Cai X, Ji L, et al. Associations between metformin use and vitamin B_{12} levels, anemia, and neuropathy in patients with diabetes: a meta-analysis. *J Diabetes.* 2019;11(9):729-743. PMID: 30615306

Porter KM, Ward M, Hughes CF, et al. Hyperglycemia and metformin use are associated with B vitamin deficiency and cognitive dysfunction in older adults. *J Clin Endocrinol Metab.* 2019;104(10):4837-4847. PMID: 30920623

7 ANSWER: B) Canagliflozin, 100 mg daily

Canagliflozin (Answer B) is the only antidiabetes agent from the 5 options listed that has the indication to reduce the risk of end-stage kidney disease, doubling of serum creatinine, cardiovascular death, and hospitalization for heart failure in adults with type 2 diabetes and diabetic nephropathy with albuminuria (>300 mg/g). This indication was approved based on the CREDENCE trial results. In this double-blind, randomized controlled trial, patients with type 2 diabetes and albuminuric chronic kidney disease were assigned to receive canagliflozin, an oral SGLT-2 inhibitor, at a dosage of 100 mg daily, or placebo. All included patients had an estimated glomerular filtration rate of 30 to 90 mL/min per 1.73 m^2 of body-surface area and albuminuria (ratio of albumin [mg] to creatinine [g], >300 to 5000) and were treated with renin-angiotensin system blockade. The primary outcome was a composite of end-stage kidney disease (dialysis, transplant, or a sustained estimated glomerular filtration rate <15 mL/min per 1.73 m^2), a doubling of the serum creatinine level, or death of renal or cardiovascular causes. Prespecified secondary outcomes (such as cardiovascular death, hospitalization for heart failure, etc) were tested hierarchically. The trial was stopped early after a planned interim analysis on the recommendation of the data and safety monitoring committee. At that time, 4401 patients had undergone randomization, with a median follow-up of 2.62 years. The relative risk of the primary outcome was 30% lower in the canagliflozin group than in the placebo group, with event rates of 43.2 and 61.2 per 1000 patient-years, respectively (hazard ratio, 0.70; 95% CI, 0.59-0.82; $P = .00001$). The relative risk of the renal-specific composite of end-stage kidney disease, a doubling of the creatinine level, or death of renal causes was lower by 34% (hazard ratio, 0.66; 95% CI, 0.53-0.81; $P < .001$), and the relative risk of end-stage kidney disease was lower by 32% (hazard ratio, 0.68; 95% CI, 0.54-0.86; $P = .002$). The canagliflozin group also had a lower risk of cardiovascular death, myocardial infarction, or stroke (hazard ratio, 0.80; 95% CI, 0.67-0.95; $P = 0.01$) and hospitalization for heart failure (hazard ratio, 0.61; 95% CI, 0.47-0.80; $P < .001$). There were no significant differences in rates of amputation or fracture.

DPP-4 inhibitors (Answer A) and oral semaglutide (oral GLP-1 receptor agonist) (Answer D) have not been shown to have a significant benefit on hard renal outcomes, although a decrease in albuminuria can be seen. Pioglitazone (Answer C) cannot be used in this patient who has a low estimated glomerular filtration rate and edema in the lower extremities, as it could increase the risk of heart failure. In addition, pioglitazone has not been shown to have a significant benefit on hard renal outcomes. Pramlintide (Answer E) is an amylin analogue added to mealtime insulin; it lowers hepatic glucose output, enhances satiety, and delays gastric emptying. It has no effect on renal outcome.

EDUCATIONAL OBJECTIVE

Explain the kidney protective effect and new renal indication of canagliflozin even for an estimated glomerular filtration rate as low as 30 mL/min per 1.73 m².

REFERENCE(S)

Perkovic V, Jardine MJ, Neal B, et al; CREDENCE Trial Investigators. Canagliflozin and renal outcomes in type 2 diabetes and nephropathy. *N Engl J Med.* 2019;380(24):2295-2306. PMID: 30990260

Rosenstock J, Perkovic V, Johansen OE, et al; CARMELINA Investigators. Effect of linagliptin vs placebo on major cardiovascular events in adults with type 2 diabetes and high cardiovascular and renal risk. *JAMA.* 2019;321(1):69-79. PMID: 304184475

Kristensen SL, Rorth R, Jhund PS, et al. Cardiovascular, mortality, and kidney outcomes with GLP-1 receptor agonists in patients with type 2 diabetes: a systematic review and meta-analysis of cardiovascular outcome trials. *Lancet Diabetes Endocrinol.* 2019;7(10):776-785. PMID: 31422062

8 ANSWER: A) Glipizide

This patient has severe hypoglycemia due to intake of glipizide (sulfonylurea) (Answer A), which stimulates β cells to release insulin, C-peptide, and proinsulin.

A plasma insulin concentration of 3 μIU/mL or higher (≥20.8 pmol/L) by immunochemiluminometric assay when the plasma glucose concentration is below 55 mg/dL (<3.1 mmol/L) indicates insulin excess and is consistent with hyperinsulinemia (either from insulinoma, exogenous insulin, or sulfonylurea). Plasma C-peptide distinguishes endogenous from exogenous hyperinsulinemia (Answer D) at a cutoff of 0.6 ng/mL (0.20 nmol/L). In patients with insulinoma or sulfonylurea intake, the C-peptide concentration is at least 0.6 ng/mL or higher (≥0.20 nmol/L) as opposed to the setting of exogenous insulin intake where the C-peptide concentration is less than 0.6 ng/mL (<0.20 nmol/L). A plasma proinsulin concentration of 44.1 pg/mL or greater (≥5 pmol/L) is seen in the setting of insulinoma or sulfonylurea intake. Because of the antiketogenic effect of insulin, plasma β-hydroxybutyrate concentrations are lower in patients with an insulinoma than in patients without. All patients with hyperinsulinemia or IGF-mediated hypoglycemia have plasma β-hydroxybutyrate values of 28 mg/dL or less (≤2700 μmol/L). Obviously, a plasma sulfonylurea screen will reveal the sulfonylurea agent causing the hypoglycemia.

In adrenal insufficiency (Answer B) and hepatic failure (Answer E), plasma insulin is less than 3 μIU/mL (<20.8 pmol/L), plasma C-peptide is less than 0.6 ng/mL (<0.2 nmol/L), plasma proinsulin is less than 44.1 pg/mL (<5 pmol/L), and plasma β-hydroxybutyrate is greater than 28 mg/dL (>2700 μmol/L). In IGF-2–secreting tumors (Answer C), plasma insulin is less than 3 μIU/mL (<20.8 pmol/L), plasma C-peptide is less than 0.6 ng/mL (<0.2 nmol/L), plasma proinsulin is less than 44.1 pg/mL (<5 pmol/L), *but* plasma β-hydroxybutyrate is 28 mg/dL or less (≤2700 μmol/L).

EDUCATIONAL OBJECTIVE

Interpret laboratory test results associated with hypoglycemia.

REFERENCE(S)

Cryer PE, Axelrod L, Grossman AB, et al; Endocrine Society. Evaluation and management of adult hypoglycemic disorders: an Endocrine Society clinical practice guideline. *J Clin Endocrinol Metab.* 2009;94(3):709-728. PMID: 19088155

Iglesias P, Diez JJ. Management of endocrine disease: a clinical update on tumor-induced hypoglycemia. *Eur J Endocrinol.* 2014;170(4):R147-R157. PMID: 24459235

Service FJ, O'Brien PC. Increasing serum betahydroxybutyrate concentrations during the 72-hour fast: evidence against hyperinsulinemic hypoglycemia. *J Clin Endocrinol Metab.* 2005;90(8):4555-4558. PMID: 15886243

9 ANSWER: C) Weight loss and exercise to prevent type 2 diabetes

The diagnostic abnormalities documented by oral glucose tolerance testing in this patient are impaired fasting glucose and impaired glucose tolerance, both signifying prediabetes. Therefore, weight loss and exercise should be recommended to prevent type 2 diabetes (Answer C). He does not have diabetes (Answer B) because the fasting glucose level is less than 126 mg/dL (<7.0 mmol/L), and the 2-hour value from the oral glucose tolerance test is less than 200 mg/dL (<11.1 mmol/L). The 1-hour value is elevated, but this can occur in persons with prediabetes, and it is not a standard parameter for the diagnosis of diabetes. Diagnosis of diabetes on the basis of fasting glucose requires 2 separate abnormal values, but repeating this measurement (Answer D) in a patient such as this one who has a nondiagnostic level is not indicated.

Common forms of maturity-onset diabetes of the young (MODY) are associated with autosomal dominant inheritance, and the presented family history (with neither parent being affected) is not consistent with this diagnosis. In addition, MODY is rare. Thus, genetic screening (Answer E) is incorrect.

Although insulin resistance can be inferred from measurement of insulin (Answer A) during an oral glucose tolerance test, this is not likely to affect management in this patient.

The American Diabetes Association criteria for the diagnosis of diabetes are as follows:

1. Hemoglobin A_{1c} ≥6.5% (≥48 mmol/mol). The test should be performed in a laboratory using a method that is certified by the National Glycohemoglobin Standardization Program and standardized to the Diabetes Control and Complications Trial assay.*

OR

2. Fasting plasma glucose ≥126 mg/dL (≥7.0 mmol/L). Fasting is defined as no caloric intake for at least 8 hours.*

OR

3. Two-hour plasma glucose value ≥200 mg/dL (≥11.1 mmol/L) during an oral glucose tolerance test. The test should be performed as described by the World Health Organization, using a glucose load containing the equivalent of 75-g anhydrous glucose dissolved in water.*

OR

4. In a patient with classic symptoms of hyperglycemia or hyperglycemic crisis, a random plasma glucose value ≥200 mg/dL (≥11.1 mmol/L).

*In the absence of unequivocal hyperglycemia, criteria 1 to 3 should be confirmed by repeated testing.

EDUCATIONAL OBJECTIVE

Diagnose prediabetes on the basis of results from oral glucose tolerance testing.

REFERENCE(S)

American Diabetes Association. 2. Classification and diagnosis of diabetes: standards of medical care in diabetes-2020. *Diabetes Care.* 2020;43(Suppl 1): S14-S31. PMID: 31862745

Kumar R, Nandhini LP, Kamalanathan S, Sahoo J, Vivekanadan M. Evidence for current diagnostic criteria of diabetes mellitus. *World J Diabetes.* 2016;7(17):396-405. PMID: 27660696

Inzucchi SE. Clinical practice. Diagnosis of type 2 diabetes. *N Engl J Med.* 2012;367(6):542-550. PMID: 22873534

10 ANSWER: E) Eye examination

In a 2-year trial (SUSTAIN-6) involving patients with type 2 diabetes and high cardiovascular risk, more events of diabetic retinopathy complications occurred in patients treated with semaglutide (3.0%) compared with placebo (1.8%). The difference was seen very early in the trial (in the first 2 to 8 weeks). The absolute risk increase for diabetic retinopathy complications was larger among patients with a history of diabetic retinopathy at baseline (semaglutide, 8.2%; placebo, 5.2%) than among patients without a known history of diabetic retinopathy (semaglutide, 0.7%; placebo, 0.4%). Rapid improvement in glucose control has been associated with a temporary worsening of diabetic retinopathy. The applicability of such an association to semaglutide and retinopathy is unclear, and a direct effect of semaglutide cannot be ruled out. The effect of long-term glycemic control with semaglutide on diabetic retinopathy complications has not been studied. Patients with a history of diabetic retinopathy should be monitored for progression. Thus, this patient should have an eye examination (Answer E) at his follow-up visit.

GLP-1 receptor agonists have a boxed warning regarding the risk of C-cell tumors observed in rodents and a warning regarding acute pancreatitis. However, measuring calcitonin (Answer B) is not recommended unless there is a suspicion for medullary thyroid carcinoma (based on thyroid biopsy, family history, or presence of multiple endocrine neoplasia type 2). Similarly, it is not recommended to measure serum amylase and lipase (Answer A) unless the patient has gastrointestinal symptoms suggestive of acute pancreatitis.

GLP-1 receptor agonists have a warning regarding renal impairment/acute kidney injury, but this is in the setting of a patient with baseline kidney dysfunction and severe gastrointestinal symptoms (diarrhea, vomiting) leading to dehydration with subsequent worsening of the renal impairment. Thus, creatinine measurement (Answer D) is not necessary now.

GLP-1 receptor agonists have not been associated with foot injuries such as amputations (as opposed to certain SGLT-2 inhibitors). Thus, monofilament testing (Answer C) is not required now.

EDUCATIONAL OBJECTIVE

Monitor for progression of diabetic retinopathy in a patient with diabetes mellitus taking a GLP-1 receptor agonist.

REFERENCE(S)

Marso SP, Bain SC, Consoli A, et al; SUSTAIN-6 Investigators. Semaglutide and cardiovascular outcomes in patients with type 2 diabetes. *N Engl J Med.* 2016;375(19):1834-1844. PMID: 27633186

Semaglutide [package insert]. Plainsboro, NJ: Novo Nordisk; 2019.

Drab SR. Glucagon-like peptide-1 receptor agonists for type 2 diabetes: a clinical update of safety and efficacy. *Curr Diabetes Rev.* 2016;12(4):403-413. PMID: 26694823

11 ANSWER: D) A3243G pathogenic variant in mitochondrial DNA

Maternally inherited diabetes and deafness (MIDD) is a rare form of diabetes first described in 1992. It is a mitochondrial disorder that is characterized by progressive insulinopenia and sensorineural hearing loss, most commonly caused by a pathogenic variant at position 3243 (A to G substitution) in the tRNA (Answer D). Mitochondrial DNA is exclusively maternally inherited, so all offspring of an affected mother inherit the genetic defect. Because egg cells, but not sperm cells, contribute mitochondria to the developing embryo, only females pass mitochondrial conditions to their children.

Mitochondrial disorders can appear in every generation of a family and can affect both males and females.

There is wide variability in the phenotypic expression of MIDD (*see box*). Onset of the diabetes phenotype usually occurs between ages 15 and 70 years, with a mean age of 32.8 to 38.8 years. The mean duration of diabetes before insulin dependence is only 3.9 years. The mean age of onset of hearing impairment is 33.2 years. Hearing loss is progressive and nearly universal. Impaired renal function and proteinuria from mitochondrial dysfunction is a known phenotype of this genetic disorder. As such, these complications may be misinterpreted as a diabetic microvascular complication. The renal lesions observed in MIDD include focal segmental glomerulosclerosis with hyalinized glomeruli and myocyte necrosis in afferent arterioles and small arteries. Macular pattern dystrophy is a retinal lesion that is commonly seen in MIDD. This has the appearance of linear pigmentation on the retina surrounding the macula and the optic disc. Patients can also have cardiac conduction defects (such as Wolff-Parkinson-White syndrome), myopathy, and exercise intolerance that improves after coenzyme Q10 supplementation.

Zinc transporter 8 (ZnT8) antibodies (Answer A) and glutamic acid decarboxylase antibodies (GAD 65) (Answer C) are used to test for type 1 diabetes/latent autoimmune diabetes in adults. Although this patient could possibly have type 1 diabetes given her BMI and rapid insulin dependence, the constellation of other findings makes MIDD much more likely. Both *GCK* (glucokinase) pathogenic variants (Answer B) and *HNF1A* (hepatocyte nuclear factor 1α) pathogenic variants (Answer E) lead to maturity-onset diabetes of the young, which occurs at an age younger than 25 years and can often be controlled with diet or a secretagogue.

EDUCATIONAL OBJECTIVE

Diagnose maternally inherited diabetes and deafness associated with the A3243G mitochondrial pathogenic variant.

Box. Reported Clinical Manifestations of the A3243G Mitochondrial Pathogenic Variant

- Diabetes
- Sensorineural hearing loss
- Cardiac issues
  - Conduction abnormalities (Wolff-Parkinson-White syndrome, atrial fibrillation, sick sinus syndrome
  - Cardiomyopathy (dilated and hypertrophic)
- Neurologic disorders
  - Mitochondrial myopathy
  - Basal ganglia calcifications
  - Cerebellar ataxia
  - Oculomotor palsy
  - Weakness and exercise intolerance
- Neuropsychiatric disorders
  - Mental disability
  - Dementia
  - Depression
  - Psychosis
- Ophthalmic disorders
  - Macular pattern degeneration
  - Cataracts
- Renal disorders
  - Focal segmental glomerulosclerosis with hyalinized glomeruli
  - Myocyte necrosis in afferent arterioles and small arteries
- Complications of pregnancy
  - Placenta accrete
  - Preterm labor

REFERENCE(S)

Naing A, Kenchaiah M, Krishnan B, et al. Maternally inherited diabetes and deafness (MIDD): diagnosis and management. *J Diabetes Complications.* 2014;28(4):542-546. PMID: 24746802

Li HZ, Li RY, Li M. A review of maternally inherited diabetes and deafness. *Front Biosci (Landmark Ed).* 2014;19:777-782. PMID: 24389221

Murphy R, Turnbull DM, Walker M, Hattersley AT. Clinical features, diagnosis and management of maternally inherited diabetes and deafness (MIDD) associated with the 3243A>G mitochondrial point mutation. *Diabet Med.* 2008;25(4): 383-389. PMID: 18294221

12 ANSWER: E) Canagliflozin

In this case, the patient's blood glucose fingerstick values are consistent with her hemoglobin A_{1c} level of 6.8% (51 mmol/mol). However, her 1,5-anhydroglucitol level is less than 10 μg/mL (which indicates suboptimal glycemic control, mostly postprandially with blood glucose peaks above 180 mg/dL [>10.0 mmol/L] after meals). This discrepancy indicates that there is some interference with 1,5-anhydroglucitol measurement in this patient. Iron supplementation (Answer B), and sickle-cell trait/disease (Answer C) can affect hemoglobin A_{1c} measurement. However, we know this patient has an accurate hemoglobin A_{1c}, as it is consistent with the blood glucose fingerstick measurements, but not 1,5-anhydroglucitol. Neither biotin (Answer A) nor cinnamon (Answer D) interferes with any of these tests.

Measurement of serum 1,5-anhydroglucitol, a naturally occurring dietary polyol (a monosaccharide that is structurally similar to glucose), is another assessment to provide information on daily glycemic variations. When blood glucose levels are well controlled, most circulating 1,5-anhydroglucitol is reabsorbed in the kidneys instead of being excreted in the urine. In healthy individuals, circulating levels of 1,5-anhydroglucitol are high, with median values exceeding 20 μg/mL.

Renal reabsorption of 1,5-anhydroglucitol is competitively inhibited by glucose. Therefore, when blood glucose levels are high (>180 mg/dL [>10.0 mmol/L]), glucosuria occurs, blocking 1,5-anhydroglucitol reabsorption, and most is excreted in the urine. Individuals with type 2 diabetes and low circulating levels of 1,5-anhydroglucitol (<10 μg/mL) have more frequent and extreme hyperglycemic excursions over the previous 2-week period. An optimal 1,5-anhydroglucitol level in patients with diabetes is greater than 10 μg/mL.

SGLT-2 inhibitors decrease plasma glucose in patients with hyperglycemia by inhibiting renal glucose reabsorption via SGLT-2 (the primary renal transporter responsible for reabsorption of glucose from the urine), thereby increasing urinary glucose excretion, as well as 1,5-anhydroglucitol excretion. Thus, interference with the 1,5-anhydroglucitol assay by SGLT-2 inhibitors (Answer E) may lead to falsely low serum 1,5-anhydroglucitol measurements in patients with improved glycemic control who are treated with this class of agent.

EDUCATIONAL OBJECTIVE

Identify SGLT-2 inhibitors as a factor in falsely low serum 1,5-anhydroglucitol measurements in patients with improved glycemic control.

REFERENCE(S)

Wang Y, Zhang YL, Wang YP, Lei CH, Sun ZL. A study on the association of serum 1,5-anhydroglucitol levels and the hyperglycaemic excursions as measured by continuous glucose monitoring system among people with type 2 diabetes in China. *Diabetes Metab Res Rev.* 2012;28(4):357-362. PMID: 22238204

Dungan KM, Buse JB, Largay J, et al. 1,5-anhydroglucitol and postpriandal hyperglycemia as measured by continuous glucose monitoring system in moderately controlled patients with diabetes. *Diabetes Care.* 2006;29(6):1214-1219. PMID: 16731998

Balis DA, Tong C, Meininger G. Effect of canagliflozin, a sodium-glucose cotransporter 2 inhibitor, on measurement of serum 1,5-anhydroglucitol. *J Diabetes.* 2014;6(4):378-381. PMID: 24330128

13 ANSWER: D) Do overnight basal testing

This patient also has fasting hyperglycemia, which should raise the suspicion that he is experiencing hypoglycemia overnight that is going undetected and is followed by rebound hyperglycemia in the morning. Therefore, increasing the basal rate 1 or 2 hours before morning hyperglycemia is typically observed (Answer A) or increasing the basal rate overnight (Answer E) are not the correct recommendations. Changing the method of insulin delivery would not be expected to correct the fasting hyperglycemia, and including long-acting insulin, as you would find in a multiple daily injection regimen (Answer C), might increase the incidence of hypoglycemia. Eliminating the bedtime snack (Answer B) would only help if the patient were hyperglycemic throughout the night, which is unknown. To determine whether this is the case, it is necessary to check the overnight glucose level by fingerstick (Answer D).

EDUCATIONAL OBJECTIVE

Recommend continuous glucose monitoring to detect hypoglycemia and devise strategies for its reduction in patients with longstanding type 1 diabetes mellitus.

REFERENCE(S)

Vloemans AF, van Beers CAJ, de Wit M, et al. Keeping safe. Continuous glucose monitoring (CGM) in persons with type 1 diabetes and impaired awareness of hypoglycaemia: a qualitative study. *Diabet Med.* 2017;34(10):1470-1476. PMID: 28731509

Oyer DS. The science of hypoglycemia in patients with diabetes. *Curr Diabetes Rev.* 2013;9(3): 195-208. PMID: 23506375

Yeh H-C, Brown TT, Maruthur N, et al. Comparative effectiveness and safety of methods of insulin delivery and glucose monitoring for diabetes mellitus: a systematic review and meta-analysis. *Ann Intern Med.* 2012;157(5):336-347. PMID: 22777524

14 ANSWER: D) Fructosamine measurement

Hemoglobin A_{1c} measurement is the criterion standard test to assess the quality of glycemic control in patients with diabetes. Unfortunately, hemoglobin A_{1c} (Answer A) cannot be used as a metric of glycemic control in all patients. Of greatest importance is its unreliability in the setting of hemoglobinopathies, such as sickle-cell disease, or other causes of increased red blood cell turnover. Because glycation of hemoglobin A increases over the life of a red cell, conditions that shorten red blood cell lifespan cause an artificially reduced hemoglobin A_{1c} level, whether measurement is point of care or done in the laboratory. In this setting, other markers of long-term glucose control should be considered. Fructosamine (Answer D), a measure of glycosylated plasma proteins, is proportional to the mean blood glucose over the previous 2 weeks and may be used in place of hemoglobin A1c in this patient because it is not dependent on red blood cell turnover.

Measuring postprandial glucose levels (Answer B) is not likely to add much in this case, as they are generally proportional to fasting values. Urinary glucose testing (Answer C) is imprecise and only estimates recent levels of circulating glucose concentrations. C-peptide (Answer E) only gives a rough estimate of β-cell function and not glycemic control.

EDUCATIONAL OBJECTIVE

Explain the relationship between hemoglobinopathy and hemoglobin A_{1c}.

REFERENCE(S)

National Glycohemoglobin Standardization Program (NGSP) Web site. Factors that interfere with HbA1c test results. www.ngsp.org/factors.asp. Accessed for verification March 2020.

Lorenzo-Medina M, De-La-Iglesia S, Ropero P, Nogueria-Salgueriro P, Santana-Benitez J. Effects of hemoglobin variants on hemoglobin A1c values measured using a high-performance liquid chromatography method. *J Diabetes Sci Technol.* 2014;8(6):1168-1176. PMID: 25355712

Sacks DB, Arnold M, Bakris GL, et al; National Academy of Clinical Biochemistry; Evidence-Based Laboratory Medicine Committee of the American Association for Clinical Chemistry. Guidelines and recommendations for laboratory analysis in the diagnosis and management of diabetes mellitus. *Diabetes Care.* 2011;34(6):e61-e99. PMID: 21617108

15 ANSWER: B) Insulin drip titrated to maintain blood glucose between 140 and 180 mg/dL (7.8-10.0 mmol/L)

This critically ill patient has severe hyperglycemia. The 2009 consensus statement from the American Association of Clinical Endocrinologists and the 2015 American Diabetes Association guidelines advise that hyperglycemic patients in the intensive care unit should receive intravenous insulin to control their glucose and that the glucose levels should be maintained between 140 and 180 mg/dL (7.8-10.0 mmol/L) (Answer B). This was based on the NICE-SUGAR study (Normoglycemia in Intensive Care Evaluation and Surviving Using Glucose Algorithm Regulation), which demonstrated no benefit from more stringent blood glucose control to less than 110 mg/dL (<6.1 mmol/L).

Insulin by intermittent subcutaneous injection (Answers A and D) has little role in the intensive care unit, since blood glucose control can be achieved more quickly and more reliably with intravenous administration. Achieving a lower target of 80 to 110 mg/dL (4.4 to 6.1 mmol/L) with intravenous insulin (Answer C) is now thought to yield no additional benefit, but, instead, it markedly increases the risk of severe hypoglycemia (more than 6-fold). A basal and prandial insulin regimen, such as insulin glargine and insulin aspart, is appropriate upon transfer out of the intensive care unit, but, as with regular insulin, it is not rapid enough in its action and is not as easily adaptable as an intravenous infusion.

EDUCATIONAL OBJECTIVE

Manage blood glucose in acutely ill hospitalized patients.

REFERENCE(S)

Moghissi ES, Korytkowski MT, DiNardo M, et al; American Association of Clinical Endocrinologists; American Diabetes Association. American Association of Clinical Endocrinologists and American Diabetes Association consensus statement on inpatient glycemic control. *Diabetes Care.* 2009;32(6):1119-1131. PMID: 19429873

American Diabetes Association. 14. Diabetes care in the hospital: standards of medical care in diabetes-2018. *Diabetes Care.* 2015;41(Suppl 1): S144-S151. PMID: 29222385

16 ANSWER: C) Tissue transglutaminase IgA antibodies

About 5% of persons with type 1 diabetes develop celiac disease. Only a minority of children and adolescents with type 1 diabetes and celiac disease present with gastrointestinal symptoms. More common initial findings include unpredictable blood glucose measurements and recurrent episodes of hypoglycemia because of erratic intestinal absorption of nutrients. Thus, elevated tissue transglutaminase IgA antibodies (Answer C) would most likely explain her hypoglycemia.

Less than 1% of children with type 1 diabetes have autoimmune adrenalitis (Addison disease) (Answer A). In one report, about 2% of children with type 1 disease had circulating antibodies to steroid 21-hydroxylase (Answer D). Although less common than celiac disease, this condition is associated with decreased insulin requirement and increased frequency of hypoglycemia, hyperpigmentation, hypotension, hyponatremia, and hyperkalemia (none of which is present in this patient). Hyperthyroidism (Answer B) is rare in patients with type 1 diabetes (1%-2%) and can lead to higher blood glucose values due to insulin resistance, not hypoglycemia. In addition, except for weight loss, this patient has no symptoms or physical findings to suggest Graves disease. Antibodies to glutamic acid decarboxylase (a 65-kD protein) (Answer E) are found in about 70% of patients with type 1 diabetes at the time of diagnosis. They could very well be high in this patient, but this would not explain her hypoglycemia.

EDUCATIONAL OBJECTIVE

Recognize hypoglycemia resulting from celiac disease in type 1 diabetes mellitus and describe its presentation.

REFERENCE(S)

Khoury N, Semenkovich K, Arbeláez AM. Coeliac disease presenting as severe hypoglycaemia in youth with type 1 diabetes. *Diabet Med.* 2014;31(12):e33-e36. PMID: 24805141

Abid N, McGlone O, Cardwell C, McCallion W, Carson D. Clinical and metabolic effects of gluten free diet in children with type 1 diabetes and coeliac disease. *Pediatr Diabetes.* 2011;12(4 Pt 1): 322-325. PMID: 21615651

Warncke K, Fröhlich-Reiterer EE, Thon A, Hofer SE, Wiemann D, Holl RW; DPV Initiative of the German Working Group for Pediatric Diabetology; German BMBF Competence Network for Diabetes Mellitus. Polyendocrinopathy in children, adolescents, and young adults with type 1 diabetes: a multicenter analysis of 28,671 patients from the German/Austrian DPV-Wiss database. *Diabetes Care.* 2010;33(9):2010-2012. PMID: 20551013

17 ANSWER: B) Allow 15 minutes between the bolus and the meal

The most important variable that affects the risk of neonatal macrosomia is the postprandial glucose level. Women with diabetes who are pregnant or are planning pregnancy should try to normalize blood glucose levels to minimize congenital anomalies and other complications. The American Diabetes Association recommends that the hemoglobin A_{1c} level be less than 6.0% to 6.5% (<42-48 mmol/mol) during early pregnancy, with a lower target (<6.0% [<42 mmol/mol]) by the second and third trimesters. The American Diabetes Association also recommends maintaining fasting and preprandial glucose levels less than 95 mg/dL (<5.3 mmol/L) with either a peak (1-hour) postprandial level less than 140 mg/dL (<7.8 mmol/L) or a 2-hour postprandial level less than 120 mg/dL (<6.7 mmol/L). Although most of the patient's preprandial glucose levels are on target, there is clearly a pattern of elevated postprandial values, which return to target at the completion of the rapid-acting insulin analogue's biologic activity (before the next check). It takes 10 to 15 minutes for a rapid-acting insulin analogue to enter the circulation from a subcutaneous depot, so allowing more time between the administration of aspart and the meal (Answer B) should correct the postprandial hyperglycemia.

Changing the sensitivity factor (Answer D) would only improve postprandial levels when preprandial levels are above target, which her log does not demonstrate. Changing the insulin-to-carbohydrate ratio to 1:15 (Answer C) would give her *less* insulin before meals, not *more,* and would therefore worsen the postprandial hyperglycemia. Increasing the detemir dosage (Answer A) would not be expected to affect postprandial glucose values specifically. Continuing the same regimen (Answer E) is not correct, as changes to her regimen are needed because there is clearly a pattern of elevated postprandial values.

EDUCATIONAL OBJECTIVE

Develop a strategy, based on knowledge of insulin action, to improve postprandial glycemic control during pregnancy.

REFERENCE(S)

American Diabetes Association. 14. Management of diabetes in pregnancy: standards of medical care in diabetes-2020. *Diabetes Care.* 2020;43(Suppl 1): S183-S192. PMID: 31862757

McCance DR. Pregnancy and diabetes. *Best Pract Res Clin Endocrinol Metab.* 2011;25(6):945-958. PMID: 22115168

Kitzmiller JL, Block JM, Brown FM, et al. Managing preexisting diabetes for pregnancy: summary of evidence and consensus recommendations for care. *Diabetes Care.* 2008;31(5):1060-1079. PMID: 18445730

18 ANSWER: C) 6.0%

The risk of type 1 diabetes in children appears to be on the rise and can be affected by a number of factors, including geography, age, sex, family history, and environment. The risk of developing type 1 diabetes increases from 0.4% in individuals with no family history of the disease to 4% to 8% in offspring of an affected parent (thus, Answer C is correct). Having an affected father confers a higher risk than having an affected mother. The risk rises to as high as 30% when both parents have type 1 diabetes.

EDUCATIONAL OBJECTIVE

Counsel patients about the magnitude of risk of type 1 diabetes mellitus developing in the offspring of an affected parent.

REFERENCE(S)

Krischer JP, Liu X, Lernmark A, et al; TEDDY Study Group. The influence of type 1 diabetes genetic susceptibility regions, age, sex, and family history on the progression from multiple autoantibodies to type 1 diabetes: a TEDDY study report. *Diabetes.* 2017;66(12):3122-2129. PMID: 28903990

van Esch SC, Cornel MC, Snoek FJ. "I am pregnant and my husband has diabetes. Is there a risk for my child?" A qualitative study of questions asked by email about the role of genetic susceptibility to diabetes. *BMC Public Health.* 2010;10:688. PMID: 21067573

Mehers KL, Gillespie KM. The genetic basis for type 1 diabetes. *Br Med Bull.* 2008;88(1):115-129. PMID: 19088009

Aly TA, Ide A, Jahromi MM, et al. Extreme genetic risk for type 1A diabetes. *Proc Natl Acad Sci U S A.* 2006;103(38):14074-14079. PMID: 16966600

19 ANSWER: B) Basal rate = 0.6 units/h; carbohydrate ratio = 1 units/15 g; sensitivity factor = 1 unit/55 mg/dL

Understanding how to convert a regimen of multiple daily injections to continuous subcutaneous insulin infusion is very important. Many articles explain the conversion, all summarized nicely in the 2014 American Association of Clinical Endocrinologists/ American College of Endocrinology Consensus Statement. References may vary slightly regarding the conversion numbers. For example, the pump total daily dose (TDD) can be 0.75 to 1 × prepump TDD depending on the patient's glycemic control. The carbohydrate ratio is 450 to 500 divided by the TDD, and the insulin sensitivity factor is 1700 to 1800 divided by the TDD. Thus, the optimal parameters are listed in Answer B.

EDUCATIONAL OBJECTIVE

Convert a regimen of multiple daily insulin injections to insulin pump therapy in a patient with type 1 diabetes mellitus.

REFERENCE(S)

Grunberger C, Abelseth JM, Bailey TS, et al. Consensus statement by the American Association of Clinical Endocrinologists/American College of Endocrinology Insulin Pump Management Task Force. *Endocr Pract.* 2014;20(5):463-489. PMID: 24816754

Bode BW, Kyllo J, Kaufman ER. *Pumping Protocol: A Guide to Insulin Pump Initiation.* Medical Education Academia. Northridge, CA: Medtronic, 2013.

20 ANSWER: D) Perform basal rate testing from breakfast until dinner

Changes to insulin pump settings should be based on identified patterns, such as the very frequent hypoglycemia that this patient is experiencing several days a week in the midafternoon. Either an excessive basal rate or a prelunch bolus may be the cause. To diagnose which component is responsible, one should perform basal rate testing (Answer D). In this case, with the hypoglycemia occurring midafternoon, the patient should fast and take no insulin bolus for at least 5 hours before the time in question. Fingerstick glucose values should be checked approximately hourly; if the value does not change by more than 30 mg/dL (1.7 mmol/L) over this period, then one can conclude that the basal rate is appropriate and that the bolus before the previous meal is causing the hypoglycemia. If the value drops by more than 30 mg/dL (1.7 mmol/L), the basal rate should be lowered at least 2 hours before the time that the hypoglycemia is occurring.

Increasing his carbohydrate intake at lunch (Answer A) or eating a carbohydrate snack at 2 or 3 PM (Answer B) may help some, but these options are not the best choices because they require the patient to ingest extra carbohydrate to counteract excessive insulin and they do nothing to help uncover or correct the cause of the hypoglycemia. Changing the prelunch carbohydrate ratio to 1:6 (Answer C) is incorrect because it would mean the patient would be getting *more*, not *less*, insulin before lunch, and this would most likely make the problem worse and/or cause the hypoglycemia to occur earlier. Lowering the basal rate to 1.2 units/h from noon to 6 PM (Answer E) is incorrect, as one does not know whether the hypoglycemia is due to a high basal rate without first doing a basal rate test.

EDUCATIONAL OBJECTIVE

Devise a strategy to identify and correct a common problem encountered with the use of continuous subcutaneous insulin infusion.

REFERENCE(S)

Bolderman KM. *Putting Your Patients on the Pump: Initiation and Maintenance Guidelines.* Alexandria, VA: American Diabetes Association; 2013.

Walsh J, Roberts R. *Pumping Insulin: Everything You Need for Success on a Smart Insulin Pump.* 5th ed. San Diego, CA: Torrey Pines Press; 2012.

Hirsch IB. Practical pearls in insulin pump therapy. *Diabetes Technol Ther.* 2010;12(Suppl 1): S23-S27. PMID: 20515302

21 ANSWER: D) Liraglutide

Of the agents listed as answer options, only liraglutide (Answer D) has been shown to significantly lower the 3-point major adverse cardiovascular events (MACE) in the LEADER trial. MACE includes the first occurrence of death of cardiovascular causes, nonfatal myocardial infarction, or nonfatal stroke. The other drugs (oral semaglutide [Answer A], once-weekly exenatide [Answer B], sitagliptin [Answer C], alogliptin [Answer E]) were neutral regarding MACE in their respective trials (PIONEER, EXSCEL, TECOS, EXAMINE).

In the LEADER trial, the primary outcome (3-point MACE) occurred in significantly fewer patients in the liraglutide group (608 of 4668 patients [13.0%]) than in the placebo group (694 of 4672 patients [14.9%]) (hazard ratio, 0.87; 95% CI, 0.78-0.97; $P < .001$ for noninferiority; $P = .01$ for superiority). Because of the LEADER trial results, an additional indication was added to liraglutide prescribing information, which reads as follows:

Liraglutide is a GLP-1 receptor agonist indicated:

- As an adjunct to diet and exercise to improve glycemic control in adults with type 2 diabetes.
- To reduce the risk of major adverse cardiovascular events in adults with type 2 diabetes and established cardiovascular disease.

EDUCATIONAL OBJECTIVE

In patients with type 2 diabetes mellitus and established cardiovascular disease, recommend an agent to decrease hemoglobin A_{1c} and reduce the risk of major adverse cardiovascular events.

REFERENCE(S)

Marso SP, Daniels GH, Brown-Frandsen K, et al; LEADER Trial Investigators. Liraglutide and cardiovascular outcomes in type 2 diabetes. *N Engl J Med.* 2016;375(4):311-322. PMID: 27295427

Liraglutide [package insert]. Plainsboro, NJ: Novo Nordisk; 2017.

Semaglutide [package insert]. Plainsboro, NJ: Novo Nordisk; 2017.

Cefalu WT, Kaul S, Gerstein HC, et al. Cardiovascular outcomes trials in type 2 diabetes: where do we go from here? Reflections from a Diabetes Care Editors' Expert Forum. *Diabetes Care.* 2018;41(1): 14-31. PMID: 29263194

22 ANSWER: D) Lower the renal threshold for glucose excretion from 220 mg/dL to less than 100 mg/dL

SGLTs cotransport sodium and glucose into cells using the sodium gradient produced by sodium-potassium ATPase pumps at the basolateral cell membranes. SGLT-2 is expressed in segments S1 and S2 of the proximal convoluted tubules and is responsible for renal reabsorption of glucose. Renal tubular reabsorption is known to undergo adaptations in the setting of uncontrolled diabetes. Particularly relevant in this context is the up-regulation of renal SGLT-2, which is an important adaptation in diabetes to maintain renal tubular glucose reabsorption. SGLT-2 is not present in the S3 segment (thus, Answer A is incorrect) or in the distal tubule (thus, Answer C is incorrect).

SGLT-2 inhibitors reduce filtered glucose reabsorption by epithelial cells of the kidney proximal tubule. The renal threshold for glucose reabsorption in patients with type 2 diabetes was reported to be between 200 and 250 mg/dL, which is higher than that of persons without type 2 diabetes (170-200 mg/dL). SGLT-2 inhibitors, by blocking SGLT-2, lower the threshold from around 220 to 240 mg/dL to less than 100 mg/dL (thus, Answer D is correct and Answer B is incorrect).

EDUCATIONAL OBJECTIVE

Explain the mechanism of action of SGLT-2 inhibitors at the kidney level.

REFERENCE(S)

Nair S, Wilding JP. Sodium glucose cotransporter 2 inhibitors as a new treatment for diabetes mellitus. *J Clin Endocrinol Metab.* 2010;95(1):34-42. PMID: 19892839

Osaki A, Okada S, Saito T, et al. Renal threshold for glucose reabsorption predicts diabetes improvement by sodium glucose cotransporter 2 inhibitor therapy. *J Diabetes Investig.* 2016;7(5):751-754. PMID: 27181936

23 ANSWER: C) Oral glucose tolerance test

Cystic fibrosis–related diabetes (CFRD) is the result of a primary defect of insulin secretion due in part to nonautoimmune destruction of β cells (mainly) and also α cells in the pancreas, so both insulin and glucagon secretion are defective. However, histologic studies have reported variability in the degree of islet-cell destruction. This indicates there are other factors contributing to the insulin deficiency in CFRD, perhaps "collateral damage" from fibrosis and fatty infiltration or islet amyloid. The presence of CFRD strongly correlates with poorer clinical status, reflected by reduced pulmonary function and nutritional status, increased frequency of acute pulmonary exacerbations, and significant sputum pathogens. Annual screening for CFRD in all patients with cystic fibrosis is recommended beginning by 10 years of age, consistent with guidelines from the American Diabetes Association, Cystic Fibrosis Foundation, Pediatric Endocrine Society, and International Society for Pediatric and Adolescent Diabetes (ISPAD). The best test for screening and diagnosis of CFRD is the oral glucose tolerance test (Answer C).

Hemoglobin A_{1c} (Answer A) and fasting plasma glucose measurement (Answer B) should not be used for screening because they have low sensitivity for detecting CFRD. This has been confirmed in several studies. In these patients, hemoglobin A_{1c} is often normal, regardless of the degree of hyperglycemia. In 1 study, only 16% of patients with cystic fibrosis had elevated hemoglobin A_{1c} values at the time of CFRD diagnosis. Also, waiting for symptoms to prompt screening for CFRD (Answer D) is not a good strategy. In a population of pediatric patients with cystic fibrosis in Toronto, only 2.7% were clinically recognized as having CFRD, but with oral glucose tolerance testing of asymptomatic adolescents (aged 10 to 18 years), 17% were found to have impaired glucose tolerance and 13% had CFRD without fasting hyperglycemia. The recommended treatment for CFRD is insulin, albeit this is based on few clinical trials. Fructosamine (Answer E) is not used for diabetes screening.

EDUCATIONAL OBJECTIVE

Recommend the best screening method for cystic fibrosis–related diabetes mellitus.

REFERENCE(S)

Moran A, Pillay K, Becker DJ, Acerini CL; International Society for Pediatric and Adolescent Diabetes. ISPAD Clinical Practice Consensus Guidelines 2014. Management of cystic fibrosis-related diabetes in children and adolescents. *Pediatr Diabetes.* 2014;15(Suppl 20):65-76. PMID: 25182308

O'Shea D, O'Connell J. Cystic fibrosis related diabetes. *Curr Diab Rep.* 2014;14(8):511. PMID: 24915888

Kelly A, Moran A. Update on cystic fibrosis-related diabetes [published correction appears in *J Cyst Fibros.* 2014;13(1):119]. *J Cyst Fibros.* 2013;12(4): 318-331. PMID: 23562217

24 ANSWER: B) Rosuvastatin, 20 mg daily

Current recommendations for statin treatment have been revised such that treatment initiation and the initial statin dosage are personalized on the basis of risk profile, rather than LDL-cholesterol levels. In patients with type 2 diabetes who are 40 years or older, moderate-intensity statin treatment, if clinically indicated, is recommended in addition to lifestyle counseling and behavioral modification. However, for patients with a high risk for cardiovascular disease such as this patient with a history of cardiovascular disease, high-intensity statin therapy is advised. Clinical trials have shown that individuals at high risk for cardiovascular disease have a significant reduction in further cardiovascular events with an aggressive regimen of high-intensity statin therapy. Currently, limited clinical trial evidence is available for statin therapy for persons older than 75 years or younger than 40 years. The only high-intensity statin therapy listed in the answer options is rosuvastatin, 20 mg daily (Answer B). Answers A, C, D and E are all moderate-intensity statin therapy options.

EDUCATIONAL OBJECTIVE

Recommend appropriate statin intensity dosing in patients with type 2 diabetes mellitus.

REFERENCE(S)

Stone NJ, Robinson JG, Lichtenstein AH, Bairey Merz CN, Blum CB, et al. 2013 ACC/AHA guideline on the treatment of blood cholesterol to reduce atherosclerotic cardiovascular risk in adults: a report of the American College of Cardiology/ American Heart Association Task Force on Practice Guidelines [published correction appears in *J Am Coll Cardiol.* 2014;63(25 Pt B):3024-3025]. *J Am Coll Cardiol.* 2014;63(25 Pt B):2889-2934. PMID: 24239923

American Diabetes Association. 9. Cardiovascular disease and risk management. Standards of medical care in diabetes-2018. *Diabetes Care.* 2018; 41(Suppl 1): S86-S104. PMID: 29222380

25 ANSWER: C) Gastric emptying study

In insulin-treated patients with diabetes, gastroparesis (delayed gastric emptying) may lead to unexplained hypoglycemia, particularly early in the postprandial period. Gastroparesis often occurs in patients with longstanding diabetes and concomitant microvascular complications. Most patients with gastroparesis present with upper gastrointestinal symptoms, although the correlation of symptoms with delayed gastric emptying is weak, and some patients are asymptomatic. The rate of gastric emptying regulates the delivery of carbohydrates to the small intestine, and it has a major impact on postprandial blood glucose. Variations in the rate of gastric emptying account for 35% of the variance in the initial rise of blood glucose after a 75-g glucose load in healthy persons and those with diabetes. Nuclear medicine scintigraphy, or gastric emptying study (Answer C), remains the criterion standard for assessing gastric emptying, although inconsistency in its use may affect its diagnostic accuracy.

Although adrenal insufficiency can be a cause of unexplained hypoglycemia in a patient with type 1 diabetes, it is a less likely diagnosis in a patient with normal blood pressure and electrolytes and without symptoms of orthostasis. Thus, a cosyntropin-stimulation test (Answer B) is incorrect. This patient is frustrated and stressed about her situation, and although psychiatric counseling (Answer A) may be helpful in dealing with any chronic condition, it is unlikely to uncover the cause of her hypoglycemia. Similarly, because she has had ongoing and recent nutrition counseling, suboptimal carbohydrate counting skills (Answer D) are unlikely to be the reason for her frequent unexplained hypoglycemia. Abdominal CT (Answer E) is incorrect, as CT will not diagnose gastroparesis. Other CT findings are irrelevant in this case.

EDUCATIONAL OBJECTIVE

Diagnose the etiology of unexplained recurrent hypoglycemia and glycemic variability.

REFERENCE(S)

Phillips LK, Deane AM, Jones KL, Rayner CK, Horowitz M. Gastric emptying and glycaemia in health and diabetes mellitus. *Nat Rev Endocrinol.* 2015;11(2):112-128. PMID: 25421372

Chang J, Rayner CK, Jones KL, Horowitz M. Diabetic gastroparesis and its impact on glycemia. *Endocrinol Metab Clin North Am.* 2010;39(4): 745-762. PMID: 21095542

Samsom M, Bharucha A, Gerich JE, Hermann K, Limmer J, Linke R, et al. Diabetes mellitus and gastric emptying: questions and issues in clinical practice. *Diabetes Metab Res Rev.* 2009;25(6): 502-514. PMID: 19610128

Ma J, Rayner CK, Jones KL, Horowitz M. Diabetic gastroparesis: diagnosis and management. *Drugs.* 2009;69(8):971-986. PMID: 19496627

26 ANSWER: B) Macular edema

Macular edema (Answer B) is a common manifestation of retinal microvascular disease. The typical symptoms are consistent with those of this patient, with gradual onset of blurred vision occurring over months. It can be bilateral. She has known retinopathy, and it is not unusual for this to progress, even with stable findings on eye examinations in the past. Macular edema can be difficult to detect on office retinal exams, but it can be detected and staged by ophthalmologists using pupillary dilation, fluorescein angiography, and optical coherence tomography. In this regard, it is unfortunate that the patient is late on her annual ophthalmologic exam.

Once confirmed, macular edema is treated with intravitreous antivascular endothelial growth factor. Focal laser photocoagulation could be considered as initial therapy in patients with clinically significant macular edema who have trouble adhering to treatment recommendations and may not return for follow-up appointments. The diagnosis of macular edema associated with diabetic retinopathy is also impetus for better glucose control. Control of blood pressure and treatment of dyslipidemia (lowering triglyceride levels with fenofibrates may have a beneficial effect) can also prevent the progression of diabetic retinopathy.

Retinal detachment (Answer A) and vitreous hemorrhage (Answer C) usually present more acutely, rarely affect both eyes, and cause focal visual deficits rather than diffuse blurred vision. Mononeuritis (Answer E) can affect the cranial nerves, but it typically causes palsy or abnormal pupillary responses when associated with blurred vision; this condition, too, does not usually affect both eyes. Cataracts (Answer D) are common and cause blurred vision that develops gradually, not at the rapid pace described here.

EDUCATIONAL OBJECTIVE

Assess vision symptoms in patients with diabetes mellitus.

REFERENCE(S)

VanderBeek BL, Shah N, Parikh PC, Ma L. Trends in the care of diabetic macular edema: analysis of a national cohort. *PLoS One.* 2016;11(2):e0149450. PMID: 26909797

Mitchell P, Wong TY; Diabetic Macular Edema Treatment Guideline Working Group. Management paradigms for diabetic macular edema. *Am J Ophthalmol.* 2014;157(3):505-513. PMID: 24269950

Schmidt-Erfurth U, Lang GE, Holz FG, et al; RESTORE Extension Study Group. Three-year outcomes of individualized ranibizumab treatment in patients with diabetic macular edema: the RESTORE extension study. *Ophthalmology.* 2014;121(5):1045-1053. PMID: 24491642

27 ANSWER: C) Pancreas transplant with or without a kidney transplant

Necrobiosis lipoidica is rare condition that occurs in 0.3% to 1.2% of patients with diabetes. It is an inflammatory granulomatous skin disorder in which microangiopathy appears to have a role in pathogenesis. Among patients with necrobiosis lipoidica, 11% to 65% have diabetes. The lesions are classically seen overlying the anterior shin, characterized by a shallow depression into the dermis that is erythematous, often with a slightly yellow hue (due to lipid deposition) and with telangiectasias. Lesion size varies considerably, ranging between 1 and several centimeters in diameter, and lesions can grow over time and are frequently bilateral. They may be subject to ulceration.

Evidence for any specific treatment is limited to case reports and small clinical trials. Pancreas transplant with or without a kidney transplant (Answer C) can resolve (not always) necrobiosis lipoidica. Kidney transplant alone (Answer A) does not. Antiplatelet therapy with dipyridamole (Answer B) alone does not resolve the lesions. Glucocorticoids may be used to treat necrobiosis lipoidica. Systemic glucocorticoids may lead to complete closure of ulcerations except for atrophic ones. However, the impact on glycemia must be considered in taking this approach. Intralesional steroids (Answer D) (injected into the borders of established lesion) and topical glucocorticoids

(Answer E), particularly for early lesions, may also be beneficial but do not lead to cure.

EDUCATIONAL OBJECTIVE

Identify dermopathies common to diabetes mellitus.

REFERENCE(S)

Feily A, Mehraban S. Treatment modalities of necrobiosis lipoidica: a concise systematic review. *Dermatol Reports.* 2015;7(2):5749. PMID: 26236446

Souza AD, El-Azhary RA, Gibson LE. Does pancreas transplant in diabetic patients affect the evolution of necrobiosis lipoidica? *Int J Dermatol.* 2009;48(9): 964-970. PMID: 19702981

Mazur MJ, Lowney AC, Prigoff J, et al. Resolution of long-standing necrobiosis lipoidica diabeticorum (NLD) lesion after restoration of euglycemia following successful pancreas after kidney (PAK) transplantation: a case report. *Transplant Proc.* 2011;43(9):3296-3298. PMID: 22099781

28 ANSWER: A) Neuropathic arthropathy

This patient presents with a classic history and signs and symptoms of a Charcot foot (neuropathic arthropathy) (Answer A). It is a specific manifestation of peripheral neuropathy that may involve autonomic neuropathy with high blood flow to the foot, leading to increased bone resorption. It may also involve peripheral somatic polyneuropathy with loss of protective sensation and high risk of acute or chronic minor trauma. In both cases, there is excess local inflammatory response to foot injury, resulting in local osteoporosis. In the Charcot foot, there are acute and chronic phases. The former is characterized by local erythema and edema, while pain is not a prominent symptom. In the latter, signs of inflammation gradually recede and deformities may develop, increasing the risk of foot ulceration. This patient presents in the interphase between the 2 phases, where there are some acute signs and some deformity, also seen on foot radiographs.

Osteoarthritis (Answer B), like a neuropathic joint, can be associated with degenerative change and joint pain. However, pain is the principal symptom associated with osteoarthritis, and it is typically exacerbated by activity and is relieved by rest. Frank inflammatory features, such as erythema or soft-tissue swelling and tenderness, are uncommon in uncomplicated osteoarthritis. Most patients with septic arthritis (Answer C) are febrile and have high white blood cell counts and erythrocyte sedimentation rates. Pseudogout (Answer D) (acute calcium pyrophosphate arthropathy) can occur at a higher incidence in the older population with longstanding diabetes, but it does not typically affect the ankle and foot (as in this case) and can be diagnosed by the presence of the characteristic positively birefringent crystals in the synovial fluid. Cellulitis (Answer E) is usually accompanied by leukocytosis and a high erythrocyte sedimentation rate.

EDUCATIONAL OBJECTIVE

Identify Charcot foot in a patient with diabetes mellitus.

REFERENCE(S)

Mascarenhas JV, Jude EB. The Charcot foot as a complication of diabetic neuropathy. *Curr Diab Rep.* 2014;14(12):561. PMID: 25354828

Papanas N, Maltezos E. Etiology, pathophysiology and classifications of the diabetic Charcot foot. *Diabetic Foot Ankle.* 2013;4. PMID: 23705058

Gouveri E, Papanas N. Charcot osteoarthropathy in diabetes: a brief review with an emphasis on clinical practice. *World J Diabetes.* 2011;2(5):59-65. PMID: 21691556

Diabetes Mellitus Section 2 Board Review

Michelle F. Magee, MD

29 **ANSWER: C) Fournier gangrene**

The abdominal CT shows significant subcutaneous air and edema in the left lateral anterior abdominal wall tracking into the left groin and extending into the perineum. These findings are consistent with Fournier gangrene. There is no apparent drainable abscess and there does not appear to be extension into the pelvic musculature/pelvic girdle.

Fournier gangrene (Answer C) is an aggressive form of necrotizing fasciitis due to mixed aerobic and anaerobic organisms. It affects the perineal and genital region. Urinary extravasation and perirectal and periurethral skin infections serve as a common nidus of infection due to a breach in the integrity of the gastrointestinal or urethral mucosa. Uncontrolled diabetes, as was present as a new diagnosis in this patient, immunosuppressed states, and obesity often contribute to its rapid progression. The Fournier Gangrene Severity Index Score (FGSI) is used to predict mortality. Specifically, there is an increase in mortality from 22% to 75% once the FGSI score rises above 9. Mortality rates have improved over the past 20 years and currently range from 7% to 10%.

Necrotizing cellulitis (Answer A) is typically caused by anaerobic pathogens that are divided into 2 types: clostridial (usually caused by *Clostridium perfringens,* less frequently by *Clostridium septicum*) and nonclostridial (caused by polymicrobial infection). In both types, crepitus is observed in the skin, but there is sparing of the fascia and deep muscles. Pain, swelling, and systemic toxicity are not prominent features.

Cellulitis (Answer B) presents with skin erythema, edema, and warmth. Fever may be present, but cellulitis is generally not associated with hemodynamic instability or exquisite tenderness. Elevations in serum creatine kinase or AST concentrations would suggest deep infection involving muscle or fascia, as opposed to cellulitis.

Pyoderma gangrenosum (Answer D) can be difficult to distinguish from necrotizing fasciitis. Pyoderma gangrenosum has a strong link with inflammatory bowel disease, does not resemble cellulitis (as Fournier gangrene may in its early stages), has a violaceous ulcer edge, does not respond to antibiotics, and is unlikely to be associated with sepsis or require intensive care. The distinction is important because inappropriate surgical debridement of pyoderma gangrenosum can cause extension of the lesion, and inappropriate administration of immunosuppressive therapy may worsen necrotizing fasciitis.

Pyomyositis (Answer E) is characterized by abscess formation in skeletal muscle, which was not a finding on this patient's CT of the abdomen and pelvis.

EDUCATIONAL OBJECTIVE

Recognize a rapidly progressive, life-threatening infection (Fournier gangrene) that is seen in association with diabetes mellitus.

REFERENCE(S)

Sparenborg JD, Brems JA, Wood AM, Hwang JJ, Venkatesan K. Fournier's gangrene: a modern analysis of predictors of outcomes. *Transl Androl Urol.* 2019;8(4):374-378. PMID: 31555561

Chernyadyev SA, Ufimtseva MA, Vishnevskaya IF, et al. Fournier's gangrene: literature review and clinical cases. *Urol Int.* 2018;101(1):91-97. PMID: 29949811

Taken K, Oncu MR, Ergun M, et al. Fournier's gangrene: causes, presentation and survival of sixty-five patients. *Pak J Med Sci.* 2016;32(3): 746-750. PMID: 27375726

30 **ANSWER: E) Ezetimibe**

Multiple large randomized controlled trials have investigated the benefits of adding nonstatin agents to statin therapy, including those that have evaluated further lowering of LDL cholesterol with ezetimibe and PCSK9 inhibitors.

For secondary prevention in adults with diabetes and atherosclerotic cardiovascular disease at very high risk, if the LDL-cholesterol concentration is 70 mg/dL or greater (≥1.81 mmol/L) on the maximally tolerated statin dosage, additional LDL-cholesterol–lowering therapy should be added. The American College of Cardiology Cholesterol Guideline for secondary prevention in patients with clinical atherosclerotic cardiovascular disease recommends adding ezetimibe (Answer E) as the next step. As noted in the American Diabetes Association 2020 Standards of Medical Care in Diabetes, an additional consideration in this choice is the fact that ezetimibe costs less than a PCSK9 inhibitor.

Evolocumab (Answer B) is a PCSK9 (proprotein convertase subtilisin kexin type 9) inhibitor antibody. In adults with established cardiovascular disease, PCSK9 inhibitors are indicated to reduce the risk of myocardial infarction, stroke, and coronary revascularization. Addition of a PCSK9 inhibitor is deemed reasonable when the maximal tolerated dosage of statin plus ezetimibe does not result in an LDL-cholesterol concentration less than 70 mg/dL (<1.81 mmol/L).

On the basis of evidence from the REDUCE-IT trial, icosapent ethyl (Answer A) is indicated as an adjunct to maximally tolerated statin therapy to reduce the risk of myocardial infarction, stroke, coronary revascularization, and unstable angina requiring hospitalization in adults with hypertriglyceridemia (>150 mg/dL [>1.70 mmol/L]) and established cardiovascular disease or diabetes mellitus and 2 or more additional risk factors for cardiovascular disease. This patient does not have hypertriglyceridemia, so icosapent ethyl is incorrect.

Coenzyme Q10 (Answer C) is one of the most commonly used dietary supplements in the United States. Due to its antioxidant and antiinflammatory effects, coenzyme Q10 has been studied extensively for possible use in managing coronary heart disease. One of the most common applications of coenzyme Q10 is to mitigate statin-associated muscle symptoms based on the theory that statin-associated muscle symptoms are caused by statin depletion of coenzyme Q10 in the muscle. Although previous studies of coenzyme Q10 for statin-associated muscle symptoms have produced mixed results, coenzyme Q10 appears to be safe. Current evidence does not support routine use of coenzyme Q10 in patients with coronary heart disease.

Compared with placebo, colchicine (Answer D), 0.5 mg daily, among patients with recent myocardial infarction has been shown to lead to a significantly lower risk of ischemic cardiovascular events. However, this woman has not had a myocardial infarction, so there is no evidence base for adding colchicine to her regimen. It also is not an LDL-cholesterol–lowering agent.

EDUCATIONAL OBJECTIVE

Discuss agents that may alter cardiovascular disease outcomes in adults with type 2 diabetes and established high risk for cardiovascular disease.

REFERENCE(S)

American Diabetes Association. 10. Cardiovascular disease and risk management: American Diabetes Association Standards of Medical Care in Diabetes-2020. *Diabetes Care.* 2020;43(Suppl 1): S111-S134. PMID: 31862753

Grundy SM, Stone NJ, Bailey AL, et al. 2018 AHA/ACC/AACVPR/AAPA/ABC/ACPM/ADA/AGS/APhA/ASPC/NLA/PCNA guideline on the management of blood cholesterol: executive summary: a report of the American College of Cardiology/American Heart Association Task Force on Clinical Practice Guidelines. *J Am Coll Cardiol.* 2019;73(24):3168-3209. PMID: 30423391

Ayers J, Cook J, Koenig RA, Sisson EM, Dixon DL. Recent developments in the role of coenzyme Q10 for coronary heart disease: a systematic review. *Curr Atheroscler Rep.* 2018;20(6):29. PMID: 29766349

Tardif JC, Kouz S, Waters DD, et al. Efficacy and safety of low-dose colchicine after myocardial infarction. *N Engl J Med.* 2019;381(26): 2497-2505. PMID: 31733140

Bhatt DL, Steg PG, Miller M, et al; REDUCE-IT Investigators. Cardiovascular risk reduction with icosapent ethyl for hypertriglyceridemia. *N Engl J Med.* 2019;380(1):11-22. PMID: 30415628

31 ANSWER: D) A change in mealtime insulin to faster-acting insulin aspart injections

Time to onset of action of subcutaneously administered regular U500 insulin may be from 30 to 45 minutes to up to 2.5 hours. The reported mean duration of action is 21 hours (range, 13-24 hours). This suggests that U500 may pose challenges when used as a premeal bolus insulin. The patient's regimen was switched to faster-acting insulin aspart (Answer D) by subcutaneous injection for his meal boluses using an insulin-to-carbohydrate ratio of 1:2. The U500 in the pump now serves solely as basal insulin. This obviates the need for taking a meal bolus via the pump well ahead of a meal, which is inconvenient to accommodate and may not be long enough to allow for onset of the U500 bolus to avoid the postmeal highs. Thus, a bolus 45 minutes before meals (Answer A) is incorrect.

The Evaluating U-500R Infusion Versus Injection in Type 2 Diabetes (VIVID) randomized controlled trial compared U500 regular delivered by continuous subcutaneous insulin infusion with U500 regular delivered by multiple daily injections in persons requiring high-dosage insulin (total daily dose >200 to ≤600 units). This study provides guidance for determination of insulin pump settings when U500 regular is used. The protocol specified how the total daily dose of U500 regular should be distributed and offered 3 bolus options. The total daily dose was divided into 50:50 bolus and basal. Basal insulin was split into 2 rates: 6 AM to 9 PM at the calculated basal rate and 9 PM to 6 AM at a 10% reduced basal rate. Up to 4 basal rates were allowed. Participants were encouraged to have a bedtime snack without an insulin bolus to prevent nocturnal hypoglycemia. The pump bolus calculator was used to determine bolus doses using 1 of 3 options: fixed bolus (40:30:30 for breakfast, lunch, and dinner), carbohydrate counting, or meal size per participant estimate (small = 30 g carbohydrate; medium = 60 g carbohydrate; large = 90 g carbohydrate). For the 2 latter options, the suggested starting insulin-to-carbohydrate ratio was programmed between 1:3 and 1:5 units/g with customization being allowed. Duration of insulin onboard was 6 hours. Mean changes from baseline hemoglobin A_{1c} were −1.27% in the continuous subcutaneous insulin infusion group and −0.87% in the multiple daily injection group ($P < .001$), and 28.7% of the continuous subcutaneous insulin infusion group compared with 18.4% of the multiple daily injection group achieved a hemoglobin A_{1c} target less than 7.0% (<53 mmol/mol) ($P = .015$). Weight changes and documented symptomatic and severe hypoglycemia were similar between groups; however, the continuous subcutaneous insulin infusion group had a higher rate of nocturnal hypoglycemia, despite the bedtime snack recommendation.

Increasing this patient's insulin-to-carbohydrate ratio (Answer B) would aggravate the trend for late postmeal hypoglycemia and may increase his time spent in the hypoglycemic range. Increasing the basal insulin from 4 PM to 12 AM (Answer C) might lead to "overbasalization" and does not specifically target attenuation of postmeal glucose excursions, which is the primary management challenge in this patient now. Reducing the basal rate from 3 AM to 8 AM (Answer E) would attenuate the trend for nocturnal blood glucose to be lower, but it would not correct the amount of time spent in hyperglycemia. It should also be noted that the time this patient spends in the hypoglycemic range is only 1% and the main issue is time spent in the hyperglycemic range (52%).

EDUCATIONAL OBJECTIVE

Explain practical aspects of use of regular U500 insulin in a continuous subcutaneous insulin infusion pump system.

REFERENCE(S)

Grunberger G, Bhargava A, Ly T, et al. Human regular U-500 insulin via continuous subcutaneous insulin infusion versus multiple daily injections in adults with type 2 diabetes: the VIVID study. *Diabetes Obes Metab.* 2020;22(3):434-441. PMID: 31865633

McCall AL. U-500 insulin pump case. In: Draznin B, ed. *Diabetes Case Studies Real Problems, Practical Solutions.* American Diabetes Association; 2015:105-108.

Danne T, Nimri R, Battelino T. International consensus on use of continuous glucose monitoring. *Diabetes Care.* 2017;40:1631-1640. PMID: 29162583

32 ANSWER: D) Hemoglobin A_{1c} target <7.0%; blood glucose targets of 120-150 mg/dL; glargine dose, 12 units once daily; prandial insulin dose of 3 units; correction factor of 1/60 if >150 mg/dL

This is a high-risk pregnancy in a woman with labile type 1 diabetes that is complicated by severe hypoglycemia with reactions resulting in unconsciousness. She has been provided with survival skills education and instructed in a consistent carbohydrate diet before hospital discharge.

It is appropriate to relax her glycemic targets to a hemoglobin A_{1c} level of 7.0% (53 mmol/mol), fasting blood glucose concentration less than 120 mg/dL (<6.7 mmol/L), and 2-hour postprandial blood glucose concentration less than 150 mg/dL (<8.3 mmol/L). On 14 units of insulin glargine, her fasting blood glucose is low, so a reduction in the glargine dose to 12 units is appropriate. Her response to 5 units of prandial insulin has been variable. On the morning of the third hospital day, it was recognized that she had been eating constantly since admission to allay her fear of another episode of loss of consciousness and she agreed to stop doing this. Nonetheless, subsequent postmeal blood glucose values were variable following administration of 5 units of prandial insulin, including 1 value of 48 mg/dL (2.7 mmol/L). Therefore, the prandial insulin dose was reduced to 3 units until she could be instructed in carbohydrate counting after hospital discharge. Finally, correction insulin doses were recommended with an insulin sensitivity factor of 1:60 to be taken only if her blood glucose concentration was greater than 150 mg/dL (>8.3 mmol/L).

Answer A is incorrect for this patient, as it is aligned with guideline-recommended stringent pregnancy glycemic targets that are more aggressive than would be appropriate for her at this time in view of her known severe hypoglycemia.

Answer B is incorrect because while the hemoglobin A_{1c} target has been relaxed, the blood glucose targets have not. A 50% reduction in the insulin glargine dose will most likely result in fasting and premeal hyperglycemia to a degree that is unacceptable in pregnancy. She has not yet learned carbohydrate counting, so she cannot use an insulin-to-carbohydrate ratio. A 1:60 correction factor for blood glucose values greater than 120 mg/dL (>6.7 mmol/L) may lead to hypoglycemia, which must be avoided.

Answer C is incorrect because a hemoglobin A_{1c} target less than 6.0% (<42 mmol/mol) is not appropriate for this patient given her risk for severe hypoglycemia. For the same reason, an insulin glargine dose of 14 units is excessive.

Answer E is incorrect. A hemoglobin A_{1c} target less than 8.0% (<64 mmol/mol) and even more relaxed blood glucose targets may be appropriate for this woman later in pregnancy if she continues to have severe hypoglycemia. However, she is now entering her second trimester. The first-trimester tendency for hypoglycemia will attenuate as total insulin requirements begin to rise. Therefore, a 40% reduction in basal insulin dose (from 12 to 7 units) and a 60% reduction in meal insulin (from 5 to 2 units) is more than is needed now, as it would lead to hyperglycemia.

EDUCATIONAL OBJECTIVE

Set appropriate glycemic targets and prescribe safe insulin dosing for patients with diabetes who have severe hypoglycemia in pregnancy.

REFERENCE(S)

American Diabetes Association. 14. Management of diabetes in pregnancy: standards of medical care in diabetes-2020. *Diabetes Care.* 2020;43(Suppl 1): S183-S192. PMID: 31862757

33 ANSWER: A) Diabetes-related muscle infarction

Diabetes-related muscle infarction (Answer A) is also referred to as muscle ischemia or spontaneous myonecrosis. Multiplanar, multisequence magnetic resonance images of the right thigh demonstrated extensive and marked edema of the right thigh adductor and quadriceps muscles. There is also a confluent signal abnormality in the vastus medialis and intermedius, patchy signal abnormality within the rectus femoris and vastus medialis musculature, and distortion of fibrillar morphology in the adductor magnus muscle belly. The imaging is suggestive of diabetes-related muscle infarction, with a heterogenous appearance with linear streaks of enhancement crossing central nonenhancing regions surrounded by regions of enhanced muscle.

Diabetes-related muscle infarction causes acute or subacute pain, swelling, and tenderness, typically in the thigh, as was seen in this patient, or in the calf. Laboratory findings are nonspecific and are normal in many patients. Some may exhibit elevated creatine kinase, elevated erythrocyte sedimentation rate, and leukocytosis. MRI may show high intensity in the involved muscle on T2-weighted sequences, as well as subcutaneous edema, subfascial fluid, and loss of the normal fatty intramuscular septa, which is optimally observed in T1-weighted images, where the affected muscles appear hypointense or isointense. The primary findings on muscle biopsy, which is diagnostic, are muscle necrosis and edema. Occlusion of arterioles and capillaries by fibrin may also be seen. Pathogenesis appears to be related to vasculopathy associated with longstanding, suboptimally controlled diabetes. Treatment of diabetes-related muscle infarction involves symptomatic management with rest, optimal glycemic control, analgesia, and low-dosage aspirin.

On this patient's imaging, there is no intrinsic T1 hyperintense signal suggestive of blood products, so intramuscular hematoma (Answer B) is incorrect.

Spontaneous gangrenous myositis (Answer C) due to streptococcal infection is characterized by gangrenous necrosis and more systemic toxicity than was seen in this patient. There were also no foci indicating soft-tissue gas present on her MRI images.

Muscle denervation (Answer D) due to diabetes-related myopathy is characterized by muscle atrophy, not swelling as was seen in this patient.

Pyomyositis (Answer E) commonly involves large muscles of the thigh. Infectious and inflammatory myositis/pyomyositis is characterized by smooth-walled intramuscular abscesses with rimlike enhancement. While pyomyositis in its early stages may be hard to distinguish from diabetes-related muscle infarction, fever, leukocytosis, well-defined intramuscular fluid collection will be seen at a more advanced stage. This patient has had a relatively indolent course over several weeks and there is no evidence of a discrete organized intramuscular fluid collection on imaging to suggest pyomyositis. Treatment for pyomyositis would require antibiotic therapy and drainage.

EDUCATIONAL OBJECTIVE

Construct the differential diagnosis of pain and swelling in a lower extremity in a patient with diabetes mellitus.

REFERENCE(S)

Yong TY, Khow KSF. Diabetic muscle infarction in end-stage renal disease: A scoping review on epidemiology, diagnosis and treatment. *World J Nephrol.* 2018;7(2):58-64. PMID: 29527509

Horton WB, Taylor JS, Ragland TJ, Subauste AR. Diabetic muscle infarction: a systematic review. *BMJ Open Diabetes Res Care.* 2015;3:e000082. PMID: 25932331

34 ANSWER: B) Dulaglutide

This man with type 2 diabetes, heart failure, and chronic kidney disease is at high risk for cardiovascular mortality and kidney disease progression. GLP-1 receptor agonists reduce the risk for 3-point MACE (nonfatal stroke, nonfatal myocardial infarction, and cardiovascular death). Their impact on renal outcomes has been assessed in large cardiovascular outcomes trials among persons with type 2 diabetes. Liraglutide, semaglutide, and dulaglutide (Answer B) reduce prespecified renal outcomes overall (including decline in estimated glomerular filtration rate, need for renal replacement therapy, and/or impact on proteinuria). Furthermore, no dosage adjustment is required for renal impairment with GLP-1 receptor agonists, so this agent would be safe to use in this man and may positively influence his risk for cardiovascular events and renal progression.

SGLT-2 inhibitors, including dapagliflozin (Answer A), reduce hospitalizations for heart failure, the need for urgent visits resulting in intravenous therapy for heart failure, and progression of chronic kidney disease, each of which would be desirable outcomes in this patient. However, the use of SGLT-2 inhibitors in persons with a low estimated glomerular filtration rate has not been studied extensively, as there were relatively few patients with lower-range estimated glomerular filtration rates in the cardiovascular outcome trials. Use of dapagliflozin is not recommended when the estimated glomerular filtration rate is less than 45 mL/min per 1.73 m^2, and its use is contraindicated at rates less than 30 mL/min per 1.73 m^2. This man's estimated glomerular filtration rate has been as low as 27 mL/min per 1.73 m^2 and is now 29 mL/min per 1.73 m^2, so prescribing an SGLT-2 inhibitor would not be advised.

The efficacy and safety of canagliflozin for glycemic control were evaluated in a trial that included patients with moderate renal impairment (estimated glomerular filtration rate 30 to less than 50 mL/min 1.73 m^2), and dosing guidance for persons with an estimated glomerular filtration rate in the range of 30 to 45 mL/min 1.73 m^2 has been approved. In addition, patients already on canagliflozin whose estimated glomerular filtration rate declines below 30 mL/min 1.73 m^2, with albuminuria greater than 300 mg daily, can continue on the 100 mg daily dosage unless dialysis is initiated.

Saxagliptin (Answer C) has been associated with an increased risk for hospitalizations due to heart failure. Linagliptin (Answer D) combined with basal insulin would be a reasonable combination treatment for this patient to attain glycemic control, as it has demonstrated safety from cardiovascular and renal perspectives across all ages and renal impairment groups. However, it does not influence cardiovascular disease outcomes.

The addition of metformin (Answer E) to this patient's regimen is contraindicated because his estimated glomerular filtration rate is less than 30 mL/min 1.73 m^2.

EDUCATIONAL OBJECTIVE

Explain the relative risks and benefits of antihyperglycemic agents for type 2 diabetes management in the setting of chronic kidney disease and heart failure.

REFERENCE(S)

Zelnicker TA, Wiviott SD, Raz I, et al. Comparison of the effects of glucagon-like peptide receptor agonists and sodium-glucose cotransporter 2 inhibitors for prevention of major adverse cardiovascular and renal outcomes in type 2 diabetes mellitus. *Circulation.* 2019;139(17): 2022-2031. PMID: 30786725

Zelniker TA, Wiviott SD, Raz I, et al. SGLT2 inhibitors for primary and secondary prevention of cardiovascular and renal outcomes in type 2 diabetes: a systematic review and meta-analysis of of cardiovascular outcome trials. *Lancet.* 2019;393(10166):31-39. PMID: 30424892

Giugliano D, Ceriello, A, De Nicola L, Perrone-Filardi P, Cosentino F, Esposito K. Primary versus secondary cardiorenal prevention in type2 diabetes: Which newer anti-hyperglycaemic drug matters? *Diabetes Obes Metab.* 2020;22(2): 149-157. PMID: 31495989

Giugliano D, Meier JJ, Esposito K. Heart failure and type 2 diabetes: from cardiovascular outcome trials, with hope. *Diabetes Obes Metab.* 2019;21(5): 1081-1087. PMID: 30609236

35 ANSWER: C) Hydralazine

Cardiovascular autonomic neuropathy is associated with mortality independent of other cardiovascular risk factors. This woman has supine hypertension and a marked orthostatic drop in blood pressure, both systolic and diastolic upon arising. This presentation is consistent with orthostatic hypotension due to autonomic neuropathy. She does not, however, have a fixed tachycardia that often accompanies autonomic neuropathy. About one-half of persons with neurogenic orthostatic hypotension are hypertensive in the supine position. Supine hypertension promotes nocturnal sodium excretion, and orthostatic hypotension and may predispose to cardiovascular and renal disease. These reasons provide a rationale for treating supine hypertension. Given the lack of evidence from clinical trials on which to base therapy, recommendations are necessarily based on expert opinion and observations in small case series.

Pharmacologic treatment must be individualized. Persons with autonomic failure are highly sensitive to vasodilators, and hydralazine (Answer C) often effectively lowers nocturnal blood pressure without exacerbating orthostatic symptoms the next morning.

Due to $\alpha2$ adrenoreceptor-mediated vasoconstriction, clonidine (Answer A) may paradoxically raise blood pressure in patients with pure autonomic failure.

β-Adrenoreceptor blockade alone (Answer B) may not lower supine blood pressure unless a drug with additional vasodilator properties is used. However, nebivolol, which is a vasodilating β-adrenergic blocker, can effectively lower nighttime hypertension.

Patients with neurogenic orthostatic hypotension and supine hypertension are highly sensitive to pressor drugs. Medications such as nonsteroidal antiinflammatory drugs (Answer D) in commonly prescribed dosages can elicit a substantial pressor response and should be avoided. Midodrine (Answer E) is a vasopressor agent that is used to treat refractory orthostatic hypotension.

Relative to nonpharmacologic treatments for neurogenic orthostatic hypotension and supine hypertension, modest orthostatic stress can substantially lower blood pressure. Therefore, raising the head of the bed by 10 to 20 degrees has been applied to ameliorate supine blood pressure. The intervention also attenuates pressure-induced natriuresis, nocturnal volume loss, and orthostatic symptoms the next day. Water drinking may elicit a profound pressor response. This "osmopressor response" has a rapid onset within minutes, reaches a maximum after approximately 30 minutes, and is sustained for 60 to 90 minutes. Therefore, patients should limit drinking water 60 to 90 minutes before bedtime depending on their sensitivity to the osmopressor response. Finally, patients with orthostatic hypotension can also exhibit postprandial hypotension. A snack before bedtime may lower supine blood pressure in such cases. Compared with other macronutrients, carbohydrates result in larger blood pressure drops. Limitations to trying this approach clearly exist for an obese woman with uncontrolled diabetes such as this patient.

Table. Management of Supine Hypertension[a]

- Avoid offending agents
  - Avoid lying down during the day
  - Avoid rest in the seated position
  - Beware of "hidden" pressor agents
    - Ibuprofen
    - Indomethacin
    - Atomoxetine
  - Limit water ingestion near bedtime
  - Avoid fludrocortisone in favor of short-acting pressor agents when possible
- Nonpharmacologic treatments
  - Tilt the whole bed head up by approximately 10 degrees; in patients who do not tolerate this measure, tilt only the head of the bed up 30 degrees
  - Carbohydrate-rich snack at bedtime
  - If alcohol is consumed, small amount at bedtime
- Pharmacologic treatments
  - Consider individualized antihypertensive treatment taken at bedtime
- Monitor nighttime blood pressure with 24-hour ambulatory blood pressure monitors
  - Monitor before starting treatment to see if patient "dips" to a normal pressure later in the night
  - Monitor to evaluate treatment efficacy

[a]These recommendations are based on expert opinion and results from small-scale studies. Larger-scale trials with hard clinical endpoints do not exist.

Table adapted from Jordan J, Fanciulli A, Tank J, et al. Management of supine hypertension in patients with neurogenic orthostatic hypotension: scientific statement of the American Autonomic Society, European Federation of Autonomic Societies, and the European Society of Hypertension. *J Hypertens.* 2019;37(8):1541-1546.

This patient is off the multiple antihypertensive agents she was taking before hospital admission. While proximally due to dehydration secondary to her intercurrent viral illness, her hypertension was most likely driven by high sodium intake, which masked her orthostatic hypotension, and blood pressure–lowering agents were added sequentially even though it is not clear that she was taking any of them regularly. Her orthostasis improved with hydration during the hospital stay. Her blood pressure should to be monitored closely following discharge. Once she has reequilibrated and is taking hydralazine, 24-hour ambulatory blood pressure monitoring would be useful to ensure her blood pressure management is optimized. Medical nutrition therapy as an outpatient should be recommended.

EDUCATIONAL OBJECTIVE

Recommend treatment options for diabetes-related cardiovascular autonomic neuropathy with supine hypertension.

REFERENCE(S)

American Diabetes Association. 11. Microvascular complications and foot care: standards of medical care in diabetes-2020. *Diabetes Care.* 2020;43(Suppl 1):S135-151. PMID: 31862754

Jordan J, Fanciulli A, Tank J, et al. Management of supine hypertension in patients with neurogenic orthostatic hypotension: scientific statement of the American Autonomic Society, European Federation of Autonomic Societies, and the European Society of Hypertension. *J Hypertens.* 2019;37(8):1541-1546. PMID: 30882602

36 ANSWER: B) Applying topical cromolyn

Acquired partial local lipodystrophies include lipohypertrophy and lipoatrophy at insulin injection sites. Insulin absorption from these sites is unpredictable and can lead to erratic glycemic control and an increased predisposition to severe hypoglycemia, which this patient needs to avoid.

He has marked lipoatrophy at the sites where he has been injecting insulin. Atrophy results from local formation of complexes between injected antigen and circulating antibody with activation of complement and infiltration of inflammatory cells, including mast cells and eosinophils. Localized overproduction of cytokines and tumor necrosis factor from mast cells inhibit adipocyte differentiation. Skin biopsy shows degenerative changes in adipose tissue with an increase in degranulated mast cells. While transient red bumps or urticarial lesions may be noted after starting insulin shots, the clinical appearance of lipoatrophy is noted for its lack of inflammatory features, as is the case in this man.

Tryptase- and chymase-positive mast cells are known to be sensitive to sodium cromolyn, which a mast-cell stabilizer. In case reports, topical application of cromolyn (Answer B) has been shown to improve or even resolve the atrophy, and ongoing use may help avoid atrophy at new injection sites. From a pragmatic perspective, lipoatrophy is relatively uncommon and local treatments have not been widely examined and are generally not necessary.

These mast cells are resistant to glucocorticoids, so adding dexamethasone to the insulin (Answer D) would not be expected to be effective as a treatment.

Failure to rotate insulin injection sites and reuse of needles (Answer C) are associated with risk for lipoatrophy. While rotation of injection sites (Answer A) and avoiding reuse of needles (Answer C) are cornerstones for the prevention of atrophy, neither would address the underlying immune response process. Anabolic steroids (Answer E) do not have a role in lipoatrophy treatment and also would not address the underlying pathophysiologic process.

Lipohypertrophy, which is more common than lipoatrophy, results from a direct local anabolic response to insulin itself, which leads to local fat and protein synthesis. This results in atrophy of fat cells and hypoplastic collagenous scar tissue. It is observed even with recombinant insulins and with use of continuous subcutaneous insulin infusion pumps. Lipohypertrophy presents as soft dermal nodules or fibrocollagenous scar tissue within the skin that can be missed by visual inspection alone and will be felt most readily via a firm stroking and sweeping motion of the hand rather than traditional light or deep palpation. Lipohypertrophy is treated by avoiding the affected areas until the tissue returns to normal, which may take months to years. It should be noted that switching from areas of lipohypertrophy to normal tissue often requires a reduction in the dose of insulin injected, as absorption will be more efficient. The preferred preventive strategies are the same as those for lipoatrophy (ie, rotation of injection sites and nonreuse of needles).

Other medications, such as glucocorticoids and antibiotics, can also cause localized lipoatrophy. Other rare causes of localized lipoatrophy include repeated pressure against any body part and lipoatrophy occurring as part of a rare syndrome called lipodystrophia centrifugalis abdominalis infantilis. Finally, some patients have localized lipoatrophy (ie, lack of adipose tissue in small areas of the trunk or parts of a limb) as an isolated abnormality. Patients with HIV infection who are treated with antiretroviral therapy, and especially HIV-1 protease inhibitors, can develop lipodystrophy, and these drugs are probably the cause.

EDUCATIONAL OBJECTIVE

Explain the pathophysiologic processes underlying acquired, partial localized insulin-induced lipodystrophies and how this understanding informs treatment of lipoatrophy.

REFERENCE(S)

Kadiyala P, Walton S, Sathyapalan T. Insulin induced lipodystrophy. *Br J Diabetes Vasc Dis.* 2014;14(4): 131-133.

Lopez X, Castells M, Ricker A, et al. Human insulin analog--induced lipoatrophy. *Diabetes Care.* 2008;31(3):442-444. PMID: 18162498

37 ANSWER: A) Now

According to the American Diabetes Association guidelines, screening for diabetes should begin at age 45 years regardless of other factors such as ethnicity, family history, BMI (Answer D), blood pressure, and dyslipidemia. As this woman is older than 45 years, she should be screened for diabetes now (thus, Answer A is correct and Answer B is incorrect). It should be noted that the US Preventive Services Task Force, the Centers for disease Control and Prevention, the Canadian Task Force on Preventive Health Care, and the International Diabetes Federation all recommend that screening start at age 40 to 45 years in asymptomatic patients.

In asymptomatic adults, diabetes screening should also be considered in those who are overweight or obese or who have 1 or more of the following risk factors: first-degree relative with diabetes (as is the case for this woman); high-risk race/ethnicity; history of cardiovascular disease; hypertension (thus, Answer C is incorrect); HDL-cholesterol concentration less than 35 mg/dL (<0.90 mmol/L) and/or triglyceride concentration greater than 250 mg/dL (>2.83 mmol/L) (not >150 mg/dL [>1.70 mmol/L]) (thus, Answer E is incorrect); polycystic ovary syndrome; and physical inactivity. Patients with prediabetes should have annual testing, and women diagnosed with gestational diabetes should have testing at least every 3 years.

EDUCATIONAL OBJECTIVE

Recommend when to screen for diabetes mellitus in an asymptomatic adult.

REFERENCE(S)

American Diabetes Association. 2. Classification and diagnosis of diabetes: standards of medical care in diabetes-2020. *Diabetes Care.* 2020;43(Suppl 1): S14-S31. PMID: 31862745

Siu AL; US Preventive Services Task Force. Screening for abnormal blood glucose and type 2 diabetes mellitus: U.S. Preventive Services Task Force Recommendation Statement. *Ann Intern Med.* 2015;163(11):861-868. PMID: 26501513

38 ANSWER: B) Reduce all insulin doses by 10% to 20%

The “honeymoon” phase in type 1 diabetes is characterized by reduced exogenous insulin requirements in the face of well-maintained glycemic control. It may develop relatively soon after the diagnosis and is a transient phase of “remission,” thought to be due either to adaptive immune tolerance or to some improvement in β-cell function. Improved residual insulin secretory function reduces the need for all exogenous insulins (thus, Answer B is correct), not only premeal or basal insulins (Answers A and C). Increasing her carbohydrate intake to at least 50 g with each meal (Answer D) is not the best choice, as it does not correct the problem of excessive insulin at mealtimes and it requires that the patient ingest extra calories.

EDUCATIONAL OBJECTIVE

Develop a strategy to manage glycemic levels during the "honeymoon" phase of type 1 diabetes.

REFERENCE(S)

Aly H, Gottlieb P. The honeymoon phase: intersection of metabolism and immunology. *Curr Opin Endocrinol Diabetes Obes.* 2009;16(4): 286-292. PMID: 19506474

Akirav E, Kushner JA, Herold KC. Beta-cell mass and type 1 diabetes: going, going, gone? *Diabetes.* 2008;57(11):2883-2888. PMID: 18971435

39 ANSWER: B) Continue metformin; add dulaglutide

Unless there is intolerance or a contraindication to its use, a combination of metformin monotherapy plus lifestyle change (eg, lifestyle counseling, weight-loss education, and exercise) is the preferred initial treatment of type 2 diabetes. If the hemoglobin A_{1c} level is not 7.0% or lower (≤53 mmol/mol) after approximately 3 months of lifestyle management and metformin, an additional agent should be initiated. In the absence of high risk for or established cardiovascular disease and in the presence of a compelling need to minimize weight gain or promote loss as is the case in this patient, a combination of metformin and GLP-1 receptor agonist or SGLT-2 inhibitor is recommended. Thus, because the patient has moderate to poor glycemic control on metformin monotherapy, the best course of action is to add the GLP-1 receptor agonist dulaglutide (Answer B) to her current regimen. Adding an SGLT-2 inhibitor to her metformin therapy would also be an option; however, this is not listed as a choice in this question. Stopping metformin and starting insulin (Answer A) or empagliflozin (Answer D) would result in monotherapy rather than the recommended dual therapy. Simply increasing the metformin dosage (Answer C) would not be adequate. Adding sitagliptin (Answer E), a DPP-4 inhibitor, would not be as likely as a GLP-1 receptor agonist to help her achieve weight management goals.

EDUCATIONAL OBJECTIVE

Guide therapy for type 2 diabetes when lifestyle efforts and metformin therapy fail to provide adequate glycemic control.

REFERENCE(S)

American Diabetes Association. 9. Pharmacologic approaches to glycemic treatment: standards of medical care in diabetes-2020. *Diabetes Care.* 2020;43(Suppl 1):S98-S110. PMID: 31862752

Buse J, Wexler D, Tsapas, et al. 2019 update to: management of hyperglycemia in type 2 diabetes, 2018. A consensus report by the American Diabetes Association (ADA) and the European Association for the Study of Diabetes. *Diabetes Care.* 2019;43(2):487-493. PMID: 31857443

40 ANSWER: C) Transferrin saturation

Whenever diabetes is diagnosed, the possibility of secondary diabetes should be considered. Secondary diabetes occurs when a separate condition leads to hyperglycemia; these are considered distinct from routine type 1 or type 2 diabetes, although clinical features are often shared. Broad categories of secondary diabetes include medication-induced (eg, corticosteroids), other endocrinopathies (eg, acromegaly), pancreatic diseases (eg, pancreatitis), infections (eg, cytomegalovirus), and genetic conditions (eg, Rabson-Mendenhall syndrome). One relatively common condition that should be considered is hemochromatosis, or iron overload. Primary hemochromatosis is the most common genetic disorder in the United States, affecting approximately 1 in every 200 to 300 Americans. It is more common in persons of Western European heritage. It results from increased absorption of iron through the gastrointestinal tract, with excess iron deposition in many tissues. Traditional teaching has been that hyperglycemia results from iron deposition in the pancreas, resulting in islet-cell dysfunction. However, recent data suggest that the pathogenesis involves primarily insulin resistance with secondary β-cell decompensation, as in routine cases of type 2 diabetes. Secondary hemochromatosis includes conditions characterized by increased red blood cell breakdown or a history of many blood transfusions (thalassemia, sideroblastic anemia, hemolytic anemia). The clues in this case include amenorrhea (due to hypogonadotropic hypogonadism from pituitary iron deposition) and hepatic dysfunction and enlargement. The initial approach to diagnosis is assessing markers of iron stores such as transferrin saturation (Answer C) and/or ferritin.

The presence of an *HNF1A* pathogenic variant (Answer A) is diagnostic of maturity-onset diabetes of the young, which does not apply to this case. Zinc transporter 8 antibodies (Answer B) would be elevated if this were type 1 diabetes or latent autoimmune diabetes of adults, but these diagnoses seem unlikely. Measuring serum ceruloplasmin (Answer D) would not be helpful since Wilson disease is unlikely in this patient (diabetes does not typically occur in Wilson disease). Mitochondrial antibodies (Answer E) are increased in primary biliary cirrhosis, but this is not associated with diabetes.

EDUCATIONAL OBJECTIVE

Diagnose hemochromatosis as a cause of secondary diabetes mellitus.

REFERENCE(S)

Barton JC, Acton RT. Diabetes in *HFE* hemochromatosis. *J Diabetes Res.* 2017;2017:9826930. PMID: 28331855

Hatunic M, Finucane FM, Brennan AM, Norris S, Pacini G, Nolan JJ. Effect of iron overload on glucose metabolism in patients with hereditary hemochromatosis. *Metabolism.* 2010;59(3): 380-384. PMID: 19815242

Bacon BR, Adams PC, Kowdley KV, Powell LW, Tavill AS; American Association for Study of Liver Diseases. Diagnosis and management of hemochromatosis: 2011 practice guideline by the American Association for the Study of Liver Diseases. *Hepatology.* 2011;54(1):328-343. PMID: 21452290

41 ANSWER: B) Ketosis-prone diabetes

Although diabetic ketoacidosis has long been the hallmark of type 1 diabetes, in recent years it has become clear that a subset of patients of African or Hispanic descent can present with ketoacidosis as the first manifestation of diabetes (Answer B). Often these patients have dramatic presentations (weight loss, severe polyuria/ polydipsia, and diabetic ketoacidosis) and require insulin treatment, but steady improvement in control over weeks to months may permit a change to long-term oral agent therapy. The pathophysiology of this syndrome is not known, but it seems to be due to a transient and reversible loss of β-cell function.

Autoimmune diabetes (type 1 diabetes or latent autoimmune diabetes in adults, LADA) (Answer A) is possible but not as likely as ketosis-prone diabetes in this vignette. The patient's strong family history of diabetes and elevated BMI are more consistent with type 2 diabetes. Moreover, relative to the degree of hyperglycemia, the ketoacidosis is not as severe as it is in most cases of type 1 diabetes. Diabetes due to LADA and maturity-onset diabetes of the young (Answer C) almost never present with ketoacidosis. Alcoholic ketoacidosis (Answer D) can be associated with moderately elevated blood glucose, but rarely with levels greater than 300 mg/dL (>16.7 mmol/L), and this man has no evidence of recent intoxication. Pancreatitis (Answer E) can present with severe hyperglycemia and ketoacidosis, but this is typically associated with more dramatic abdominal signs and symptoms, as well as high amylase and lipase.

EDUCATIONAL OBJECTIVE

Diagnose ketosis-prone diabetes mellitus.

REFERENCE(S)

Saxon D, Rasouli N. Ketosis-prone diabetes. In: Draznin B, ed. *Diabetes Case Studies.* American Diabetes Association; 2015:36-38.

Seok H, Jung CH, Kim SW, et al. Clinical characteristics and insulin independence of Koreans with new-onset type 2 diabetes presenting with diabetic ketoacidosis. *Diabetes Metab Res Rev.* 2013;29(6): 507-513. PMID: 23653323

Balasubramanyam A, Yajnik CS, Tandon N. Non-traditional forms of diabetes worldwide: implications for translational investigation. *Transl Endocrinol Metab.* 2011;2(1):43-67.

42 ANSWER: C) Acarbose

Late postbariatric hypoglycemia is seen most commonly in patients who have undergone Roux-en-Y gastric bypass. Spikes in glucose due to rapid gastric emptying, vigorous insulin secretion, reduced insulin clearance and insulin-independent glucose uptake, and high levels of GLP-1 all contribute to the phenomenon. If medical nutrition therapy with a low–glycemic index meal plan does not enable control of the hypoglycemia, other medications can be added to the regimen. α-Glucosidase inhibitors (Answer C) slow postprandial glucose absorption and reduce postmeal blood glucose spikes and insulin secretion. Slow introduction and escalation in dosage can help to avoid the adverse effects of gastrointestinal discomfort.

Octreotide (Answer A), which reduces incretin and insulin secretion, can also be administered; however, its use may be limited by high cost and adverse effects, including diarrhea, steatorrhea, and acute hypoglycemia, most likely due to inhibition of insulin secretion. Diazoxide (Answer B) reduces insulin secretion, so it may also be used, but it can lead to fluid retention and headaches. Reports on the efficacy of GLP-1 receptor agonists (Answer D) in this setting have been variable. Finally, metformin (Answer E) absorption and bioavailability seem to be higher after gastric bypass, and this may have implications on dosing and toxicity risk.

Note: Continuous glucose monitoring image reprinted from Patti ME. Hypoglycemia after bariatric surgery. Meet the Professor Endocrine Case Management. Presented at ENDO in Chicago, Illinois. March 2018.

EDUCATIONAL OBJECTIVE

Explain the rationale and strategies for management of late postbariatric hypoglycemia.

REFERENCE(S)

Goldfine AB, Patti ME. How common is hypoglycemia after gastric bypass? *Obesity.* 2016;24(6):1210-1211. PMID: 27225595

Suhl E, Anderson-Haynes SE, Mulla C, Patti ME. Medical nutrition therapy for post-bariatric hypoglycemia: practical insights. *Surg Obes Relat Dis.* 2017;13(5):888-896. PMID: 28392017

Patti ME. Hypoglycemia after bariatric surgery. Meet the Professor Endocrine Case Management. Presented at ENDO in Chicago, Illinois. March 2018.

43 ANSWER: D) Insulin degludec; take it at his convenience once daily

The duration of action of insulin degludec (Answer D) is longer than 42 hours; the half-life is approximately 25 hours and it reaches steady state in 2 to 3 days. It may be given safely and effectively with a minimum of 8 hours and maximum of 40 hours between doses. This makes it well suited to being used during travel, as long as the patient takes it once daily.

NPH insulin at bedtime, given at the same time when traveling (Answer A), is an impractical regimen as it is difficult to give it at the same time when crossing multiple time zones. Insulin detemir may be given once daily at bedtime, but reducing the dose by 50% when traveling (Answer B) will lead to hyperglycemia. The half-life of U300 insulin glargine (Answer C) is about 23 hours. It reaches a steady state in 4 days, and the duration of action is less than or equal to 36 hours. Data regarding U300 insulin support its safety and efficacy up to a ± 3-hour window for administration, so this also may not be ideal for dosing when traveling.

EDUCATIONAL OBJECTIVE

Optimize basal insulin therapy for travel across time zones.

REFERENCE(S)

Ritzel R, Rouseel R, Bolli GB, et al. Patient-level meta-analysis of the EDITION 1, 2 and 3 studies: glycaemic control and hypoglycaemia with new insulin glargine 300 U/ml versus glargine 100 U/mL in people with type 2 diabetes. *Diabetes Obes Metab.* 2015;17(9):859-867. PMID: 25929311

Matheiu C, Hollander P, Miranda-Palma B, et al. Efficacy and safety of insulin degludec in a flexible dosing regimen vs insulin glargine in patients with type 1 diabetes (BEGIN: Flex T1): a 26-week randomized, treat-to-target trial with a 26-week extension. *J Clin Endocrinol Metab.* 2013;98(3): 1154-1162. PMID: 23393185

44 ANSWER: E) Continue the intravenous insulin drip and maintain nothing-mouth-status

At this time, the patient's anion gap is not in fact closed and she is still vomiting and having abdominal pain, so transition from the intravenous insulin drip to subcutaneous insulin (Answers A, B, and C) is not appropriate. Her albumin is low, most likely related to nutritional intake and her ongoing hyperemesis. Anion gap is underestimated in the setting of hypoalbuminemia; if albumin decreased by 1 g/L, then the anion gap decreases by 0.25 mmol. To overcome the effects of the hypoalbuminemia on the anion gap, the corrected anion gap can be used: anion gap + 0.25 × (40-albumin) expressed in g/L. When corrected for hypoalbuminemia, this patient's anion gap at the time of the proposed transition was 14.5.

If her anion gap had been closed and she met criteria for resolution of diabetic ketoacidosis (a serum glucose level <200 mg/dL [<11.1 mmol/L] and 2 of the following: serum bicarbonate >15 mEq/L [>15 mmol/L]; pH >7.3; anion gap <12 for 8 to 12 hours), transitioning to insulin detemir (Answer B) would have been the only appropriate option.

Regular insulin (U100 and U500), insulin aspart, insulin lispro (U100 and U200), NPH, and insulin detemir are all designated as pregnancy category B medications. Insulin glargine (Answer A) no longer has a pregnancy category, and its package insert states there are "no well-controlled clinical studies in pregnant women." Insulin degludec (Answer C) should only be used during pregnancy if "potential benefits justify the potential risk to the fetus." The patient has continued to be nauseated and have ongoing abdominal pain, so it is not yet appropriate for her to eat (Answer D). The best option is to continue the intravenous drip and maintain nothing-by-mouth status (Answer E).

Ultimately, the patient's corrected anion gap closed, and her regimen was transitioned from intravenous insulin to subcutaneous insulin using detemir and aspart.

EDUCATIONAL OBJECTIVE

Recommend an in-hospital insulin regimen for a pregnant patient with diabetic ketoacidosis.

REFERENCE(S)

Gosmanov AR, Gosmanova EO, Dillard-Cannon E. Management of adult diabetic ketoacidosis. *Diabetes Metab Syndr Obes.* 2014;7:255-264. PMID: 25061324

American Diabetes Association. 14. Management of diabetes in pregnancy: *standards of medical care in diabetes-2020. Diabetes Care.* 2020;43(Suppl 1): S137-S143. PMID: 31862757

Blum AK. Insulin use in pregnancy: an update. *Diabetes Spectr.* 2016;29(2):92-97. PMID: 27182178

45 ANSWER: A) Replace the sliding scale with a fixed and reduced dose of insulin with each meal

This case highlights the need for simplification strategies in pharmacotherapy for older patients with diabetes. This patient is still overinsulinized. It is not clear what insulin doses he is taking with each meal. When there may be errors in the insulin scale being used, the strategies that can be undertaken, especially in older adults such as this patient, include avoid insulin sliding scales and replacing them with fixed-dose insulin (Answer A) before meals.

Simplification strategies should be applied when barriers to diabetes self-care are present in older adults and will be matched to the barrier identified during the needs assessment process. Some examples of solutions that may be considered under these circumstances include:

- Discontinuing mealtime injections and substituting a noninsulin agent that acts to address postprandial blood glucose excursions (eg, a meglitinide) for a patient who forgets to take mealtime insulin injections

- Changing the time of day basal insulin is administered to a time the patient thinks will be easier to remember (eg, with breakfast or the evening meal instead of bedtime if the patient has been missing injections due to falling asleep right after dinner)
- Stopping meal insulin scales and starting a fixed insulin meal dose (strategy used in this case) if the patient is having trouble with numbers (health numeracy)
- Engaging family members or caregivers to give injections and minimizing number of insulin injections daily by substituting noninsulin alternative antihyperglycemic agents for those patients who cannot self-administer insulin
- Maximizing use of once-daily and/or once-weekly antihyperglycemic agents when medication doses are being missed; for older patients with multiple medications, use of a pill box or multidose pill pack pharmacy program may also be helpful if medication adherence is an issue

The patient's C-peptide level is low, so replacing his mealtime insulin with an oral agent (Answer B) to simplify his regimen is not an option, as he will need mealtime insulin onboard to control postmeal glucose levels. This is, however, often a useful strategy in older adults with adequate β-cell reserve who forget to take their mealtime insulin doses, particularly when they are on low doses (ie, <10 units of insulin per dose). His total daily dose of insulin is 47 units, so a concentrated insulin such as U500 is not indicated. While he may require a higher dosage of basal insulin as evidenced by his high overnight glucose values, the first priority is to reduce the insulin, which is leading to hypoglycemia. Thus, moving basal insulin to the morning and titrating the dose up to control fasting hyperglycemia (Answer C) is incorrect. Finally, active engagement of caregivers (Answer D) is required when cognitive function testing reveals that deficits are present, which was not the case in this man after his hypoglycemia was corrected. It is not clear based on the information provided whether this older man could effectively use an insulin pump (Answer E), so it would not be the preferred modality of therapy at this time.

The patient was advised to reduce his mealtime insulin dose to 9 units. His continuous glucose monitoring after this regimen change is shown (*see image*).

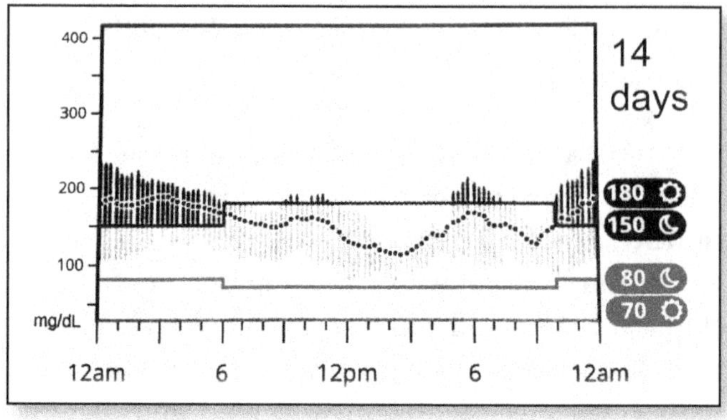

He found the continuous glucose monitoring so useful in helping to avoid hypoglycemic episodes that he obtained a personal continuous glucose monitor. At a future follow-up visit, he and his wife both observed that he was feeling a lot better, he was less tired, and his mind was sharper. Concerning the status of his diabetes, it was deemed appropriate for him to return to work.

EDUCATIONAL OBJECTIVE

Guide the strategy for simplification of the insulin regimen in older patients with hypoglycemia.

REFERENCE(S)

Munshi M. Cognitive dysfunction in older adults with diabetes: what a clinician needs to know. *Diabetes Care.* 2017;40(4):461-467. PMID: 28325796

Munshi, M, Slyne C, Segal AR, Saul N, Lyons C, Weinger K. Simplification of insulin regimen in older adults and risk of hypoglycemia. *JAMA Intern Med.* 2016;176(7):1023-1025. PMID: 27273335

Kirkman MS, Briscoe VJ, Clark N, et al. Diabetes in older adults. *Diabetes Care.* 2012;35(12): 2650-2664. PMID: 23100048

Munshi MN, Segal AR, Suhl E, et al. Frequent hypoglycemia among elderly patients with poor glycemic control. *Arch Intern Med.* 2011;171(4): 362-364. PMID: 21357814

Hay LC, Wilmshurst EG, Fulcher G. Unrecognized hypo- and hyperglycemia in well-controlled patients with type 2 diabetes mellitus: the results of continuous glucose monitoring. *Diabetes Technol Ther.* 2003;5(1):19-26. PMID: 12725703

46 ANSWER: A) Consider lifting weights for a short period before jogging to reduce the chance of hypoglycemia

With an appropriate concentration of insulin on board, aerobic activity is most often associated with a slight increase, no change, or a mild decrease in blood glucose during or shortly after the activity. Anaerobic exercise, however, often induces a rise in blood glucose levels because of an associated increase in release of catecholamines (14- to 18-fold rise). Aerobic exercise is associated with a more modest rise (2- to 4-fold) in catecholamines. Hypoglycemia is certainly still possible with aerobic exercise such as jogging, especially if the jogging is strenuous, and there is no magic number for the ideal pre-jog glucose value that will guarantee against it (thus, Answer C is incorrect). Evidence has shown that engaging in small amounts of anaerobic activity (eg, weight lifting) prior to aerobic exercise may reduce the tendency for a drop in blood glucose associated with moderate-intensity aerobic exercise (thus, Answer A is correct). It should also be noted that following anaerobic exercise, a delayed drop in blood glucose can occur. This manifests as a reduction in mean glucose 4.5 to 6 hours after exercise. This can increase the risk for hypoglycemia after weight lifting. This phenomenon can be addressed by adding an alternative lower basal insulin delivery rate during the postexercise period when blood glucose levels are lower. Increasing her basal rate during jogging (Answer B) could heighten the risk for hypoglycemia by increasing the insulin onboard during the activity. Physical activity is recommended for patients with type 1 diabetes because regular exercise is associated with a longer life and a lower frequency of complications. Thus, avoiding aerobic activity to avoid hypoglycemia (Answer D) is incorrect.

EDUCATIONAL OBJECTIVE

Advise patients with type 1 diabetes about the effects of exercise on the risk of hypoglycemia.

REFERENCE(S)

Lumb AN, Gallen IW. Diabetes management for intense exercise. *Curr Opin Endocrinol Diabetes Obes.* 2009;16(2):150-155. PMID: 19300093

Yardley JE, Sigal RJ, Perkins BA, Riddell MC, Kenny GP. Resistance exercise in type 1 diabetes. *Can J Diabetes.* 2013;37(6):420-426. PMID: 24321724

Yardley JE, Kenny GP, Perkins BA. Resistance versus aerobic exercise: acute effects on glycemia in type 1 diabetes. *Diabetes Care.* 2013;36(3):537-542. PMID: 23172972

Cryer PE. Mechanisms of hypoglycemia-associated autonomic failure in diabetes. *N Engl J Med.* 2013;369(4):362-372. PMID: 23883381

Davis SN, Tate D, Hedrington MS. Mechanisms of hypoglycemia and exercise-associated autonomic dysfunction. *Trans Am Clin Climatol Assoc.* 2014;125:281-291. PMID: 25125745

47 ANSWER: E) >90%

The annual incidence of diabetic retinopathy ranges from 2.2% to 12.7%, and the incidence of progression ranges from 3.4% to 12.3%. Progression to proliferative diabetic retinopathy is higher in individuals with mild disease than in those with no disease at baseline. Understanding the available treatment options for persons with diabetic retinopathy is key because targeted glycemic, blood pressure, and lipid control has been shown to reduce both the incidence and progression of retinopathy.

The American Diabetes Association recommends retinopathy screening by an eye specialist within 5 years of the diagnosis of type 1 diabetes in adults. Patients with type 2 diabetes should have an initial dilated and comprehensive eye examination by an ophthalmologist or optometrist at the time of the diabetes diagnosis, as microvascular changes can begin before diagnosis if prediabetes has been present. Female patients should be advised to have a dilated eye exam before conception or during the first trimester of pregnancy, and then every trimester and for 1 year postpartum. If any level of diabetic retinopathy is present, subsequent dilated retinal examinations for patients with type 1 (or type 2) diabetes should be repeated at least annually by an ophthalmologist or optometrist. If retinopathy is progressive or sight-threatening, examinations are required more frequently.

Management recommendations call for optimizing glycemic control, blood pressure, and lipids to reduce the risk or slow the progression of retinopathy. It is important to emphasize to the patient that attention to lifestyle and pharmacotherapeutic measures to optimize blood glucose, blood pressure, and lipids can be highly effective and would indeed reduce risk of progression of her eye changes by more than 90% (Answer E). Effective metabolic control will significantly reduce her risk of progression to proliferative retinopathy, macular edema, and the need for laser or alternative treatments, thus protecting sight.

If retinopathy does advance, current therapeutic options can be remarkably effective at preventing severe vision loss when administered in an appropriate and timely manner.

EDUCATIONAL OBJECTIVE

Counsel a patient on the impact of appropriate medical care on the risk of vision loss in type 1 diabetes.

REFERENCE(S)

American Diabetes Association. 11. Microvascular complications and foot care: standards of medical care in diabetes-2020. *Diabetes Care.* 2020;43(Suppl 1): S135-S151. PMID: 31862754

Sabanayagam C, Banu R, Chee ML, et al. Incidence and progression of diabetic retinopathy: a systematic review. *Lancet Diabetes Endocrinol.* 2019;7(2):140-149. PMID: 30005958

Bloomgarden ZT. Screening for and managing diabetic retinopathy: current approaches. *Am J Health Syst Pharm.* 2007;64(17 Suppl 12):S8-S14. PMID: 17720893

48 ANSWER: A) Diabetic radiculopathy

Diabetic neuropathy is generally more common in patients with long disease duration and poor glycemic control. Classification is subdivided into somatosensory, motor, and autonomic.

Diabetes-related radiculopathy (Answer A) manifests as acute sensory and/or motor neuropathy characterized by sudden pain and dysesthesias and/or muscle weakness in the distribution of 1 or more individual peripheral nerves or nerve roots. The patient in this vignette has right-sided facial pain and muscle weakness in the distribution of the facial (seventh cranial) nerve. This is an acute mononeuropathy or radiculitis. There is no specific therapy for this complication. The patient can be reassured that it typically resolves after 2 to 3 months. Neuropathy pain relief medications such as tricyclic antidepressants or selective serotonin and norepinephrine reuptake inhibitors may be given in the interim. The most common presentation of neuropathy with diabetes involves damage to sensory nerve fibers and typically affects the distal extremities in a "stocking-glove" distribution as this patient has on examination. Affected patients describe numbness, paresthesias, and occasionally sharp pains.

Autonomic dysfunction (Answer B) may affect 1 or several organ systems including the vasculature (orthostatic hypotension), the heart (silent ischemia, abnormal cardiac rhythms), the gastrointestinal tract (gastroparesis, constipation, diarrhea from bacterial overgrowth), and the urinary bladder (atonic bladder, chronic urinary tract infections, overflow incontinence). It does not cause pain syndromes.

Herpes zoster (Answer C) can cause localized pain in a pattern similar to that described here, and pain can precede the typical rash but not usually for about 1 week after the onset of pain. Otitis media (Answer D) can spread to the facial nerve and inflame it, causing compression of the nerve in its canal; however, there is no evidence of otitis on his exam. Findings on his head CT do not suggest cerebrovascular accident (Answer E).

EDUCATIONAL OBJECTIVE

Diagnose less common manifestations of diabetic neuropathy.

REFERENCE(S)

Tesfaye S, Boulton AJ, Dyck PJ, et al; Toronto Diabetic Neuropathy Expert Group. Diabetic neuropathies: update on definitions, diagnostic criteria, estimation of severity, and treatments. *Diabetes Care.* 2010;33(10):2285-2293. PMID: 20876709

Casellini CM, Vinik AI. Clinical manifestations and current treatment options for diabetic neuropathies. *Endocr Pract.* 2007;13(5):550-566. PMID: 17872358

49 ANSWER: C) Glucagonoma syndrome

The development of type 2 diabetes, particularly in a relatively abrupt fashion, is unusual and should prompt consideration of a secondary cause. The presence of new-onset diabetes and necrotizing migratory erythema accompanied by weight loss suggests glucagonoma syndrome (Answer C), which has a mean age of presentation of 55 years. Other clinical features can include anemia, stomatitis, thromboembolism (as seen in this patient), and gastrointestinal and neuropsychiatric disturbances.

Necrolytic migratory erythema is the typical rash associated with glucagonoma syndrome (present in 80% of cases), as observed in this patient. It can be itchy and painful, and it often affects the genital and anal region, groin, buttocks, and lower legs, but any site may be involved. Necrolytic migratory erythema is nontender with irregular borders, sometimes associated with scaling or crusting, and it progresses through an initial ring-shaped red area that blisters, erodes, then crusts over and leaves behind a brown mark.

Glucagonomas are rare neuroendocrine tumors of the pancreas (others include insulinomas, somatostatinomas, carcinoid, and nonsecreting neuroendocrine tumors). In this setting, hyperglycemia, which is typically quite severe, results predominantly through the counterregulatory effects of glucagon. In larger tumors, destruction of nearby islet cells and pancreatic insulin secretion may also have an etiologic role.

Glucagonomas are often malignant and frequently present already metastatic to the liver. If localized, surgical resection is necessary. Unless large portions of the pancreas are sacrificed, hyperglycemia typically resolves relatively rapidly postoperatively. If metastatic or residual tumor is demonstrated after surgery, somatostatin receptor agonist therapy (eg, octreotide, lanreotide) should be considered.

Other etiologies of secondary diabetes include medication-induced (eg, corticosteroids), other endocrinopathies (eg, acromegaly [Answer A]), Cushing disease [Answer D]), pancreatic diseases (eg, pancreatitis), infections (eg, cytomegalovirus), and genetic conditions (eg, Rabson-Mendenhall syndrome [Answer B]). Latent autoimmune diabetes (Answer E) is not a secondary cause of diabetes and is not associated with skin lesions at the time of presentation.

EDUCATIONAL OBJECTIVE

Diagnose glucagonoma as a secondary cause of diabetes mellitus.

REFERENCE(S)

Jabbour SA. Skin manifestations of hormone-secreting tumors. *Dermatol Ther.* 2010;23(6): 643-650. PMID: 21054708

Warner RR. Enteroendocrine tumors other than carcinoid: a review of clinically significant advances. *Gastroenterology.* 2005;128(6):1668-1684. PMID: 15887158

Chastain MA. The glucagonoma syndrome: a review of its features and discussion of new perspectives. *Am J Med Sci.* 2001;321(5):306-320. PMID: 11370794

50 ANSWER: A) Both temperature and altitude

Several physical factors influence the accuracy of blood glucose strips; the most common are altitude and temperature (thus, Answer A is correct and Answers B, C, and D are incorrect).

Persons with diabetes who intend to participate in activities at high altitude or at low temperature, should be informed that blood glucose meters may give unreliable false low or high readings. The partial pressure of oxygen in a plane cabin is 16 kPa compared with 21 kPa at sea level. Thus, there is a risk that a glucose meter could indicate false hypoglycemia or normoglycemia while in the air, when the true value in fact could be higher. Glucose dehydrogenase–based meters perform better than the glucose oxidase–based meter at high altitude. However, at low temperature, all tested meters perform with similar magnitudes of discrepancy.

Temperature can also indirectly affect readings by influencing circulation to the skin (cold temperature), which may particularly influence results of alternate site testing.

EDUCATIONAL OBJECTIVE

Identify environmental factors that can affect the accuracy of blood glucose meter readings.

REFERENCE(S)

Jendle J, Adolfsson P. Impact of high altitudes on glucose control. *J Diabetes Sci Technol.* 2011;5(6) 1621-1622. PMID: 22226288

Öberg D, Östenson CG. Performance of glucose dehydrogenase-and glucose oxidase-based blood glucose meters at high altitude and low temperature. *Diabetes Care.* 2005;28(5):1261. PMID: 15855608

Olansky L, Kennedy L. Finger-stick glucose monitoring: issues of accuracy and specificity. *Diabetes Care.* 2010;33(4):948-949. PMID: 20351231

51 ANSWER: C) Nonadherence to insulin therapy

Hospitalizations for diabetic ketoacidosis are increasing in the United States. Diabetic ketoacidosis is a common, life-threatening complication of diabetes, accounting for as many as 4% to 9% of all hospital admissions in patients with diabetes. Diabetic ketoacidosis is the leading cause of mortality among children and young adults with type 1 diabetes, accounting for 50% of all deaths in this population. Most cases of diabetic ketoacidosis are associated with type 1 diabetes, but 1 in 5 cases of diabetic ketoacidosis are associated with a history of type 2 diabetes.

There are many precipitating causes of diabetic ketoacidosis, with one of the most common being undertreatment or omission of insulin doses (Answer C). There are higher prevalence rates of eating disorders among persons with type 1 diabetes, as compared with their peers without diabetes. Given the detailed meal planning, precision in food portions, and constant monitoring of food intake (carbohydrates in particular) related to insulin doses recommended for diabetes management, persons with diabetes may be inherently more prone to issues revolving around food. Eating disorders and disordered eating behaviors—especially insulin omission—are associated with suboptimal glycemic control and serious risk for increased morbidity, including diabetic ketoacidosis and mortality. Insulin omission is sometimes viewed as a weight-control strategy. This patient has euglycemic diabetic ketoacidosis because she has been taking correction insulin doses since she developed hyperglycemia symptoms.

Although this patient's serum creatinine concentration is elevated, there is clear evidence of volume depletion, and this is a more likely reason for her azotemia than acute kidney injury (Answer A).

Atypical antipsychotic agents (Answer B) have been linked to weight gain and rarely to diabetic ketoacidosis, but these instances have been in the setting of type 2 diabetes.

Unrecognized pregnancy (Answer D) is also a precipitating factor for diabetic ketoacidosis, but this patient is taking an oral contraceptive. Nonetheless, a pregnancy test is needed to rule out this possibility.

EDUCATIONAL OBJECTIVE

Identify eating disorders and omission of insulin doses as a cause of diabetic ketoacidosis in type 1 diabetes.

REFERENCE(S)

Vellanki P, Umpierrez GE. Increasing hospitalizations for DKA: a need for prevention programs. *Diabetes Care.* 2018;41(9):1839-1841. PMID: 301135197

Hanlan ME, Griffith J, Patel N, Jaser SS. Eating disorders and disordered eating in type 1 diabetes: prevalence, screening, and treatment options. *Curr Diab Rep.* 2013. PMID: 24022608

Steenkamp DW, Alexanian SM, McDonnell ME. Adult hyperglycemic crisis: a review and perspective. *Curr Diab Rep.* 2013;13(1):130-137. PMID: 23115048

Guenette MD, Hahn M, Cohn TA, Teo C, Remington GJ. Atypical antipsychotics and diabetic ketoacidosis: a review. *Psychopharmacology (Berl).* 2013;226(1):1-12. PMID: 23344556

Kitabchi AE, Umpierrez GE, Miles JM, Fisher JN. Hyperglycemic crises in adult patients with diabetes. *Diabetes Care.* 2009;32(7): 1335-1343. PMID: 19564476

52 ANSWER: A) Insulin autoantibody assessment

Hypoglycemia in patients without diabetes mellitus has a broad differential. In unprovoked hypoglycemia in patients with preexisting autoimmune disease (such as Graves disease), the possibility of insulin autoantibody syndrome (Hirata disease) should be strongly considered. In this condition, first described by Hirata et al in 1970, autoantibodies (IgG) are produced that bind insulin with variable affinity, which may result in glucose intolerance. Sudden dissociation of prebound insulin from the antibody results, however, in unpredictable episodes of hypoglycemia. This can be seen as a rare adverse reaction to methimazole, and almost all cases of methimazole-induced insulin autoimmune syndrome are reported in East Asia, especially in Japan. This association is due to the DRB1*0406 genotype, which is relatively common in persons of East Asian descent, and it is exclusively associated with an elevated risk of developing methimazole-induced insulin autoimmune syndrome. Additionally, the specific allelic combination of HLA-Bw62/Cw4/DR4 carrying DRB1*0406 is a major genetic risk factor. Thus, the best next step in this vignette is an insulin autoantibody assessment (Answer A).

All the other answer choices are unlikely to reveal the precise cause of the hypoglycemia. A sulfonylurea screen (Answer B) is appropriate in all cases in which endogenous insulin and C-peptide hypersecretion are demonstrated. It is an unlikely culprit here, however, given the strong history of autoimmunity and the lack of apparent access to antihyperglycemic drugs. Both C-peptide and insulin levels should be obtained. In Hirata disease, increased insulin levels are usually demonstrated, particularly if the insulin assay cannot distinguish between bound and unbound insulin. C-peptide levels are variable, but usually detectable. There is nothing in the history to suggest hypoadrenalism. Although cortisol (Answer C) should be measured routinely in the evaluation of hypoglycemia, it is most likely to be normal (or high if obtained when the patient has hypoglycemia). Overexpression of insulinlike growth factor 2 (Answer D) in β cells leads to β-cell dysfunction and makes islet cells more vulnerable to β-cell damage, which can result in diabetes rather than hypoglycemia. Metanephrines (Answer E) secreted by a pheochromocytoma are likely to increase blood glucose levels.

EDUCATIONAL OBJECTIVE

Investigate causes of hypoglycemia not related to treatment of diabetes mellitus.

REFERENCE(S)

Lupsa BC, Chong AY, Cochran EK, Soos MA, Semple RK, Gorden P. Autoimmune forms of hypoglycemia. *Medicine (Baltimore).* 2009;88(3): 141-153. PMID: 19440117

Uchigata Y, Kuwata S, Tsushima T, et al. Patients with Graves' disease who developed insulin autoimmune syndrome (Hirata disease) possess HLA-Bw62/Cw4/DR4 carrying DRB1*0406. *J Clin Endocrinol Metab.* 1993;77(1):249-254. PMID: 8325948

53 ANSWER: C) Ask him to demonstrate how he self-administers insulin injections

This patient is overweight and is taking 288 units of insulin daily, corresponding to 2.8 units/kg per day. This is a large dose for a man of his size (BMI = 26 kg/m^2). When the patient was asked to demonstrate how he self-administers an injection of insulin aspart (Answer C), he dialed the dose into the pen correctly and administered the shot in his upper arm. The dose appeared to have been delivered (as the pen read "zero"); however, there was a stream of insulin dribbling down his arm from the injection site. Thus, it was not clear what insulin dose he had actually received. This patient clearly needs instruction in insulin self-administration technique, and this emergency department visit represents an opportunity to initiate basic diabetes self-management education.

Many patients with diabetes do not receive adequate diabetes self-management education to support optimal self-care outcomes. Despite evidence that diabetes self-management education reduces the number of emergency department visits and hospitalizations, lowers hemoglobin A_{1c}, and improves other outcomes, less than 55% of US patients with diabetes receive this type of education over the course of their illness and less than 7% receive it within the first year of diagnosis.

This patient's blood glucose has responded well to hydration and subcutaneous insulin. He is therefore clinically stable for discharge home. Thus, admitting him to the hospital (Answer A) is incorrect.

U500 regular insulin (Answer B) is used to treat patients with insulin resistance. If he had been taking all of the insulin prescribed and his blood glucose values were indeed persistently high, then this concentrated insulin would be a reasonable choice for his glycemic management. He was actually receiving an insulin dose that would be high for him if the entire dose were being delivered correctly. He does not require such a high total daily dose of insulin.

Increasing the insulin doses by 30% (Answer D) is the rule of thumb that his endocrinologist has been following when making insulin adjustments. However, in view of his body size and the high number of units of insulin per kg body weight—and yet still no response in terms of blood glucose lowering—something else is going on.

EDUCATIONAL OBJECTIVE

Evaluate the need for diabetes self-management and skills education in patients with suboptimally controlled diabetes mellitus.

REFERENCE(S)

Powers MA, Bardsley J, Cypress M, et al. Diabetes self-management education and support in type 2 diabetes: a joint position statement of the American Diabetes Association, the American Association of Diabetes Educators, and the Academy of Nutrition and Dietetics. *Diabetes Care.* 2015;38(7):1372-1382. PMID: 26048904

Magee MF, Nassar CN, Reyes-Castano J, McDonnell ME. In: Draznin B, ed. Emergency Department Management of Diabetes Patients with Non-crisis Hyperglycemia. *Managing Diabetes and Hyperglycemia in the Hospital Setting.* American Diabetes Association; 2016.

Lowery JB, Donihi AC, Korytkowski MT. U-500 insulin as a component of basal bolus insulin therapy in type 2 diabetes. *Diabetes Technol Ther.* 2012;14(6):505-507. PMID: 22364143

Rodriguez K, Meneghini L, Seley JJ, Magee MF. In: Draznin B, ed. Patient Education. *Managing Diabetes and Hyperglycemia in the Hospital Setting.* American Diabetes Association; 2016.

54 ANSWER: B) Insulin glargine U100, 8 units twice daily plus regular insulin every 6 hours

When selecting a subcutaneous insulin regimen for this man with diabetes mellitus, an effort should be made to prescribe a physiologic basal-bolus regimen that will meet both his basal insulin requirements and nutritional insulin needs.

The underlying principles of subcutaneous insulin therapy for patients receiving enteral nutrition call for use of judicious basal insulin therapy, so that if the tube feedings are interrupted the patient will not become hypoglycemic. For the basal insulin dosing, a weight-based starting dose of 0.2 units/kg per day (16 units daily in this case) (Answer B) or 40% of the total daily dose of insulin administered via insulin infusion before the transition (22 units/day in this case) are the rules of thumb. This may be administered as insulins glargine or detemir once daily or in a split dose twice daily, or as short (regular U100 insulin) every 6 hours—the latter can also provide a steady 24-hour basal action profile. Use of NPH insulin (2 to 3 times daily) has also been reported in this clinical setting. However, NPH insulin once daily (Answer A) is incorrect because this would not provide continuous basal insulin coverage.

Regular insulin administered every 4 hours (Answer C) would lead to insulin stacking and hypoglycemia. Insulin glargine U300 (Answer D) has not been evaluated for use in the inpatient setting. Nutritional insulin needs will be met using regular insulin via a scaled dose of either regular U100 insulin every 6 hours or rapid-acting insulin analogue every 4 hours.

Only 1 published randomized controlled trial has examined specific subcutaneous insulin regimens in patients with diabetes receiving enteral nutrition. Fifty patients were randomly assigned to sliding-scale regular insulin alone or sliding-scale regular insulin plus glargine. By the end of the insulin titration period, 48% of the patients randomly assigned to sliding-scale regular insulin alone required the addition of NPH insulin to the regimen for persistent hyperglycemia (blood glucose >180 mg/dL [>10 mmol/L]).

The Endocrine Society Clinical Practice Guideline on management of hyperglycemia in the hospital outlines approaches depending on which type of enteral nutrition is being given (*see table*).

Enteral nutrition administration method	Potential approach to subcutaneous insulin therapy
Continuous	• Basal insulin once daily (glargine or detemir) or twice-daily detemir or NPH • Short- or rapid-acting every 4 hours (rapid) or every 6 hours (regular)
Cycled	• Basal insulin once daily (glargine, detemir, or NPH) with short- or rapid-acting at start of enteral nutrition • Repeat the rapid-acting every 4 hours or the regular every 6 hours
Bolus	• Short- or rapid-acting insulin before each bolus*

*With judicious dose of basal insulin as described above if indicated (eg, if on insulin therapy before hospital admission and/or there is persistent hyperglycemia across a 24-hour period).

EDUCATIONAL OBJECTIVE

Order a physiologic basal-bolus insulin regimen for patients receiving enteral nutrition.

REFERENCE(S)

Korytkowski MT, Salata RJ, Koerbel GL, et al. Insulin therapy and glycemic control in hospitalized patients with diabetes during enteral nutrition therapy. *Diabetes Care.* 2009;32(4):594-596. PMID: 19336639

Umpierrez GE, Hellman R, Korytkowski MT, et al; Endocrine Society. Management of hyperglycemia in hospitalized patients in non-critical care setting: an Endocrine Society clinical practice guideline. *J Clin Endocrinol Metab.* 2012;97(1):16-38. PMID: 22223765

Low Wang CC, Hawkins M, Gianchandani R, Dungan K. Glycemic control in the setting or parenteral nutrition or enteral nutrition via tube-feeding. In: Draznin B, ed. *Managing Diabetes and Hyperglycemia in the Hospital Setting.* American Diabetes Association; 2016.

55 ANSWER: B) Vascular segmental pressures and pulse volume recordings

This patient has multiple risk factors for atherosclerosis, including diabetes, retinopathy, chronic kidney disease, hypertension, and hyperlipidemia. His diabetes, blood pressure, and lipids are well controlled on his current regimen. Diagnosing peripheral vascular disease is clinically important for several reasons: (1) to identify whether the patent is at high risk for cardiovascular disease and stroke; (2) to reduce the risk for foot ulcers, functional disability, and limb amputations; and (3) to ensure that revascularization may be considered in cases where the limb is threatened or a foot ulcer fails to heal.

He may have peripheral arterial disease with intermittent claudication. It should be noted that dorsalis pedis pulses are reported to be absent in 8.1% of healthy individuals, and the posterior tibial pulse is absent in 2.0%. Nevertheless, the absence of both pedal pulses strongly suggests the presence of vascular disease.

His ankle brachial index is 1.4. The diagnostic criteria for peripheral arterial disease based on the ankle brachial index are as follows:

0.91-1.30 = normal
0.70-0.90 = mild obstruction
0.40-0.69 = moderate obstruction
<0.40 = severe obstruction
>1.30 = poorly compressible

An ankle brachial index greater than 1.3 suggests poorly compressible arteries at the ankle due to the presence of calcification, which is a common finding in patients with diabetes and atherosclerosis. Calcification makes the diagnosis of peripheral arterial disease by ankle brachial index alone less reliable, so the diagnosis should be confirmed by sending this patient to the vascular lab to have his vascular segmental pressures and pulse volumes checked (Answer B). In patients with confirmed peripheral arterial disease, these tests are used to localize disease and determine its severity. As in this patient's case, these tests are also helpful when poorly compressible vessels are present. Finally, these tests are also used when the ankle brachial index is normal and when there is high suspicion of peripheral arterial disease. Segmental pressures help with lesion localization. Pulse volume recordings provide segmental waveform analysis for a qualitative assessment of blood flow.

The other listed assessments are used in different case scenarios or at intermediate points in the workup of peripheral arterial disease. Treadmill functional testing (Answer D) is used if the patient has a normal ankle brachial index with typical symptoms of claudication. Further noninvasive studies are used to guide clinical decision-making regarding potential for revascularization to be done when a patient has a nonhealing foot ulcer or rest ischemic pain. Transcutaneous oxygen pressure (Answer A) is used to predict capacity to heal a foot ulcer. A value less than 30 mm Hg is associated with poor wound healing or amputations. Systolic toe pressure (Answer C) less than 40 mm Hg or toe waveform less than 4 mm also predicts poor wound healing. Systolic toe pressure may be also be used as an adjunctive test to evaluate patients who have medial arterial calcification, for whom the ankle brachial index is less accurate. Angiography (Answer E) would be undertaken only if evidence of circulatory impairment is found on noninvasive testing.

EDUCATIONAL OBJECTIVE

Order appropriate initial tests when a patient is suspected to have peripheral arterial disease.

REFERENCE(S)

American Diabetes Association. Peripheral arterial disease in people with diabetes. *Diabetes Care.* 2003;26(12):3333-3341. PMID: 14633825

56 ANSWER: D) Maturity-onset diabetes of the young

Maturity-onset diabetes of the young (MODY) (Answer D) is a monogenic form of diabetes, inherited in an autosomal dominant manner, and it accounts for 1% to 5% of all cases of diabetes in the United States. Unlike type 1 or type 2 diabetes, MODY is caused by a single-gene pathogenic variant that primarily affects β-cell function. Correctly diagnosing monogenic forms of diabetes is important because an incorrect diagnosis of type 1 or type 2 diabetes can result in suboptimal treatment and delays in diagnosing other family members. The most common form, MODY 3, is associated with pathogenic variants in genes encoding hepatic transcription factors (hepatocyte nuclear factor 1α or transcription factor 1). The second most common form, MODY 2, is associated with pathogenic variants in the glucokinase gene.

A diagnosis of MODY should be considered in patients who present with the following findings: (1) mild fasting hyperglycemia (100-150 mg/dL [5.6-8.3 mmol/L]), especially if nonobese, as is the case in this young woman; (2) lack of typical features of type 2 diabetes, including obesity; (3) lack of diabetes-associated autoantibodies; (4) multiple family members with diabetes not clearly type 1 or type 2 diabetes; and (5) diabetes diagnosed within the first 6 months of life. These characteristics distinguish MODY from type 1 diabetes (Answer A), type 2 diabetes (Answer B), and latent autoimmune diabetes in adults

(Answer E). Given this patient's personal and strong family history, MODY is the most likely diagnosis. Commercial genetic testing is now available. Gestational diabetes (Answer C) would not be diagnosed until the late second or early third trimester.

EDUCATIONAL OBJECTIVE

Diagnose maturity-onset diabetes of the young and contrast this condition with type 1 and type 2 diabetes.

REFERENCE(S)

American Diabetes Association. 2. Classification and diagnosis of diabetes: standards of medical care in diabetes-2020. *Diabetes Care.* 2016;43(Suppl 1): S14-S31. PMID: 31862745

Sanyoura M, Philipson LH, Naylor R. Monogenic diabetes in children and adolescents: recognition and treatment options. *Curr Diab Rep.* 2018;18(8): 58. PMID: 29931562

Rubio-Cabezas O, Hattersley AT, Njølstad PR, et al; International Society for Pediatric and Adolescent Diabetes. ISPAD Clinical Practice Consensus Guidelines 2014. The diagnosis and management of monogenic diabetes in children and adolescents. *Pediatr Diabetes.* 2014;15(Suppl 20):47-64. PMID: 25182307

Female Reproduction Board Review

Kathryn A. Martin, MD

1 ANSWER: C) Reassurance; no evaluation needed

Amenorrhea is a common occurrence in women taking certain oral contraception regimens. It is due to the development of an atrophic endometrium (progestin effect). Amenorrhea eventually develops in most women on continuous preparations (hormone pills only, no placebos), but it also can occur in women using cyclic preparations, most commonly the 20-mcg pills, which are more progestin-dominant than the 30- to 35-mcg preparations. Women should be reassured that the pill is effective and that no further evaluation is needed (Answer C). As long as they have not missed pills or started medications that interfere with estrogen's metabolism, monthly pregnancy tests (Answer D) are unnecessary. Some women prefer to switch to a different preparation with a higher dose of estrogen that is less likely to result in an atrophic endometrium, in order to restore menstrual bleeding each month. Many clinicians worry that a new endocrine disorder has developed when amenorrhea occurs in this setting, but the amenorrhea is a reflection of the endometrial response to the exogenous estrogen and progestin. Thus, serum prolactin measurement (Answer A), FSH measurement (Answer B), and endometrial biopsy (Answer E) are not necessary.

EDUCATIONAL OBJECTIVE

Recommend the best course of action for women who develop amenorrhea on low-dosage oral estrogen-progestin contraceptives.

REFERENCE(S)

Hillard PA. Menstrual suppression: current perspectives. *Int J Womens Health.* 2014;6:631-637. PMID: 25018654

Archer DF. Menstrual-cycle-related symptoms: a review of the rationale for continuous use of oral contraceptives. *Contraception.* 2006;74(5): 359-366. PMID: 17046376

2 ANSWER: A) No further testing needed

A number of different criteria have been proposed for the diagnosis of polycystic ovary syndrome (PCOS). Most often used are the Rotterdam criteria, which require 2 of the following 3 findings: hyperandrogenism, oligomenorrhea, and polycystic ovarian morphology on ultrasonography. This patient already meets 2 criteria (oligomenorrhea and hyperandrogenism [hirsutism]). Therefore, ultrasonography to demonstrate polycystic ovarian morphology (Answer E) is not essential. No additional evaluation is needed (Answer A). The LH-to-FSH ratio (Answer C) and free testosterone measurement (Answer B) are not part of the diagnostic criteria for PCOS. Serum antimullerian hormone (Answer D) is increased in most women with PCOS, but it has not been validated as a diagnostic test.

Many women with irregular menses and hyperandrogenic symptoms can be diagnosed based on the history and physical examination findings alone. However, the diagnosis of PCOS is only confirmed when other conditions that mimic PCOS are excluded (eg, disorders that cause oligoovulation, anovulation, and/or hyperandrogenism, such as thyroid disease, nonclassic congenital adrenal hyperplasia, hyperprolactinemia, and androgen-secreting tumors).

A figure explaining the Ferriman-Gallwey hirsutism scoring system can be found in the Endocrine Society Clinical Practice Guideline: Evaluation and Treatment of Hirsutism in Premenopausal Women.

EDUCATIONAL OBJECTIVE

Identify the diagnostic criteria for polycystic ovary syndrome.

REFERENCE(S)

Martin KA, Anderson RR, Chang RJ, et al. Evaluation and treatment of hirsutism in premenopausal women: an Endocrine Society clinical practice guideline. *J Clin Endocrinol Metab.* 2018;103(4): 1233-1257. PMID: 29522147

Teede HJ, Misso ML, Costello MF, et al; International PCOS Network. Recommendations from the international evidence-based guideline for the assessment and management of polycystic ovary syndrome. *Fertil Steril.* 2018;110(3): 364-379. PMID: 30033227

Ahmad AK, Quinn M, Kao CN, et al. Improved diagnostic performance for the diagnosis of polycystic ovary syndrome using age-stratified criteria. *Fertil Steril.* 2019;111(4):787-793. PMID: 30871762

Alsamarai S, Adams JM, Murphy MK, et al. Criteria for polycystic ovarian morphology in polycystic ovary syndrome as a function of age. *J Clin Endocrinol Metab.* 2009;94(12):4961-4970. PMID: 19846740

3 ANSWER: D) Oral estrogen-progestin contraceptive (ethinyl estradiol, 20 mcg/norethindrone acetate, 1 mg)

This patient has oligomenorrhea and significant hyperandrogenism (hirsutism), and she desires contraception. The best option would be a combined oral contraceptive containing a low dose of ethinyl estradiol (eg 20 mcg), with a neutral or nonandrogenic progestin (in this case, norethindrone acetate) (Answer D). This approach is consistent with the Endocrine Society clinical practice guidelines. Although she is 38 years old, she appears to be at low risk for adverse events. She has a low risk of cardiovascular disease and has no history of migraine headaches, gallbladder disease, or personal or family history of venous thromboembolism. Her calculated 5-year risk of breast cancer is similar to that of other women her age.

A levonorgestrel-releasing intrauterine device would provide contraception, and laser hair removal would benefit her hirsutism (Answer B). However, the laser therapy would be more successful if she were also on pharmacologic therapy to suppress her androgens (a combined oral contraceptive or antiandrogen such as spironolactone). If not, she will continue to regrow terminal hairs and require frequent laser treatments. There are also reports of levonorgestrel-releasing intrauterine devices causing alopecia and exacerbating depression, particularly in women with polycystic ovary syndrome.

Spironolactone and barrier contraception (Answer C) would help her hirsutism and provide some degree of contraception but would not treat her irregular menses. This would leave her at risk for endometrial hyperplasia due to unopposed endogenous estrogen.

Combined oral contraceptives with a higher dose of ethinyl estradiol (50 mcg) (Answer A) are now rarely used because they are associated with higher risks of thromboembolism and stroke.

The combination of a levonorgestrel-releasing intrauterine device and flutamide (an antiandrogen) (Answer E) would not be an optimal choice. The Endocrine Society specifically recommends against the use of flutamide because of its potential hepatotoxicity.

EDUCATIONAL OBJECTIVE

Recommend treatment for a patient with multiple clinical manifestations of polycystic ovary syndrome.

REFERENCE(S)

Martin KA, Anderson RR, Chang RJ, et al. Evaluation and treatment of hirsutism in premenopausal women: an Endocrine Society clinical practice guideline. *J Clin Endocrinol Metab.* 2018;103(4): 1233-1257. PMID: 29522147

Somani N, Turvy D. Hirsutism: an evidence-based treatment update. *Am J Clin Dermatol.* 2014;15(3): 247-266. PMID: 24889738

4 ANSWER: B) 46,XX

This patient most likely has mullerian agenesis. Mullerian agenesis or hypoplasia leads to variable uterine development and congenital absence of the vagina, termed the Mayer-Rokitansky-Kuster-Hauser syndrome. The uterus may be underdeveloped or absent. Affected persons have a normal female phenotype at birth, are raised as girls, have functioning ovaries, normal external genitalia, and a 46,XX karyotype (Answer B). Breast development and growth of pubic hair are also normal.

Patients with complete androgen insensitivity who are diagnosed during their teenage years present with primary amenorrhea, absence of axillary or pubic hair, serum testosterone within or above the normal range for boys and men, high LH, and normal FSH. Mullerian structures are absent (blind vaginal pouch and absent uterus and cervix), and the karyotype is 46,XY (Answer C). This disorder is due to a defect in the androgen receptor that results in complete resistance to androgens. Women with Turner syndrome have short stature, primary hypogonadism, a high rate of cardiovascular anomalies, a number of comorbidities, and a 45,X karyotype (Answer A). A 46,XXY karyotype (Answer D) is seen in patients with Klinefelter syndrome and such individuals have a male, not female, phenotype.

EDUCATIONAL OBJECTIVE

Distinguish between complete androgen insensitivity syndrome and mullerian agenesis in young women who present with primary amenorrhea.

REFERENCE(S)

Doehnert U, Bertelloni S, Werner R, Dati E, Hiort O. Characteristic features of reproductive hormone profiles in late adolescent and adult females with complete androgen insensitivity syndrome. *Sex Dev.* 2015;9(2):69-74. PMID: 25613104

Grimbizis GF, Gordts S, Di Spiezio Sardo A, et al. The ESHRE/ESGE consensus on the classification of female genital tract congenital anomalies. *Hum Reprod.* 2013;28(8):2032-2044. PMID: 23771171

5 ANSWER: D) In vitro fertilization with donor oocytes

This woman has spontaneous primary ovarian insufficiency. Her primary ovarian insufficiency is not due to Turner syndrome, fragile X premutation, or autoimmune oophoritis. Fertility strategies for women with ovulatory infertility (without ovarian insufficiency) are ovulation induction agents. For example, women with polycystic ovary syndrome are treated with either letrozole (Answer E) or clomiphene citrate (Answer A). However, neither would work in patients with ovarian insufficiency. Low-dosage estradiol therapy (Answer B), exogenous gonadotropins, and GnRH agonists followed by exogenous gonadotropins (Answer C) have all been used to induce ovulation in women with primary ovarian insufficiency, but none have been successful. One successful strategy has been in vitro fertilization with donor oocytes (Answer D). Other options include embryo donation and adoption. If this patient had Turner syndrome, a careful cardiovascular evaluation would be required before considering in vitro fertilization with donor oocytes, as death from aortic dissection has been reported during pregnancy.

EDUCATIONAL OBJECTIVE

Recommend treatment options for women with primary ovarian insufficiency and infertility.

REFERENCE(S)

Practice Committee of American Society for Reproductive Medicine. Increased maternal cardiovascular mortality associated with pregnancy in women with Turner syndrome. *Fertil Steril.* 2012;97(2):282-284. PMID: 22192347

Ameratunga D, Weston G, Osianlis T, Catt J, Vollenhoven B. In vitro fertilisation (IVF) with donor eggs in post-menopausal women: are there differences in pregnancy outcomes in women with premature ovarian failure (POF) compared with women with physiological age-related menopause? *J Assist Reprod Genet.* 2009;26(9-10):511-514. PMID: 19847640

6 ANSWER: A) Increase in oily skin

This transgender man has been started on testosterone therapy. He can anticipate masculinizing effects, many of which are not seen until after 6 to 12 months of therapy, including deepening of the voice (Answer B) and increased muscle strength (Answer E). In contrast, an increase in oily skin (Answer A) (and sometimes acne) can occur within the first 6 months of treatment. Androgen administration is associated with an increase in lean body mass and body weight, not weight loss (Answer D). Testosterone therapy is not associated with breast growth (Answer C); it more typically results in a decrease in glandular tissue.

EDUCATIONAL OBJECTIVE

Identify the early masculinizing features of gender-affirming hormone therapy in transgender men.

REFERENCE(S)

Hembree WC, Cohen-Kettenis PT, Gooren L, et al. Endocrine treatment of gender dysphoric/gender-incongruent persons: an Endocrine Society clinical practice guideline. *J Clin Endocrinol Metab.* 2017;102(11):3869-3903. PMID: 28945902

Deutsch MB, Feldman JL. Updated recommendations from the world professional association for transgender health standards of care. *Am Fam Physician.* 2013;87(2):89-93. PMID: 23317072

Wierckx K, Van de Peer F, Verhaeghe E, et al. Short- and long-term clinical skin effects of testosterone treatment in trans men. *J Sex Med.* 2014;11(1):222-229. PMID: 24344810

7 ANSWER: A) Daily prospective symptom diary for 2 cycles

This patient appears to have premenstrual dysphoric disorder. However, it is necessary to have prospective documentation of the timing of her symptoms to confirm the diagnosis (Answer A). Unlike other mood disorders, premenstrual dysphoric disorder symptoms should resolve in the follicular phase. In some cases, perimenopause must be ruled out with a cycle day 3 measurement of serum FSH and serum antimullerian hormone (Answers C and D), as there can be some overlap in clinical mood symptoms. Patients with thyroid disease may also have similar mood changes, but their symptoms would not be cyclic. Thus, TSH measurement (Answer B) is not the best next step. Unipolar depression that worsens before menses is not considered to be premenstrual dysphoric disorder. Therefore, depression screening (Answer E) is not the best next step.

EDUCATIONAL OBJECTIVE

Identify the symptoms of premenstrual dysphoric disorder and diagnose this condition.

REFERENCE(S)

Cohen LS, Soares CN, Otto MW, Sweeney BH, Liberman RF, Harlow BL. Prevalence and predictors of premenstrual dysphoric disorder (PMDD) in older premenopausal women. The Harvard Study of Moods and Cycles. *J Affect Disord.* 2002;70(2):125-132. PMID: 12117624

Freeman EW, Halberstadt SM, Rickels K, Legler JM, Lin H, Sammel MD. Core symptoms that discriminate premenstrual syndrome. *J Womens Health (Larchmt).* 2011;20(1):29-35. PMID: 21128818

8 ANSWER: A) Transvaginal ultrasonography

Postmenopausal hirsutism or virilization of recent onset with a serum testosterone level greater than 150 ng/dL (>5.2 nmol/L) or a serum DHEA-S level greater than 700 to 800 µg/dL (18.9 to 21.7 µmol/L) suggests a neoplastic source of hyperandrogenism. Signs of virilization include deepening of the voice, increased muscle mass and clitoromegaly. Clitoromegaly is determined by clitoral length or by the clitoral index (length × width). A clitoral length greater than 10 mm or a clitoral index greater than 35 mm^2 is considered to be clitoromegaly. Virilization is only seen with more severe hyperandrogenemia (serum testosterone >150 ng/dL [>5.2 nmol/L]). Postmenopausal women with polycystic ovary syndrome do not have serum testosterone levels in this range, nor are they virilized.

Women with ovarian hyperthecosis typically develop symptoms gradually, but some with severe hyperthecosis have a more rapid course with severe hyperandrogenemia that mimics androgen-secreting tumors. Women with androgen-secreting adrenal tumors often present with symptoms of Cushing syndrome in addition to virilization. Unlike ovarian tumors, adrenal androgen-secreting tumors often, but not always, cause elevation in serum levels of the adrenal androgen DHEA-S. However, DHEA-S can be normal in androgen-secreting adrenal tumors. Androgen-secreting ovarian tumors include Sertoli-Leydig–cell tumors, arrhenoblastomas, or hilus-cell tumors.

The first step in the evaluation of severe hyperandrogenism in postmenopausal women is transvaginal ultrasonography (Answer A) to look for a tumor or asymmetry of the ovaries, as the tumors are typically very small. If ultrasonography is negative, adrenal CT (Answer D) should be performed, because there are occasional cases of adrenal tumors that secrete only testosterone. However, adrenal CT would not be the first test one would do. In addition, ultrasonography is a better imaging test than abdominal CT for visualizing the ovaries.

Dexamethasone-suppression testing (Answer B) is used in the workup of Cushing syndrome and might be indicated if an adrenal mass were detected. With adrenal Cushing syndrome, the presentation would be different from this patient's and the testosterone level would not be as high as it is in this vignette.

Serum inhibin (Answer C) is a marker for some ovarian tumors, including granulosa-cell tumors and sex-cord stromal tumors, but ultrasonography is the more important next step. Serum 17-hydroxyprogesterone (Answer E) would be measured when there are concerns for nonclassic congenital adrenal hyperplasia due to 21-hydroxylase deficiency (which is associated with hirsutism, but not virilization).

EDUCATIONAL OBJECTIVE

Evaluate postmenopausal hyperandrogenism.

REFERENCE(S)

Alpañés M, González-Casbas JM, Sánchez J, Pián H, Escobar-Morreale HF. Management of postmenopausal virilization. *J Clin Endocrinol Metab.* 2012;97(8):2584-2588. PMID: 22669303

Petersons CJ, Burt MG. The utility of adrenal and ovarian venous sampling in the investigation of androgen-secreting tumours. *Intern Med J.* 2011;41(1a):69-70. PMID: 21265966

Pugeat M, Déchaud H, Raverot V, Denuzière A, Cohen R, Boudou P; French Endocrine Society. Recommendations for investigation of hyperandrogenism. *Ann Endocrinol (Paris).* 2010;71(1): 2-7. PMID: 20096825

Carmina E, Dewailly D, Escobar-Morreale HF, et al. Non-classic congenital adrenal hyperplasia due to 21-hydroxylase deficiency revisited: an update with a special focus on adolescent and adult women. *Hum Reprod Update.* 2017;23(5): 580-599. PMID: 28582566

9 ANSWER: B) Combined estrogen-progestin contraceptive (ethinyl estradiol, 20 mcg, with norethindrone, 1 mg, given continuously [ie, no placebos])

The best option in this healthy, 45-year-old, perimenopausal woman at low risk for venous thromboembolism is a continuous low-dosage oral contraceptive (Answer B). It will provide contraception, as well as relieve her hot flashes and night sweats. In addition, it will suppress her hypothalamic-pituitary-ovarian axis (thereby controlling her cycles and bleeding). The 20-mcg oral contraceptives were originally developed for this population—they can be continued until the age of menopause if needed or desired. The rationale for giving the oral contraceptive in a continuous rather than cyclic regimen is to prevent hot flashes during the placebo week or pill-free interval.

The transdermal low-dosage estradiol patch and oral micronized progesterone (Answer A) is a possibility, but the estrogen dosage is low and may not relieve her symptoms. In addition, in a perimenopausal woman, continuous administration of progestin is likely to result in persistent breakthrough bleeding. A cyclic progestin regimen would be preferred.

A levonorgestrel-releasing intrauterine device (Answer C) would manage her bleeding, but the gabapentin would not be nearly as effective as estrogen for her hot flashes. Medroxyprogesterone (Answer D) would provide some control of her bleeding, but no relief of her hot flashes.

A levonorgestrel-containing intrauterine device would help with her heavy bleeding, but it would not help her hot flashes or difficulty sleeping.

EDUCATIONAL OBJECTIVE

Identify the best treatment options in a perimenopausal woman with severe hot flashes (in the late transition).

REFERENCE(S)

Stuenkel CA, Davis SA, Gompel A, et al. Treatment of symptoms of the menopause: an Endocrine Society clinical practice guideline. *J Clin Endocrinol Metab.* 2015;100(11):3975-4011. PMID: 26444994

The NAMS 2017 Hormone Therapy Position Statement Advisory Panel. The 2017 hormone therapy position statement of The North American Menopause Society. *Menopause.* 2017;24(7):728-753. PMID: 28650869

Taylor HS, Manson JE. Update in hormone therapy use in menopause. *J Clin Endocrinol Metab.* 2011;96(2):255-264. PMID: 21296989

Jensen JT, Nelson AL, Costales AC. Subject and clinician experience with the levonorgestrel-releasing intrauterine system. *Contraception.* 2008;77(1):22-29. PMID: 18082662

10 ANSWER: E) Cardiac MRI

Turner syndrome occurs in 1 in 2500 live births and is associated with growth failure, pubertal delay, and cardiac abnormalities. Current recommendations include comprehensive cardiovascular evaluation by a cardiology specialist, consisting of echocardiography in infants and children and MRI (Answer E) in older girls and women. Other initial testing should include renal ultrasonography; screening for celiac disease and diabetes mellitus; and hearing, orthodontic, and psychosocial evaluations. TSH measurement (Answer C) to screen for autoimmune thyroiditis should also be performed as part of the initial evaluation, but cardiac MRI is the most important test because congenital cardiac abnormalities are present in up to 50% of patients and include coarctation of the aorta, bicuspid aortic valve, and partial anomalous pulmonary venous return. Cardiac MRI follow-up is recommended on a routine schedule based on the presence of abnormalities at baseline, as well as the aortic severity index.

There is no need to perform transvaginal ultrasonography (Answer A) unless Y-chromosomal material is present, in which case ultrasonography would be needed to assess for the risk of gonadoblastoma (5% to 30%). Patients with Turner syndrome are at increased risk for diabetes, and screening (Answer B) is indicated, but cardiac MRI is the most important and urgent test to perform. Patients with Turner syndrome have an increased risk of autoimmune thyroid disease, but appropriate screening would be TSH and thyroid antibody assessment, not thyroid ultrasonography (Answer D).

EDUCATIONAL OBJECTIVE

Recommend appropriate evaluation for girls with gonadal dysgenesis.

REFERENCE(S)

Gravholt CH, Andersen NH, Conway GS, et al; International Turner Syndrome Consensus Group. Clinical practice guidelines for the care of girls and women with Turner syndrome: proceedings from the 2016 Cincinnati International Turner Syndrome Meeting. *Eur J Endocrinol.* 2017;177(3): G1-G70. PMID: 28705803

Davenport ML. Approach to the patient with Turner syndrome. *J Clin Endocrinol Metab.* 2010;95(4): 1487-1495. PMID: 20375216

Ross JL, Quigley CA, Cao D, et al. Growth hormone plus childhood low-dose estrogen in Turner's syndrome. *N Engl J Med.* 2011;364(13):1230-1242. PMID: 21449786

Pinsker JE. Clinical review: Turner syndrome: updating the paradigm of clinical care. *J Clin Endocrinol Metab.* 2012;97(6):994-1003. PMID: 22472565

11 ANSWER: C) Intrauterine adhesions (Asherman syndrome)

In the evaluation of amenorrhea, one must consider whether the problem is due to a hormonal or mechanical problem. This young woman had normal menarche and was able to conceive. She has no signs of hyperandrogenism. The most likely cause of her amenorrhea is intrauterine adhesions (Asherman syndrome) (Answer C) related to vigorous curettage of the endometrial lining after a miscarriage or with endometrial ablation.

Hyperprolactinemia due to mild thyroid dysfunction, medications, or tumors can suppress hypothalamic GnRH secretion and present as amenorrhea. However, in these situations, estradiol would be low (eg, 20 pg/mL rather than 70 pg/mL). A prolactinoma (Answer A) would be associated with elevated prolactin and low estradiol. Excessive stress, exercise, and low weight can result in amenorrhea (known as functional hypothalamic amenorrhea [Answer B]). However, functional hypothalamic amenorrhea would be associated with low estradiol. Her TSH concentration is slightly elevated, but this would be unlikely to cause amenorrhea. Primary ovarian insufficiency (Answer E) would be associated with high FSH and LH and low estradiol. In addition, the patient would most likely be experiencing hot flashes.

EDUCATIONAL OBJECTIVE

Determine the most likely cause of amenorrhea in a woman with normal hormone levels.

REFERENCE(S)

Zupi E, Centini G, Lazzeri L. Asherman syndrome: an unsolved clinical definition and management. *Fertil Steril.* 2015;104(6):1380-1381. PMID: 26484781

12 ANSWER: C) Reproductive history, including age at menarche and age at first pregnancy

Although estrogen therapy or combined estrogen and progestin hormone therapy was once offered to many menopausal women, results of studies such as the Women's Health Initiative have suggested that the risks outweigh the benefits in many women, especially those without symptoms. Clinical considerations include age, time since menopause, current vascular health, risk for breast cancer, and genetic and family risk profile.

The Endocrine Society guidelines suggest that clinicians calculate women's cardiovascular and breast cancer risks before considering menopausal hormone therapy. This woman does not report any cardiovascular risk factors. However, her menarche was slightly early, and she has never been pregnant (Answer C)—both of which are factors associated with an increased risk of breast cancer.

A family history of Parkinson disease (Answer A) is not associated with any adverse hormone therapy outcomes. A family history of a maternal aunt with breast cancer (Answer B) does not impact breast cancer risk in most calculators. Neither a history of autoimmune thyroid disease (Answer D) nor kidney stones (Answer E) is considered in the risk vs benefit assessment of hormone therapy in symptomatic postmenopausal women.

EDUCATIONAL OBJECTIVE

Evaluate the risks and benefits of postmenopausal hormone therapy.

REFERENCE(S)

Stuenkel CA, Davis SR, Gompel A, et al. Treatment of symptoms of the menopause: an Endocrine Society clinical practice guideline. *J Clin Endocrinol Metab.* 2015;100(11):3975-4011. PMID: 26444994

Pinkerton JV. Hormone therapy for postmenopausal women. *N Engl J Med.* 2020;382(5): 446-455. PMID: 31995690

Gompel A, Santen RJ. Hormone therapy and breast cancer risk 10 years after the WHI. *Climacteric.* 2012;15(3):241-249. PMID: 22612610

13 ANSWER: A) Oral 17β-estradiol, 2 mg daily

This patient is an excellent candidate for estrogen. The results of the Women's Health Initiative are not relevant to her, as the mean patient age was 63 years and she is only 41. She should be approached like any woman with primary ovarian insufficiency and be treated with estrogen until the average age of menopause (50/51 years). She has severe symptoms that are interfering with her quality of life and her ability to function, so estrogen is indicated. Women with primary ovarian insufficiency are prescribed higher dosages of estrogen than other women. Progestin therapy is not indicated in a patient after hysterectomy, as its only role is to prevent endometrial hyperplasia. The best answer is oral 17β-estradiol, 2 mg daily (Answer A). She could also use unopposed transdermal estrogen, but it is not necessary (and was not offered as an option).

One combination estrogen-progestin option is listed (Answer D), which she does not need. Venlafaxine (Answer C) and gabapentin (Answer B) are nonhormonal alternatives—these are options for some patients with breast cancer who cannot take estrogen. However, she is an excellent candidate for estrogen.

EDUCATIONAL OBJECTIVE

Recommend the optimal approach to managing severe hot flashes in a 41-year-old woman after total hysterectomy and bilateral salpingo-oophorectomy.

REFERENCE(S)

Stuenkel CA, Davis SR, Gompel A, et al. Treatment of symptoms of the menopause: an Endocrine Society clinical practice guideline. *J Clin Endocrinol Metab.* 2015;100(11):3975-4011. PMID: 26444994

The NAMS 2017 Hormone Therapy Position Statement Advisory Panel. The 2017 hormone therapy position statement of The North American Menopause Society. *Menopause.* 2017;24(7):728-753. PMID: 28650869

Committee on Gynecologic Practice. Committee opinion No. 698: hormone therapy in primary ovarian insufficiency. *Obstet Gynecol.* 2017;129(5):e134-e141. PMID: 28426619

14 ANSWER: A) Pregnancy

It is always critical to exclude pregnancy (Answer A) in a woman of childbearing years who presents with irregular menses or amenorrhea. Pregnancy can be detected by an elevated serum hCG value before the time of a missed menses or in a urine pregnancy test soon afterward. During early pregnancy, estrogen levels rise and suppress gonadotropins.

The pattern of high LH, low FSH, and normal estradiol is seen in many women with polycystic ovary syndrome (Answer B) if they are not severely obese, although it is not essential for the diagnosis. Patients with nonclassic congenital adrenal hyperplasia due to 21-hydroxylase deficiency (Answer C) have normal FSH and LH, low or normal estradiol, and elevated androgens, and they present with hirsutism and irregular menses. A high FSH, high LH, and low estradiol would be seen in a patient with primary ovarian insufficiency (Answer D). A patient with a prolactinoma (Answer E) would present with low FSH, low LH, and low estradiol because prolactin suppresses the GnRH pulse generator.

EDUCATIONAL OBJECTIVE

Describe the laboratory changes seen in an amenorrheic patient who is pregnant.

REFERENCE(S)

Melmed S, Casanueva FF, Hoffman AR, et al; Endocrine Society. Diagnosis and treatment of hyperprolactinemia: an Endocrine Society clinical practice guideline. *J Clin Endocrinol Metab.* 2011;96(2):273-288. PMID: 21296991

Mesian S. The endocrinology of human pregnancy and fetoplacental neuroendocrine development. In: Strauss JF, Barbieri RL, eds. *Yen & Jaffe's Reproductive Endocrinology: Physiology, Pathophysiology, and Clinical Management.* 6th ed. Saunders; 2009:249-281.

15 ANSWER: C) Sleep study

Polycystic ovary syndrome is a common disorder that occurs in 6% to 13% of women. Affected patients usually present with hirsutism, acne, and irregular menses. Sixty percent of affected women become obese. In addition to being at increased risk for impaired glucose tolerance and type 2 diabetes with a risk 5 to 10 times that of age-matched control women, women with polycystic ovary syndrome are also at high risk for sleep apnea. Given this patient's history, the next step would be to do a sleep study (Answer C).

Although she has gained weight and reports fatigue, she has no other features to suggest hypercortisolism (Answer A). An oral glucose tolerance test (Answer B) is indeed the most sensitive test for the diagnosis of type 2 diabetes in women with polycystic ovary syndrome, but she has a normal hemoglobin A_{1c} value and her symptoms are most suggestive of sleep apnea. A serum total testosterone measurement (Answer D) is part of the evaluation for hirsutism and polycystic ovary syndrome, but it is unlikely to help determine the cause of her sleepiness. Serum TSH measurement (Answer E) is a reasonable test to perform, but her history is more consistent with sleep apnea than hypothyroidism.

EDUCATIONAL OBJECTIVE

Identify the high risk of sleep apnea associated with polycystic ovary syndrome.

REFERENCE(S)

McCartney CR, Marshall JC. Clinical practice. Polycystic ovary syndrome. *N Engl J Med.* 2016;375(1):54-64. PMID: 27406348

Legro RS, Arslanian SA, Ehrmann DA, et al; Endocrine Society. Diagnosis and treatment of polycystic ovary syndrome: an Endocrine Society clinical practice guideline. *J Clin Endocrinol Metab.* 2013;98(12):4565-4592. PMID: 24151290

Ehrmann DA. Metabolic dysfunction in PCOS: relationship to obstructive sleep apnea. *Steroids.* 2012;77(4):290-294. PMID: 22178788

Tasali E, Chapotot F, Leproult R, Whitmore H, Ehrmann DA. Treatment of obstructive sleep apnea improves cardiometabolic function in young obese women with polycystic ovary syndrome. *J Clin Endocrinol Metab.* 2011;96(2):365-374. PMID: 21123449

16 ANSWER: B) Start escitalopram, 10 mg daily

This patient has hot flashes and perimenopausal depression. Her hot flashes are now relieved with estrogen therapy, but she continues to have mood symptoms. Approximately 40% to 50% of perimenopausal women experience depression and/or anxiety symptoms during the menopausal transition. The symptoms are responsive to estrogen, but many women need both estrogen and an antidepressant (a selective serotonin reuptake inhibitor) (Answer B).

It is unlikely that a further increase in the estrogen dosage (Answer A) will help her mood symptoms since she has reached the therapeutic dosage for her hot flashes. A continuous oral contraceptive (Answer C) might help mood, but it would contain more estrogen than is needed. Tricyclic antidepressants (Answer D) are less well studied for perimenopausal depression; therefore, selective serotonin reuptake inhibitors are the preferred class of drugs. Cognitive behavioral therapy (Answer E) has not been well studied in this population. If her symptoms do not improve with the selective serotonin reuptake inhibitor, another consideration would be to remove the levonorgestrel intrauterine device, as some women with depression have difficulty tolerating progestins, including these intrauterine devices. However, another strategy to protect the endometrium would then be required.

EDUCATIONAL OBJECTIVE

Identify and treat depression during the menopausal transition.

REFERENCE(S)

Stuenkel CA, Davis SA, Gompel A, et al. Treatment of symptoms of the menopause: an Endocrine Society clinical practice guideline. *J Clin Endocrinol Metab.* 2015;100(11):3975-4011. PMID: 26444994

Gordon JL, Girdler SS. Hormone replacement therapy in the treatment of perimenopausal depression. *Curr Psychiatry Rep.* 2014;16(12): 517. PMID: 25308388

17 ANSWER: E) No testing required

Women older than 45 years who present with characteristic menopausal signs and symptoms are more likely to be in the menopausal transition than to have a new endocrine problem such as hyperprolactinemia or thyroid disease. Pregnancy must always be ruled out, but this patient's hCG was negative. Although she has no hot flashes, poor sleep and musculoskeletal symptoms are suggestive of perimenopause, as these symptoms occur in up to 40% to 50% of women during the transition. While most perimenopausal women's sleep disturbances are related to hot flashes, others have poor sleep because of new-onset primary sleep disorders. Depression and anxiety can also contribute. Therefore, for women older than 45 years who present with irregular menstrual cycles with menopausal symptoms such as hot flashes, mood changes, joint aches, or sleep disturbances, biochemical evaluation or imaging is not necessary to make the diagnosis. Thus, no further testing is required (thus, Answer E is correct and Answers A, B, C, and D are incorrect). In fact, serum FSH measurement can be misleading because it is often normal (if measured after ovulation or when serum estradiol is high). An endocrine evaluation should be performed for women younger than 45 years who present with oligomenorrhea, with or without menopausal symptoms.

EDUCATIONAL OBJECTIVE
Guide the evaluation and diagnosis of the menopausal transition.

REFERENCE(S)

Harlow SD, Gass M, Hall JE, et al; STRAW + 10 Collaborative Group. Executive summary of the Stages of Reproductive Aging Workshop + 10: addressing the unfinished agenda of staging reproductive aging. *J Clin Endocrinol Metab.* 2012;97(4):1159-1168. PMID: 22344196

Randolph JF Jr, Crawford S, Dennerstein L, et al. The value of follicle-stimulating hormone concentration and clinical findings as markers of the late menopausal transition. *J Clin Endocrinol Metab.* 2006;91(8):3034-3040. PMID: 16720656

18 ANSWER: D) No treatment

No treatment is necessary for this patient now (Answer D) because it appears that she is recovering from functional hypothalamic amenorrhea. Her laboratory values are consistent with a recent ovulation (she appears to be in the mid to late luteal phase and will have a period soon). The serum progesterone concentration of 7.0 ng/mL (22.3 nmol/L) confirms that she has ovulated. Progesterone levels are also high in pregnancy, but they are considerably higher than 7 ng/mL (>22.3 nmol/L). Serum LH and FSH vary across the cycle but are relatively low in the late luteal phase (just before the important small rise in serum FSH that is responsible for the recruitment of the cohort of follicles for the subsequent menstrual cycle). Serum estradiol concentrations peak just before the midcycle surge, but there is also a secondary rise in the luteal phase that corresponds with the rise in serum progesterone (both hormones secreted by the corpus luteum).

If there were no evidence of recovery, the next step would be to start a physiologic dosage of estrogen (Answer A), rather than a pharmacologic dosage (Answer C). Bisphosphonates (Answer B) should not be given in this setting. The best option is to reassure her that she is recovering and is likely to have a period.

EDUCATIONAL OBJECTIVE
Identify a postovulatory pattern of gonadotropin and gonadal steroid levels.

REFERENCE(S)

Perkins RB, Hall JE, Martin KA. Aetiology, previous menstrual function and patterns of neuro-endocrine disturbance as prognostic indicators in hypothalamic amenorrhoea. *Hum Reprod.* 2001;16(10):2198-2205. PMID: 11574516

Filicori M, Santoro N, Merriam GR, Crowley WF Jr. Characterization of the physiological pattern of episodic gonadotropin secretion throughout the human menstrual cycle. *J Clin Endocrinol Metab.* 1986;62(6):1136-1144. PMID: 3084534

Male Reproduction Board Review

Frances J. Hayes, MB BCh, BAO

1 ANSWER: A) Substitute finasteride for tamsulosin

Ejaculation is the discharge of semen from the male reproductive tract usually accompanied by orgasm. Retrograde ejaculation occurs when semen, which would normally be ejaculated via the urethra, is instead redirected to the bladder. Normally, the sphincter of the bladder contracts before ejaculation, which acts to both inhibit the release of urine and prevent a reflux of seminal fluids into the bladder during ejaculation. Any condition, medication, or surgical procedure that interferes with central control of ejaculation or the autonomic innervation to the seminal tract can cause ejaculatory dysfunction. Use of α-adrenergic blockers such as tamsulosin to treat symptoms of benign prostatic hyperplasia is a common cause of retrograde ejaculation given that they relax the bladder sphincter. Other drug classes used to treat benign prostatic hyperplasia, such as 5α-reductase inhibitors, do not have this adverse effect, so substituting finasteride for tamsulosin (Answer A) would be a helpful strategy for this patient.

While cross-sectional studies show an association between low testosterone levels and ejaculatory dysfunction, testosterone replacement (Answer B) has not been shown to be beneficial to such patients. In any case, the patient described does not meet criteria for hypogonadism given that his testosterone level is in the normal range.

This patient can get and sustain an erection adequate for intercourse, and phosphodiesterase-5 inhibitors have no impact on ejaculatory function. Therefore, initiating treatment with a phosphodiesterase-5 inhibitor (Answer C) would not be helpful. In addition, an agent such as tadalafil can interact with tamsulosin and result in hypotension.

A diuretic might not be an ideal choice for a patient with benign prostatic hyperplasia. Nonetheless, hydrochlorothiazide is a safe, effective, and inexpensive agent that is doing a good job controlling this patient's blood pressure at a low dosage. While it may contribute to erectile dysfunction, it does not cause ejaculatory dysfunction. Therefore, substituting eplerenone for hydrochlorothiazide (Answer D) is not indicated, as it is a more expensive drug and would not be expected to confer any additional benefit. Use of eplerenone is typically reserved for men with aldosterone-mediated hypertension, in preference to the less selective mineralocorticoid antagonist spironolactone, which could cause gynecomastia.

EDUCATIONAL OBJECTIVE

Explain the association between use of α-adrenergic blockers and retrograde ejaculation in men.

REFERENCE(S)

Mehta A, Sigman M. Management of the dry ejaculate: a systematic review of aspermia and retrograde ejaculation. *Fertil Steril.* 2015;104(5):1074-1081. PMID: 26432530

Paduch DA, Polzer PK, Ni X, Basaria S. Testosterone replacement in androgen-deficient men with ejaculatory dysfunction: a randomized controlled trial. *J Clin Endocrinol Metab.* 2015;100(8);2956-2962. PMID: 26158605

2 ANSWER: B) Leuprolide, 3.75 mg intramuscularly, plus estradiol, 50 mcg by transdermal patch

As is the case in postmenopausal women, use of estrogen in transgender patients is associated with an increased risk of venous thromboembolism.

In the case described, the patient is already at increased risk of venous thromboembolism by virtue of having an inherited thrombophilia. Therefore, the priority when selecting the most appropriate hormone regimen is to identify the one with the lowest thrombogenic potential.

Risk of venous thromboembolism from estrogen depends on the dosage, formulation, and route of administration. Incorporating a GnRH agonist into the hormone regimen for a transgender female patient has the advantage of causing profound suppression of endogenous testosterone, so that only physiologic doses of estrogen need to be administered. Of the 2 hormone regimens that include a GnRH agonist, the option with the estrogen patch (Answer B) is correct, as transdermal estrogen is associated with a lower clotting risk than oral formulations (Answer A) due to the fact that it bypasses the liver and therefore leads to less of an increase in clotting factors.

Unlike GnRH analogues, use of antiandrogens such as spironolactone causes more modest suppression of testosterone, so higher estrogen dosages are needed to achieve the desired degree of testosterone suppression. Therefore, a regimen consisting of spironolactone without estrogen would not be potent enough to suppress testosterone even if combined with a 5α-reductase inhibitor such as finasteride (Answer D). Of the different types of estrogen available, risk of venous thromboembolism is highest with ethinyl estradiol (Answer C), which should therefore be avoided.

EDUCATIONAL OBJECTIVE

Guide the initiation of hormone therapy in a transgender woman at increased risk of venous thromboembolism.

REFERENCE(S)

Hembree WC, Cohen-Kettenis PT, Gooren L, et al. Endocrine treatment of gender dysphoric/gender incongruent persons: an Endocrine Society clinical practice guideline. *J Clin Endocrinol Metab.* 2017;102(11):3869-3903. PMID: 28945902

T'Sjoen G, Arcelus J, Gooren L, Klink DT, Tangpricha V. Endocrinology of transgender medicine. *Endocr Rev.* 2019;40(1):97-117. PMID: 30307546

Safer JD, Tangpricha V. Care of transgender persons. *N Engl J Med.* 2019;381(25):2451-2460. PMID: 31851801

3 ANSWER: D) Estradiol valerate, 40 mg intramuscularly weekly

There are several different formulations of estrogen from which to choose. Conjugated equine estrogens (Answer A) comprise a mixture of estrogens, largely estrone sulfate, derived from the urine of pregnant mares. They are not detected in a standard radioimmunoassay, which is designed to measure estradiol, so this would not explain the patient's high estradiol level.

Use of ethinyl estradiol (Answer C), which is a potent synthetic estrogen found in most oral contraceptive pills, could explain the patient's breast tenderness but it would also not be detected by the estradiol assay. In fact, the estradiol level in someone taking a birth control pill would be undetectable because endogenous estradiol secretion would be suppressed by this high estrogen dosage.

17β-Estradiol (Answer B) is a bioidentical hormone akin to the estrogen normally secreted by the body. While it would therefore be detected in the estradiol assay, a dosage of 4 mg daily would not result in estradiol levels in the range of 500 to 600 pg/mL (1836-2203 pmol/L).

Estradiol valerate (Answer D) is a long-acting form of estrogen, which is dissolved in oil and is metabolized in the body to estradiol, so that it is measurable in the estradiol assay. Recommended dosages are typically 10 to 20 mg every 2 weeks. Thus, a dosage of 40 mg weekly would be expected to cause supraphysiologic levels as described in the vignette.

EDUCATIONAL OBJECTIVE

Interpret the estradiol assay when monitoring patients receiving male-to-female hormone therapy.

REFERENCE(S)

Safer JD, Tangpricha V. Care of transgender persons. *N Engl J Med.* 2019;381(25):2451-2460. PMID: 31851801

Hembree WC, Cohen-Kettenis PT, Gooren L, et al. Endocrine treatment of gender-dysphoric/gender-incongruent persons: an Endocrine Society clinical practice guideline. *J Clin Endocrinol Metab.* 2017;102(11):1-35. PMID: 28945902

4 ANSWER: C) Microdissection testicular sperm extraction followed by intracytoplasmic sperm injection

Klinefelter syndrome is the most common chromosomal abnormality in men. While there may be some phenotypic variability, hypergonadotropic hypogonadism characterized by small testes and azoospermia is seen in more than 95% of patients with nonmosaic Klinefelter syndrome. While there have been rare case reports of men with Klinefelter syndrome impregnating their partners naturally, this is the exception rather than the rule, and one would not expect the patient to be able to father children without treatment (Answer A).

In men with hypogonadotropic hypogonadism, treatment with hCG (Answer B) can increase systemic and intratesticular testosterone levels and, by doing so, stimulate spermatogenesis. However, in the case described, endogenous LH levels are already elevated, so administration of hCG would be of no benefit.

With the advent of the technique of microdissection testicular sperm extraction in the late 1990s, fertility options for men with Klinefelter syndrome changed dramatically and were no longer limited to use of donor sperm or adoption. Using this technique, normal-sized seminiferous tubules, likely to contain spermatozoa, are selectively removed with microscissors and the removed tissue is immediately examined for the presence of sperm. Sperm are reportedly retrieved in up to 50% of cases (Answer C). This technique offers affected patients the possibility of biologic paternity when combined with a modification of in vitro fertilization called intracytoplasmic sperm injection, whereby an embryologist directly injects a single sperm into the cytoplasm of an egg.

Because any surviving spermatozoa from men with Klinefelter syndrome originate in euploid germ cells, use of assisted reproduction in these patients is not associated with a higher risk of having a son with Klinefelter syndrome compared with men with a 46,XY karyotype. There is a case report of a 47,XXY fetus conceived after intracytoplasmic sperm injection of spermatozoa from a patient with Klinefelter syndrome. However, given that Klinefelter syndrome occurs in about 1 in 600 boys in the background population, a few cases of 47,XXY should be expected.

Clomiphene citrate (Answer D) is a selective estrogen receptor modulator that is approved by the US FDA to induce ovulation in women but is not for use in men. Nonetheless, it is sometimes used off-label to increase testosterone levels in men with hypogonadism, as it is orally active and, unlike testosterone, does not suppress spermatogenesis. Clomiphene can increase testosterone levels in men with hypogonadotropic hypogonadism by reducing estrogen-mediated negative feedback, thus allowing an increase in endogenous LH levels. However, in the patient described who has primary hypogonadism and LH levels that are already elevated, giving clomiphene would be of no benefit.

EDUCATIONAL OBJECTIVE

Counsel patients with Klinefelter syndrome about their fertility potential.

REFERENCE(S)

Gravholt CH, Chang S, Wallentin M, Fedder J, Moore P, Skakkebaek A. Klinefleter syndrome: integrating genetics, neuropsychology, and endocrinology. *Endocr Rev.* 2018;39(4):389-423. PMID: 29438472

Corona G, Pizzocaro A, Lanfranco F, et al; Klinefelter ItaliaN Group (KING). Sperm recovery and ICSI outcomes in Klinefelter syndrome: a systematic review and meta-analysis. *Hum Reprod Update.* 2017;23(3):265-275. PMID: 28379559

5 ANSWER: B) Total testosterone, high; free testosterone, low or low-normal; estradiol, high; LH, normal

Gynecomastia is a benign enlargement of the male breast due mainly to the proliferation of ductal tissue. Gynecomastia develops when there is an increase in the ratio of estrogen to androgens, with the former having a stimulatory effect on breast tissue, while the latter antagonize this effect. A small degree of breast enlargement is a relatively common finding, especially in older men, and generally does not require any workup when asymptomatic. However, breast enlargement that is prominent, painful, progressive, or of recent onset, as in this case, requires thorough evaluation.

The patient described is clinically and biochemically hyperthyroid, a condition known to cause gynecomastia. In men with hyperthyroidism, there is increased hepatic production of SHBG, which results in high levels of total but low or low-normal levels of free testosterone, high estradiol, and normal LH (Answer B). Because of the greater affinity of SHBG for testosterone than for estradiol, there is a relative increase in the amount of free estradiol compared with testosterone. There is also increased aromatization of testosterone to estradiol and of androstenedione to estrone in extraglandular tissues.

Elevated serum estradiol with low testosterone and LH levels (Answer A) can be seen with exogenous estrogen use or with an estrogen-secreting testicular tumor of the Leydig or Sertoli cells.

High levels of testosterone, estradiol, and LH (Answer D) are typical of patients with partial androgen insensitivity.

A hormone profile characterized by normal testosterone levels, high estradiol, and low LH (Answer C) can be seen in patients with a testicular or extragonadal hCG-secreting tumor. In these patients, hCG stimulates production of both testosterone and estradiol, but because of its stimulatory effect on the aromatase enzyme, there is preferential estradiol production leading to a lower than normal testosterone-to-estradiol ratio.

EDUCATIONAL OBJECTIVE

Describe the presentation of gynecomastia due to hyperthyroidism.

REFERENCE(S)

Ali SN, Jayasena CN. Sam AH. Which patients with gynaecomastia require more detailed investigation? *Clin Endocrinol (Oxf).* 2018:88(3):360-363. PMID: 29193251

Narula HS, Carlson HE. Gynaecomastia--pathophysiology, diagnosis and treatment. *Nat Rev Endocrinol.* 2014;10(11):684-698. PMID: 25112235

Braunstein GD. Clinical practice. Gynecomastia. *N Engl J Med.* 2007;357(12):1229-1237. PMID: 17881754

6 ANSWER: B) *FGFR1*

Once congenital hypogonadotropic hypogonadism has been diagnosed, targeted genetic testing can be considered. In the last decade, considerable advances have been made in unraveling the genetic basis of congenital hypogonadotropic hypogonadism, and to date, pathogenic variants have been identified in approximately 40% of patients. While in familial cases the mode of inheritance can be used to guide genetic testing, most cases of congenital hypogonadotropic hypogonadism are sporadic, as in the patient described in this vignette. However, a careful clinical evaluation can be helpful in prioritizing genetic testing. In an analysis of 219 patients with congenital hypogonadotropic hypogonadism, the following clinical features were highly associated with specific gene defects: synkinesia (*ANOS1* [formerly *KAL1*]), dental agenesis (*FGF8/FGFR1*), digital bony abnormalities (*FGF8/FGFR1*), and hearing loss (*CHD7*). In the case described where the patient has evidence of syndactyly, genetic testing for an *FGFR1* pathogenic variant (Answer B) would be the appropriate next step.

Pathogenic variants in the *PROP1* gene (Answer C) are one of the most common causes of both familial and sporadic congenital combined pituitary hormone deficiency (GH, TSH, LH, FSH). While this patient has low levels of both testosterone and IGF-1, this is not unusual in patients with isolated hypogonadotropic hypogonadism due to the normal stimulatory effect of testosterone on GH secretion, which is why IGF-1 levels normalize after testosterone replacement without the need for GH therapy.

Pathogenic variants in the *GNRHR* gene (Answer A) cause hypogonadism but not anosmia or syndactyly.

While pathogenic variants in *CHD7* (Answer D) cause Kallmann syndrome, the absence of deafness and the presence of syndactyly in this patient make it make more likely that the genetic basis for his disease is a pathogenic variant in *FGFR1* rather than in *CHD7.*

Pathogenic variants in *NR0B1* (Answer E), formerly known as *DAX1*, cause congenital hypogonadotropic hypogonadism and adrenal insufficiency and do not cause anosmia.

EDUCATIONAL OBJECTIVE

Guide the appropriate workup in a patient with congenital hypogonadotropic hypogonadism.

REFERENCE(S)

Young J. Approach to the male patient with hypogonadotropic hypogonadism. *J Clin Endocrinol Metab.* 2012;97(3):707-718. PMID: 22392951

Costa-Barbosa FA, Balasubramanian R, Keefe KW, et al. Prioritizing genetic testing in patients with Kallmann syndrome using clinical phenotypes. *J Clin Endocrinol Metab.* 2013;98(5):E943-E953. PMID: 23533228

7 ANSWER: B) Congenital bilateral absence of the vas deferens

This couple's infertility is due to azoospermia. Absence of sperm in the ejaculate may occur because of an obstruction in the reproductive tract (obstructive azoospermia) or inadequate production of spermatozoa (nonobstructive azoospermia). The volume and pH of the seminal fluid can be used to determine in which category a patient's azoospermia falls. In this case, the low volume (normal >1.5 mL) and low pH (normal >7.2) indicate an obstructive etiology. Obstructive azoospermia may be congenital (congenital absence of the vas deferens, idiopathic epididymal obstruction) or acquired (from infections, vasectomy, or other iatrogenic injuries to the male reproductive tract).

Congenital bilateral absence of the vas deferens (Answer B) is one of the most common causes of obstructive azoospermia. It can be diagnosed by a careful clinical examination, as the vas is normally palpable as a thin ropelike structure within the spermatic cord. The diagnosis can be confirmed by transrectal ultrasonography. Genetic testing should be performed in patients with congenital bilateral absence of the vas deferens who do not have the typical pulmonary and pancreatic manifestations of cystic fibrosis, as it is associated with compound heterozygosity for a classic (severe) *CFTR* pathogenic variant and a mild *CFTR* pathogenic variant.

All of the other options cause nonobstructive azoospermia, in which case testis volume would be reduced because the bulk of the testis is composed of seminiferous tubules.

If this patient's azoospermia were due to anabolic steroid use (Answer A), his testosterone and gonadotropin levels would be suppressed.

Microdeletions of the Y chromosome (Answer C) are an important cause of nonobstructive azoospermia and typically result in reduced testicular size due to disruption of spermatogenesis and an elevated FSH level. The male-specific region on the long arm of the Y chromosome has a locus known as the azoospermia factor (AZF) that contains genes needed for spermatogenesis. This AZF locus contains 3 regions: AZFa, AZFb, and AZFc. Deletions of the entire AZFa region result in complete atrophy of the tubular compartment, with only Sertoli cells seen on testicular biopsy, making retrieval of sperm for intracytoplasmic sperm injection virtually impossible. Large deletions in the AZFb region also result in Sertoli-cell–only syndrome. Pathogenic variants in the AZFc region are the most common and account for 80% of Y-chromosome microdeletions. AZFc deletions are compatible with residual spermatogenesis, with oligospermia being a common presentation.

Patients with mosaic Klinefelter syndrome (Answer D) can present with infertility, but the patient's completely normal hormone profile, absence of gynecomastia, normal testicular size, and semen characteristics would not be consistent with this diagnosis.

Patients with a mild degree of androgen insensitivity (Answer E) can present with a low sperm count, but both testosterone and gonadotropin levels are elevated in such cases.

EDUCATIONAL OBJECTIVE

Diagnose obstructive azoospermia due to absence of the vas deferens as a cause of infertility.

REFERENCE(S)

Cooper TG, Noonan E, von Eckardstein S, et al. World Health Organization reference values for human semen characteristics. *Hum Reprod Update.* 2010;16(3):231-245. PMID: 19934213

Anawalt BD. Approach to male infertility and induction of spermatogenesis. *J Clin Endocrinol Metab.* 2013;98(9):3532-3542. PMID: 24014811

8 ANSWER: D) hCG-producing germ-cell tumor

This well-virilized man presents with a short history of tender gynecomastia, high-normal testosterone, very high estradiol, and suppressed gonadotropin concentrations. This combination can be due to exogenous testosterone use or abuse, endogenous or exogenous testosterone precursors (eg, dehydroepiandrosterone from an adrenal tumor), endogenous or exogenous hCG (eg, hCG from a germ-cell tumor [Answer D]), or exogenous LH (rhLH).

Endogenous or exogenous hCG has LH activity and stimulates testicular production of testosterone and estradiol that, in turn, suppresses endogenous gonadotropin concentrations. Endogenous or exogenous hCG increases aromatization of testosterone to estradiol and leads to a relatively lower testosterone-to-estradiol ratio than normal. The reduced testosterone-to-estradiol ratio results in breast tissue proliferation and tender gynecomastia. The absence of a testicular mass on this patient's physical examination suggests that (1) the patient has a small (impalpable) testicular tumor that is producing hCG or (2) there is possibly an extragonadal tumor that is producing hCG. The next step in this patient's evaluation would be to measure hCG and then do testicular ultrasonography to determine whether the source is testicular or extragonadal.

Leydig-cell tumors (Answer B) may produce testosterone or estradiol. In testosterone-secreting Leydig-cell tumors, testosterone concentrations are often high-normal or even elevated; the autonomous secretion of testosterone suppresses pituitary gonadotropin concentrations. In Leydig-cell tumors that produce estradiol, gonadotropin secretion is suppressed by the excess estradiol, and testosterone concentrations decrease as a result.

Ingestion of a nonaromatizable androgen (Answer C) would cause suppressed rather than high testosterone and estradiol levels.

Hyperprolactinemia (Answer A) is an uncommon cause of gynecomastia and does so by causing central hypogonadism as a result of suppression of GNRH hormone secretion. It would therefore not explain the patient's high normal testosterone level. In this case, the modestly elevated prolactin is most likely a consequence of estrogen stimulation of the lactotrophs.

In a patient with gynecomastia due to hyperthyroidism (Answer E), total testosterone and estradiol levels would be high, but LH would be normal and not suppressed as in this case.

EDUCATIONAL OBJECTIVE

Suspect an hCG-producing tumor based on clinical and biochemical features.

REFERENCE(S)

Anawalt BD. Gynecomastia. In: Jameson JL, De Groot LJ, eds. *Endocrinology: Adult and Pediatric.* 7th ed. Saunders Elsevier; 2015:2421-2430.

Braunstein GD. Clinical practice. Gynecomastia. *N Engl J Med.* 2007;357(12):1229-1237. PMID: 17881754

Daniels IR, Layer GT. Testicular tumours presenting as gynaecomastia. *Eur J Surg Oncol.* 2003;29(5): 437-439. PMID: 12798747

McLachlan RI, de Kretser DM. Hypogonadotropism with elevated serum testosterone: reversible causes of secondary infertility. *Nat Clin Pract Urol.* 2006;3(1):560-565. PMID: 17031381

Rieu M, Reznik Y, Vannetzel JM, Mahoudeau J, Berrod JL, Kuhn JM. Testicular steroidogenesis in adult men with human chorionic gonadotropin-producing tumors. *J Clin Endocrinol Metab.* 1995;80(8):2404-2409. PMID: 7629236

9 ANSWER: A) Measure free testosterone

This patient's clinical presentation with decreased libido, erectile dysfunction, and fatigue is highly suggestive of hypogonadism. His physical examination also reveals gynecomastia. Despite this, 2 total testosterone values, both measured by liquid chromatography tandem mass spectrometry, are in the high-normal range. In such clinical scenarios, where the clinical phenotype is incongruent with biochemical results, clinicians should consider alterations in SHBG levels as a potential explanation. Certain clinical conditions are associated with elevated serum SHBG levels, including aging, liver disease, hyperthyroidism, medications (anticonvulsant drugs, estrogen), and HIV infection.

Thus, in cases such as this where the history is suggestive of hypogonadism and the patient has a disorder (in this case hepatitis) that is known to impact SHBG levels, measurement of free testosterone (Answer A) is required to diagnose androgen deficiency. Reliable methods of free testosterone measurement include (1) measurement by equilibrium dialysis (considered the gold standard but is not routinely available in commercial laboratories), and (2) calculated free testosterone (derived from total testosterone and SHBG measurements using law of mass action equations). This patient's free testosterone level (measured by equilibrium dialysis) was low at 48 pg/mL (1.7 nmol/L) because of a markedly elevated SHBG level of 20.0 μg/mL (178 nmol/L), allowing a diagnosis of hypogonadism to be confirmed.

This patient has no clinical features of glucocorticoid excess, so there is no indication to screen for Cushing syndrome by measuring late-night salivary cortisol (Answer D).

Men with partial androgen insensitivity syndrome resulting from pathogenic variants in the gene encoding the androgen receptor (Answer C) can also present with symptoms and signs of hypogonadism in association with elevated serum testosterone. However, patients with partial androgen insensitivity syndrome tend to have additional clinical manifestations, including perineoscrotal hypospadias and infertility. Importantly, gonadotropin levels in such patients are elevated due to impaired testosterone negative feedback, unlike the gonadotropin profile of patients with HIV infection who typically have secondary hypogonadism.

Epitestosterone is a biologically inactive 17-epimer of testosterone that is cosecreted by the Leydig cells of the testes. The urinary testosterone-to-epitestosterone ratio (Answer B) is measured in the evaluation of men suspected of androgen abuse. However, exogenous use of testosterone by this patient would be associated with suppressed gonadotropin levels.

EDUCATIONAL OBJECTIVE

Identify the biochemical profile of men with liver disease who experience alterations in the concentration of serum SHBG.

REFERENCE(S)

Bhasin S, Brito JP, Cunningham GR, et al. Testosterone therapy in men with hypogonadism: an Endocrine Society clinical practice guideline. *J Clin Endocrinol Metab.* 2018;103(5):1715-1744. PMID: 29562364

10 ANSWER: A) Schedule a sleep study

Testosterone esters, including enanthate and cypionate, have been used for the treatment of male hypogonadism for more than 7 decades. They have the advantage of being the least expensive of the testosterone replacement modalities and they predictably restore testosterone levels to the normal range. However, they have unfavorable pharmacokinetics characterized by significant fluctuation in serum testosterone between peak and trough values. When administered by a deep intramuscular injection, testosterone is slowly released from this oily suspension into the circulation over a period of weeks. The esters are typically injected at 2-week intervals with levels reaching peak concentrations 24 to 48 hours after the injection followed by a gradual decline to the low-normal range before the next injection is due. When the interval between injections is extended to every 3 weeks, peak concentrations tend to be supraphysiologic and testosterone levels may fall to the hypogonadal range by the time the next injection is administered. Such wide excursions in serum testosterone concentrations can, in turn, cause undesirable swings in mood, libido, and energy levels. Given the pharmacokinetics of testosterone esters, they also tend to increase hematocrit more than transdermal testosterone preparations, especially when high dosages are given at less frequent intervals.

Increasing the testosterone dosage (Answer D) in a patient whose hematocrit is already high is not appropriate, especially given that the patient's testosterone level is in the desired range for a trough level (namely, the lower end of the normal range).

The pharmacokinetics of testosterone enanthate are similar to those of testosterone cypionate. Hence, switching esters (Answer B) will not address his problem.

Before initiating testosterone therapy, baseline hematocrit should be measured. Baseline hematocrit greater than 48% (and greater than 50% for men living at higher altitudes) is a relative contraindication to testosterone therapy because these men are more likely to develop a hematocrit level greater than 54% when treated with testosterone. The baseline hematocrit of 50% for this hypogonadal, nonsmoking patient is high. The Endocrine Society clinical practice guidelines recommend that the underlying cause of erythrocytosis be investigated before androgen therapy is prescribed. Given the patient's obesity and history of daytime somnolence, the possibility of obstructive sleep apnea should be considered and a sleep study should be arranged (Answer A).

Occasionally, phlebotomy (Answer C) may be necessary for testosterone therapy to be continued in a hypogonadal patient, but it is important to exclude other causes of erythrocytosis such as sleep apnea, chronic obstructive pulmonary disease, or polycythemia rubra vera before doing so.

EDUCATIONAL OBJECTIVE

Describe the pharmacokinetics of injectable testosterone esters and manage potential adverse effects.

REFERENCE(S)

Bhasin S, Brito JP, Cunningham GR, et al. Testosterone therapy in men with hypogonadism: an Endocrine Society clinical practice guideline. *J Clin Endocrinol Metab.* 2018;103(5):1715-1744. PMID: 29562364

Dobs AS, Meikle AW, Arver S, Sanders SW, Caramelli KE, Mazer NA. Pharmacokinetics, efficacy, and safety of a permeation-enhanced testosterone transdermal system in comparison with bi-weekly injections of testosterone enanthate for the treatment of hypogonadal men. *J Clin Endocrinal Metab.* 1999;84(10):3469-3478. PMID: 1052298

11 ANSWER: D) Refer him to a urologist

The diagnosis of hypogonadism made by the patient's primary care physician is correct based on the presence of symptoms of hypogonadism in association with 2 low morning testosterone measurements. The issue at hand is whether the patient is an appropriate candidate for testosterone replacement. While the patient is eager to initiate testosterone therapy in the hope of improving his symptoms, it is the physician's responsibility to ensure that he is an appropriate candidate and that the risk-to-benefit ratio favors treatment. The Endocrine Society clinical practice guidelines recommend that clinicians assess prostate cancer risk in men being considered for testosterone therapy. As a general rule, it is recommended that patients who have a palpable prostate nodule or induration or PSA level greater than 4.0 ng/mL (>4.0 µg/L) need further urologic evaluation before testosterone therapy is initiated. However, in subgroups of men considered to be at increased risk for prostate cancer, such as African American patients or men with a first-degree relative with prostate cancer, the baseline PSA level at which referral to a urologist is recommended is greater than 3.0 ng/mL (>3.0 µg/L). Thus, in this African American man with 2 baseline PSA measurements greater than 3.0 ng/mL (>3.0 µg/L), referral to a urologist (Answer D) is the best next step in his management. Should findings from this urologic workup be reassuring, one could then proceed with testosterone replacement (Answer B).

While a phosphodiesterase-5 inhibitor (Answer A) would most likely help the patient's erectile dysfunction, it would not improve his libido. In addition, use of a phosphodiesterase-5 inhibitor is contraindicated in this patient who is taking a nitrate given the risk of severe hypotension with this drug combination.

Measurement of free testosterone (Answer C) is recommended when total testosterone levels are low-normal or just below the reference range and a low SHBG level is suspected. This patient already meets criteria for hypogonadism given that he has symptoms consistent with androgen deficiency in association with two unequivocally low total testosterone levels. Therefore, measurement of free testosterone would not yield any additional information.

EDUCATIONAL OBJECTIVE

List indications for urologic evaluation before initiating testosterone therapy.

REFERENCE(S)

Bhasin S, Brito JP, Cunningham GR, et al. Testosterone therapy in men with hypogonadism: an Endocrine Society clinical practice guideline. *J Clin Endocrinol Metab.* 2018;103(5):1715-1744. PMID: 29562364

12 ANSWER: C) Reevaluate his hypothalamic-pituitary-gonadal axis in 6 months

Although the incidence of pituitary dysfunction after traumatic brain injury varies widely in published studies, it appears that pituitary dysfunction occurs commonly in men who experience moderate to severe traumatic brain injury. Low GH and testosterone concentrations are the most common abnormalities. Indeed, hypogonadism has been reported in up to 80% of men in the acute phase of posttraumatic brain injury. However, it is unclear whether treatment with GH and/or testosterone is beneficial. Furthermore, longitudinal follow-up has demonstrated that many men recover function of these axes within the first year after the traumatic brain injury. In this man who appears to be recovering well from his brain injury, the best option is therefore to reassess his gonadal axis 6 months after the initial injury (Answer C).

Treatment with hCG (Answer A) would raise his testosterone concentration and stimulate spermatogenesis; however, he does not wish to start a family for at least 1 year, so there is no urgency in starting treatment until it is clear that his hypothalamic-pituitary-gonadal axis has not recovered. Given that his libido is already beginning to improve and he has no problem with erections, there is no indication to start testosterone (Answer B). A phosphodiesterase-5 inhibitor (Answer D) would not be appropriate for a patient with low libido but normal erectile function.

EDUCATIONAL OBJECTIVE

Counsel a patient regarding the time course of secondary hypogonadism following traumatic brain injury.

REFERENCE(S)

Schneider HJ, Schneider M, Saller B, et al. Prevalence of anterior pituitary insufficiency 3 and 12 months after traumatic brain injury. *Eur J Endocrinol.* 2006;154(2):259-265. PMID: 16452539

Tanriverdi F, Senyurek H, Unluhizarci K, Selcuklu A, Casanueva FF, Kelestimur F. High risk of hypopituitarism after traumatic brain injury: a prospective investigation of anterior pituitary function in the acute phase and 12 months after trauma. *J Clin Endocrinol Metab.* 2006;91(6):2105-2111. PMID: 16522687

Agha A, Thompson C. High risk of hypogonadism after traumatic brain injury: clinical implications. *Pituitary.* 2005;8(3-4):245-249. PMID: 16470352

13 ANSWER: D) Serum total testosterone measurement in 3 months

Severe systemic illness suppresses the hypothalamic-pituitary-gonadal axis and results in a hormonal profile of secondary hypogonadism. Testing for hypogonadism should ideally be done at a time representative of an individual's baseline health status. Measurement of serum testosterone and gonadotropins should generally not be done in men with acute illness or an acute flare of chronic illness. For this man who was recently hospitalized for pneumonia, the best course of action would be to repeat the assessment of his gonadal access when he has fully recovered from the acute illness and has returned to his baseline health (Answer D).

Measuring transferrin saturation (Answer B) and serum prolactin (Answer C) is not indicated until the diagnosis of hypogonadism has been confirmed, which is not the case here. Younger men with secondary hypogonadism should be tested for iron overload. The diagnostic value of assessing iron saturation in older men with secondary hypogonadism is much lower because most older men with hemochromatosis tend to present with cirrhosis or heart failure, not isolated hypogonadotropic hypogonadism. Assessment for hyperprolactinemia should be performed in all men with secondary hypogonadism. Free testosterone (Answer A) is helpful in diagnosing hypogonadism in situations where an altered SHBG level is suspected; however, this patient does not have any conditions that one would expect to alter SHBG concentrations.

Pituitary imaging by MRI (Answer E) should be considered only after a diagnosis of hypogonadotropic hypogonadism has been confirmed. According to the Endocrine Society clinical practice guidelines, indications to do an MRI include (1) total testosterone concentration <150 ng/dL [<5.0 nmol/L]; (2) presence of hyperprolactinemia; (3) headache or visual field disturbance; and (4) presence of another anterior pituitary hormone deficiency.

EDUCATIONAL OBJECTIVE

Identify severe systemic illness as a cause of reversible suppression of the gonadal axis.

REFERENCE(S)

Bhasin S, Brito JP, Cunningham GR, et al. Testosterone therapy in men with hypogonadism: an Endocrine Society clinical practice guideline. *J Clin Endocrinol Metab.* 2018;103(5):1715-1744. PMID: 29562364

14 ANSWER: B) Anabolic steroid use

The fact that this patient is asymptomatic and has elevated hematocrit despite having a hormone profile showing profound hypogonadotropic hypogonadism suggests that he is being exposed to androgens other than testosterone that are not being detected in the testosterone assay. Therefore, use of androgenic anabolic steroids (Answer B) is the most likely diagnosis.

Answers A, C, D, and E would be expected to be associated with symptoms of androgen deficiency given the degree of hypogonadism. In addition, the fact that the patient is normally virilized and has testes of 12 mL would not be consistent with a diagnosis of congenital hypogonadotropic hypogonadism (Answer A).

In patients with marked hyperprolactinemia due to a large macroadenoma, serum prolactin levels can be read as normal unless serial dilution of serum is done to assess for the "hook effect." However, if hyperprolactinemia (Answer C) were responsible for this patient's hypogonadism, MRI would show a large pituitary adenoma as opposed to the 5-mm lesion seen in this case, which is most likely an incidentaloma.

While opioid use (Answer D) is an increasingly common cause of hypogonadism and could lead to the degree of gonadotropin suppression described in the vignette, it would not explain either the patient's lack of symptoms or his elevated hematocrit.

Hereditary hemochromatosis (Answer E) is in the differential diagnosis for acquired hypogonadotropic hypogonadism, but it would not typically cause such profoundly low testosterone and gonadotropin levels. In addition, patients with this disorder are not asymptomatic and typically have other manifestations, including arthralgias, chondrocalcinosis, and hyperpigmentation. Later in the disease course, patients may experience heart failure, cirrhosis, and diabetes mellitus. Hemochromatosis is inherited in an autosomal recessive manner and has a prevalence of about 0.4% in populations of northern European descent, but it has much lower clinical penetrance and disease severity is highly variable. Pathogenic variants in the *HFE* gene are responsible, and the most common genotype is homozygosity for the Cys282Tyr (C282Y) variant.

EDUCATIONAL OBJECTIVE

Diagnose anabolic steroid use as a cause of secondary hypogonadism.

REFERENCE(S)

Anawalt BD. Diagnosis and management of anabolic androgenic steroid use. *J Clin Endocrinol Metab.* 2019;104(7):2490-2500. PMID: 30753550

15 **ANSWER: D) Erythrocytosis**

When considering testosterone replacement therapy, particularly in older men, the risks and benefits should be discussed before initiating therapy. Erythrocytosis (Answer D) is the most common adverse effect of testosterone therapy in older men. Meta-analyses of randomized controlled trials have shown that older men on testosterone are 4 to 5 times more likely to experience erythrocytosis than those on placebo. Testosterone-related erythrocytosis is dosage-dependent and is more frequently encountered in older men and in patients on injectable testosterone preparations. Androgens stimulate erythropoiesis via various mechanisms: (1) direct stimulation of erythroid cell line in the bone marrow, (2) stimulation of erythropoietin synthesis and release from the kidneys, and (3) increasing iron availability for erythropoiesis. Although the mechanism(s) explaining why older men are predisposed to erythrocytosis remains unclear, reduced metabolic clearance rate of testosterone has been posited as a cause. Anecdotal reports also suggest that men with underlying hypoxic conditions may also be more predisposed to erythrocytosis during testosterone therapy.

Before initiating testosterone therapy, baseline hematocrit should be measured. The Endocrine Society clinical practice guidelines recommend against initiating testosterone therapy in patients with a baseline hematocrit level greater than 48% (greater than 50% for men living at higher altitudes) and suggest that the underlying cause of erythrocytosis be investigated before androgen therapy is prescribed. Once testosterone therapy is initiated, it is suggested that hematocrit be assessed in 3 to 6 months and then annually. If the hematocrit level is above 54% (>0.54), testosterone therapy should be discontinued until hematocrit normalizes (and testosterone therapy can then be initiated at a reduced dosage). Such patients should be evaluated for hypoxia and sleep apnea.

PSA elevation above 4 ng/mL (>4 µg/L) (Answer C) is seen more frequently in older men on testosterone compared with rates observed in men taking placebo, but meta-analyses of randomized controlled trials show that this risk is much less common than erythrocytosis (odds ratio, 1.22). Similarly, randomized controlled trials have not shown a higher frequency of urinary retention (Answer B) in older men. There are no data to suggest that physiologic testosterone replacement causes aggressive behavior (Answer A) in men. Elevated liver enzymes (Answer E) can occur in patients taking synthetic oral androgens such as methyltestosterone, which can cause jaundice, peliosis hepatitis, and hepatomas. However, hepatotoxicity is not an adverse effect of transdermal or intramuscular testosterone formulations.

EDUCATIONAL OBJECTIVE

Identify the most likely adverse effect of testosterone therapy in older men.

REFERENCE(S)

Snyder PJ, Bhasin S, Cunningham GR, et al; Testosterone Trials Investigators. Effects of testosterone treatment in older men. *N Engl J Med.* 2016;374(7):611-624. PMID: 26886521

Roy CN, Snyder PJ, Stephens-Shields AJ, et al. Association of testosterone levels with anemia in older men: a controlled clinical trial. *JAMA Intern Med.* 2017;177(4):480-490. PMID: 28241237

Calof OM, Singh AB, Lee ML, et al. Adverse events associated with testosterone replacement in middle-aged and older men: a meta-analysis of randomized, placebo-controlled trials. *J Gerontol A Biol Sci Med Sci.* 2005;60(11):1451-1457. PMID: 16339333

Shahani S, Braga-Basaria M, Maggio M, Basaria S. Androgens and erythropoiesis: past and present. *J Endocrinol Invest.* 2009;32(8):704-716. PMID: 19494706

16 ANSWER: B) hCG

This patient has acquired hypogonadotropic hypogonadism and azoospermia due to a pituitary macroadenoma. His normal seminal fluid volume and pH indicate nonobstructive azoospermia. His normal testicular volumes suggest that he developed hypogonadotropic hypogonadism after puberty. He has an excellent chance (80%-90%) of initiating spermatogenesis with gonadotropin therapy. Men with hypogonadotropic hypogonadism may have spermatogenesis restored with the administration of LH (usually in the form of hCG) and FSH (usually as rhFSH). Both gonadotropins may be administered subcutaneously and are administered 2 to 3 times weekly. Men with hypogonadotropic hypogonadism that has been acquired after puberty and testes that are 12 mL or larger often respond to hCG alone and typically respond within 6 to 12 months. Because rhFSH is very expensive (>$10,000 per year) and this patient has a good chance of responding to hCG alone, hCG monotherapy would be the best initial option (thus, Answer B is correct and Answer C is incorrect). Men with congenital or other causes of prepubertal hypogonadotropic hypogonadism and small testes (<6 mL) typically require LH and FSH replacement therapy; it may take 12 to 18 months for optimal spermatogenic response to gonadotropin therapy in these men.

Testosterone therapy should be stopped because exogenous testosterone inhibits gonadotropin secretion and spermatogenesis in men. GnRH therapy (Answer A) is ineffective in men with pituitary disease. Furthermore, GnRH therapy requires the use of a subcutaneous pump for continual administration every 2 hours and is not widely available.

Treatment with clomiphene (Answer D) requires an intact hypothalamus and pituitary given that it increases LH by blocking estrogen-mediated negative feedback, so it would not be effective in a patient with hypopituitarism.

Referral to an assisted reproductive technology specialist (Answer E) is unlikely to be necessary, as there is a high chance that spermatogenesis will be restored with gonadotropin therapy given the patient's good pretreatment testicular size. Such referral should be delayed until this patient has been treated appropriately with gonadotropin therapy; if spermatogenesis does not improve or the patient and his wife fail to conceive, referral would then be appropriate.

EDUCATIONAL OBJECTIVE

Recommend appropriate gonadotropin therapy in a man with hypogonadotropic hypogonadism who desires fertility.

REFERENCE(S)

Bhasin S. Approach to the infertile male. *J Clin Endocrinol Metab.* 2007;92(6):1995-2004. PMID: 17554051

Anawalt BD. Approach to male infertility and induction of spermatogenesis. *J Clin Endocrinol Metab.* 2013;98(9):3532-3542. PMID: 24014811

17 ANSWER: D) Sperm cryopreservation before chemotherapy

After 1 year of follow-up, azoospermia is seen in 90% of men with Hodgkin lymphoma who are treated with more than 3 courses of chemotherapy that includes an alkylating agent. In many of these patients, semen analysis is abnormal even before treatment and only approximately 30% of patients meet traditional criteria for sperm cryopreservation for intrauterine insemination. Nevertheless, cryopreservation of sperm (Answer D) remains the most reliable option for preserving male fertility in men about to undergo gonadotoxic chemotherapy with cyclophosphamide. Cryopreservation of human sperm does not decrease its capability for fertilization, and studies have demonstrated successful pregnancies with cryopreserved sperm. Optimal semen collection procedures for cryopreservation include obtaining at least 3 samples after abstinence for a minimum of 48 hours.

Leydig cells are less sensitive to the gonadal toxicity of chemotherapeutic agents than the germinal epithelium, which is why testosterone levels are generally preserved as in this vignette. While aromatase inhibitors (Answer A) can increase testosterone levels by blocking estrogen negative feedback leading to an increase in LH, increasing testosterone within the normal range does not help preserve spermatogenesis.

Infertility related to chemotherapy is due to loss of spermatogonial stem cells, and the recovery of spermatogenesis occurs via recolonization of the seminiferous tubules by these stem cells. Currently, cryopreservation and subsequent transplant of spermatogonial stem cells (Answer C) is considered experimental.

It has been hypothesized that hormonal suppression and the resulting disruption of gametogenesis renders the gonad less sensitive to damage by the cytotoxic drugs. However, in clinical trials, hormonal suppression with GnRH agonists (Answer B) has not been shown to reliably afford gonadal protection, and its use has led to recovery of spermatogenesis in only 20% of patients.

This patient's testosterone level is just below the lower end of the normal range during a time of an acute systemic illness. Starting testosterone therapy (Answer E) is not appropriate at this juncture, as he does not meet criteria for hypogonadism and it would not help to preserve spermatogenesis.

EDUCATIONAL OBJECTIVE

Recommend the best strategy for fertility preservation in a man about to undergo treatment for Hodgkin lymphoma.

REFERENCE(S)

Howell SJ, Shalet SM. Spermatogenesis after cancer treatment: damage and recovery. *J Natl Cancer Inst Monogr.* 2005;34:12-17. PMID: 15784814

Jahnukainen K, Ehmcke J, Hou M, Schlatt S. Testicular function and fertility preservation in male cancer patients. *Best Pract Res Clin Endocrinol Metab.* 2011;25(2):287-302. PMID: 21397199

Levine J, Canada A, Stern CJ. Fertility preservation in adolescents and young adults with cancer. *J Clin Oncol.* 2010;28(32):4831-4841. PMID: 20458029

18 ANSWER: C) Cough and shortness of breath following the injection

A long-acting intramuscular formulation comprising testosterone undecanoate was approved for the treatment of male hypogonadism in the United States in 2014. This preparation has the advantage of having a superior pharmacokinetic profile compared with other injectable formulations such as enanthate and cypionate, and it has the ability to maintain testosterone levels more consistently in the normal range over a 10-week period. The absence of marked swings in serum testosterone levels means that fluctuations in mood and energy (Answer A) are not typical adverse effects.

The US FDA has stipulated that all injections of testosterone undecanoate must be administered in an office or hospital setting by a trained health care provider and that the patient be monitored for adverse effects for 30 minutes after the injection. The restrictions associated with use of this drug result from reported cases of pulmonary oil microembolism (1.5 cases/10,000 injections) and anaphylaxis (0.4 cases/10,000 injections). Symptoms of pulmonary oil microembolism include the urge to cough, dyspnea (Answer C), throat tightening, chest pain, dizziness, and syncope. These symptoms have been reported with all testosterone injections but are more common with testosterone undecanoate because of the larger injection volume (3 mL compared with 1 mL or less for the shorter-acting formulations). Flu-like symptoms (Answer E) have not been reported with testosterone undecanoate injections.

Skin irritation (Answer D) can occur in as many as 50% of patients whose hypogonadism is treated with a testosterone patch, but this adverse effect is not seen with intramuscular testosterone undecanoate.

When ingested orally, testosterone is broken down by the liver and has the potential to cause liver damage, including cholestatic jaundice, peliosis hepatis, and hepatomas. However, testosterone formulations administered intramuscularly are not hepatotoxic, so jaundice (Answer B) is incorrect.

EDUCATIONAL OBJECTIVE

Counsel patients about potential adverse effects of the long-acting intramuscular formulation of testosterone undecanoate.

REFERENCE(S)

Wang C, Harnett M, Dobs AS, Swerdloff RS. Pharmacokinetics and safety of long-acting testosterone undecanoate injections in hypogonadal men: an 84-week phase III clinical trial. *J Androl.* 2010;31(5):457-465. PMID: 20133964

Bhasin S, Brito JP, Cunningham GR, et al. Testosterone therapy in men with hypogonadism: an Endocrine Society clinical practice guideline. *J Clin Endocrinol Metab.* 2018;103(5):1715-1744. PMID: 29562364

Obesity & Lipids Board Review

Andrea D. Coviello, MD

1 ANSWER: D) Increased LDL cholesterol

Low-carbohydrate ketogenic diets have become very popular due to the amount of weight loss observed over short periods, usually less than 6 months. The mechanistic theory behind the success of "ketonic diets" is that fuel use switches from carbohydrates to fats with increased lipolysis generating ketone bodies. To achieve this, patients generally need to restrict carbohydrate intake to less than 10% of their daily energy intake, which equates to less than 50 g of carbohydrate daily, or a more stringent target of less than 20 g of carbohydrate daily for most people following a hypocaloric diet (500 kcal a day reduction minimally). The shift to very low intake of carbohydrate to less than 10% is accompanied by 10% to 25% intake of protein and 70% to 80% intake of fats. Typically, there is a loss of lean body weight, as well as fat mass, particularly if patients do not focus on ingesting adequate amounts of protein.

This patient did adopt a low-carbohydrate ketogenic diet and had the following changes in her lipid profile 3 months later (*see table*). Concentrations of total and LDL cholesterol increased (thus, Answer D is correct and Answers B and E are incorrect). The HDL-cholesterol concentration increased, and the triglyceride concentration decreased (thus, Answers A and C are incorrect). Typically, glucose levels also improve. Persons with hyperlipidemia, particularly those not already on lipid-lowering therapy, should have their cholesterol rechecked while following a low-carbohydrate diet that significantly shifts macronutrient content.

Analyte	Baseline	After 3 months on ketogenic diet
Total cholesterol	252 mg/dL (SI: 6.53 mmol/L)	277 mg/dL (SI: 7.17 mmol/L)
LDL cholesterol	151 mg/dL (SI: 3.91 mmol/L)	201 mg/dL (SI: 5.21 mmol/L)
HDL cholesterol	42 mg/dL (SI: 1.09 mmol/L)	55 mg/dL (SI: 1.42 mmol/L)
Triglycerides	296 mg/dL (SI: 3.34 mmol/L)	105 mg/dL (SI: 2.72 mmol/L)

EDUCATIONAL OBJECTIVE

Explain the impact of low-carbohydrate ketogenic diets on lipid metabolism in patients with hyperlipidemia.

REFERENCE(S)

Bueno NB, de Melo IS, de Oliveira SL, da Rocha Ataide T. Very-low-carbohydrate ketogenic diet v. low-fat diet for long-term weight loss: a meta-analysis of randomised controlled trials. *Br J Nutr.* 2013;110(7):1178-1187. PMID: 23651522

Schwingshackl L, Hoffmann G. Low-carbohydrate diets and cardiovascular risk factors. *Obes Rev.* 2013;14(2):183-184. PMID: 23294905

Mansoor N, Vinknes KJ, Veierod MB, Retterstol K. Low-carbohydrate diets increase LDL-cholesterol, and thereby indicate increased risk of CVD. *Br J Nutr.* 2016;115(12):2264-2266. PMID: 27376624

Mansoor N, Vinknes KJ, Veierod MB, Retterstol K. Effects of low-carbohydrate diets v. low-fat diets on body weight and cardiovascular risk factors: a meta-analysis of randomised controlled trials. *Br J Nutr.* 2016;115(3):466-479. PMID: 26768850

Sackner-Bernstein J, Kanter D, Kaul S. Dietary intervention for overweight and obese adults: comparison of low-carbohydrate and low-fat diets. A meta-analysis. *PLoS One.* 2015;10(10): e0139817. PMID: 26485706

2 ANSWER: C) Roux-en-Y gastric bypass

Overweight and obesity now affects approximately 75% of the US population. It is estimated that by 2030, 50% of adults in the United States will be obese. The type 2 diabetes epidemic in the United States is following the obesity epidemic. Weight loss in general is associated with improvements glycemic control in persons with type 2 diabetes. Greater weight loss is achieved with bariatric surgery procedures than through medical weight loss. Bariatric surgery is FDA approved for patients with a BMI of 40 kg/m^2 or greater or patients with a BMI of 35 kg/m^2 or greater who have a comorbid illness such as type 2 diabetes.

Over the last 5 years, an increasing body of data has emerged on the benefits of bariatric surgery on glucose control in patients with type 2 diabetes. The STAMPEDE trial (Surgical Therapy and Medications Potentially Eradicate Diabetes Efficiently) is one of the first prospective randomized controlled trials to compare traditional medical therapy for type 2 diabetes with either gastric bypass surgery or sleeve gastrectomy. The patients enrolled had a BMI of 27 to 43 kg/m^2 at baseline and type 2 diabetes. The investigators defined remission a priori as a hemoglobin A_{1c} level less than 6.0% (<42 mmol/mol) on no glucose-lowering medications. Five-year follow-up data (February 2017) were available on 134 of the 150 participants with type 2 diabetes in the original cohort. Fourteen patients who underwent Roux-en-Y gastric bypass (RYGB) (29%) and 11 who underwent sleeve gastrectomy (23%) remained in remission from type 2 diabetes compared with 2 (5%) in the medical therapy group. In the surgical groups, 89% remained off insulin with an average hemoglobin A_{1c} level of 7.0% (53 mmol/mol) compared with 61% of patients in the medical therapy group with an average hemoglobin A_{1c} level of 8.5% (69 mmol/mol).

Of the currently performed bariatric procedures, RYGB (Answer C) has been shown to be superior to sleeve gastrectomy (Answer B) for the regression of type 2 diabetes in a randomized, blinded study in Norway. At 1 year, more patients who had undergone RYGB had remission of type 2 diabetes (hemoglobin A_{1c} <6.0% [<42 mmol/mol] without medications) than those who had sleeve gastrectomy. However, effect on β-cell function was the same in both groups. Effects on remission are thought to be due in part to the amount of weight loss and in part to the shift in gut hormones after RYGB vs sleeve gastrectomy.

Gastric banding (Answer A) is a restrictive procedure that produces the least weight loss of all invasive procedures. Insertion of a balloon into the stomach (Answer D) is also a restrictive procedure that induces some weight loss (12%-13%), but it has not been shown to result in remission of diabetes. Some fatalities with the gastric balloon have curbed use of this medical device. It is most often used as a bridge to either sleeve gastrectomy or RYGB in patients with severe obesity (BMI ≥40 kg/m^2).

EDUCATIONAL OBJECTIVE

Describe the effect of bariatric procedures on glycemic control and regression of type 2 diabetes.

REFERENCE(S)

Mullally JA, Febres GJ, Bessler M, Korner J. Sleeve gastrectomy and Roux-en-Y gastric bypass achieve similar early improvements in beta-cell function in obese patients with type 2 diabetes. *Sci Rep.* 2019;9(1):1880. PMID: 30755673

Hofso D, Fatima F, Borgeraas H, et al. Gastric bypass versus sleeve gastrectomy in patients with type 2 diabetes (Oseberg): a single-centre, triple-blind, randomised controlled trial. *Lancet Diabetes Endocrinol.* 2019;7(12):912-924. PMID: 31678062

Borgeraas H, Hjelmesaeth J, Birkeland KI, et al. Single-centre, triple-blinded, randomised, 1-year, parallel-group, superiority study to compare the effects of Roux-en-Y gastric bypass and sleeve gastrectomy on remission of type 2 diabetes and beta-cell function in subjects with morbid obesity: a protocol for the Obesity Surgery in Tonsberg (Oseberg) study. *BMJ Open.* 2019;9(6): e024573. PMID: 31167860

Zhou K, Wolski K, Malin SK, et al. Impact of weight loss trajectory following randomization to bariatric surgery on long-term diabetes glycemic and cardiometabolic parameters. *Endocr Pract.* 2019;25(6):572-579. PMID: 30865529

Schauer PR, Bhatt DL, Kirwan JP, et al. Bariatric surgery versus intensive medical therapy for diabetes - 5-year outcomes. *N Engl J Med.* 2017;376(7):641-651. PMID: 28199805

3 ANSWER: D) Add ezetimibe

The goal LDL-cholesterol concentration for secondary prevention is less than 70 mg/dL (<1.81 mmol/L), no matter which vascular bed is affected. A recent trial targeting an LDL-cholesterol concentration less than 70 mg/dL (<1.81 mmol/L) vs 90 to 110 mg/dL (2.33-2.85 mmol/L) with lipid-lowering therapy after stroke demonstrated a lower risk of cardiovascular events (composite endpoint comprised of ischemic stroke, myocardial infarction, coronary or carotid revascularization, or cardiovascular death) in the less than 70 mg/dL (<1.81 mmol/L) group (8.5% vs 10.9%; hazard ratio, 0.78; 95% CI, 0.61-0.98).

This patient has known cerebrovascular disease and significant additional risk factors for cardiovascular disease, including high blood pressure, prediabetes, fatty liver disease, and previous cigarette smoking. He is already on a statin and tolerating a high-intensity dosage of 40 mg daily, but he did not tolerate a higher dosage of atorvastatin. He needs about a 10% reduction in LDL cholesterol to achieve a concentration less than 70 mg/dL (<1.81 mmol/L). Ezetimibe (Answer D) is a reasonable addition that will lower his LDL cholesterol 10% to 15%. Ezetimibe blocks intestinal absorption of cholesterol through the Niemann-Pick C1-like 1 cholesterol transfer protein, which in turn upregulates LDL-receptor expression on hepatocytes leading to greater clearance of LDL cholesterol. The REDUCE-IT trial showed a 2% reduction in cardiovascular events when ezetimibe was added to simvastatin with a mean LDL-cholesterol concentration on treatment of 54 mg/dL (1.40 mmol/L) compared with 70 mg/dL (1.81 mmol/L) in the placebo group. Ezetimibe is very well tolerated and is not likely to cause return of the patient's myalgias.

Changing atorvastatin to pitavastatin (Answer A) may help preserve this patient's glycemic control and prevent progression to type 2 diabetes, but it would most likely not lower his LDL cholesterol more than atorvastatin, 40 mg daily, would. Neither niacin (Answer B) nor fenofibrate (Answer C) is likely to lower his risk of another cardiovascular event, and niacin may in fact increase his risk of another stroke. There is no reason to stop his atorvastatin, as he is tolerating his current dosage and the mild elevation in his liver enzymes (ALT and AST) in the setting of fatty liver disease is not a contraindication to statin use. Ezetimibe is the recommended second-line treatment in this scenario for secondary prevention before consideration of a PCSK9 inhibitor (evolocumab or alirocumab) (Answer E).

There was some concern over a report that very low LDL-cholesterol levels (<50 mg/dL [<1.30 mmol/L]) may be associated with higher risk of hemorrhagic stroke, but this has not been confirmed in follow-up studies of LDL targets for ischemic stroke. The LDL-cholesterol goal for secondary prevention of cerebrovascular events remains less than 70 mg/dL (<1.81 mmol/L) for now, as it appears to be a safe goal that is associated with reduced risk of future cardiovascular disease.

EDUCATIONAL OBJECTIVE

Identify the LDL-cholesterol target for secondary prevention of stroke through lipid-lowering therapy.

REFERENCE(S)

Amerenco P, Kim JS, Labreuche J, et al; Treat Stroke to Target Investigators. A comparison of two LDL cholesterol targets after ischemic stroke. *N Engl J Med.* 2020;382(1):9. PMID: 31738483

Michos ED, McEnvoy JW, Blumenthal RS. Lipid management for the prevention of atherosclerotic cardiovascular disease. *N Engl J Med.* 2019;381(16): 1557-1567. PMID: 31618541

Schade DS, Eaton RP. A simplified approach to reducing cardiovascular risk. *J Clin Endocrinol Metab.* 2019;104(12):6033-6039. PMID: 30785997

Ose L. Pitavastatin: finding its place in therapy. *Ther Adv Chronic Disease.* 2011;2(2):101-117. PMID: 23251745

4 ANSWER: A) Red yeast rice

Many supplements have been used to lower cholesterol. Red yeast rice (Answer A) and red yeast rice extract have been used historically in China to lower cholesterol. Red yeast rice is produced by fermentation of a fungus (Monascus purpureus) grown on rice, which makes a substance called monacolin K (similar to lovastatin) that lowers total and LDL cholesterol by competitively binding HMG-CoA reductase with very high affinity (as statins do). A byproduct is a red pigment that gives the rice its red color. Several small studies of short duration (1-12 months) have demonstrated its lipid-lowering effects, and a meta-analysis of 13 trials showed a significant reduction in both total and LDL cholesterol. In a placebo-controlled trial for secondary prevention in 5000 patients in China, red yeast rice taken for 4.5 years showed a 45% relative risk reduction in nonfatal myocardial infarction and cardiovascular death compared with placebo (5.7% vs 10.4%) and a 35% reduction in cardiovascular death, which suggests some efficacy. In general, data have not reached sufficient quality that red yeast rice can be recommended from an evidence-based perspective compared with the amount of data on FDA-approved statin medications. Since this patient is statin intolerant, the use of a supplement that has a similar mechanism of action as statin medications (ie, HMG-CoA reductase inhibition) would convey similar adverse effects.

The supplement berberine (Answer B), an alkaloid derived from the bark of a shrub found in the Himalayas called *Berberis aristata,* is thought to lower cholesterol by inhibiting PSCK9 production (thus functioning like a PCSK9 inhibitor antibody) and by stimulating AMPK. Folate (Answer D) functions to methylate homocysteine, but treatment with folate has failed to show beneficial effects on cardiovascular disease. Coenzyme Q10 (Answer C) is an antioxidant supplement that is believed to be beneficial due to its ability to prevent LDL oxidation, but which is depleted by HMG-CoA reductase inhibitor therapy (ie, by statin use). Many people anecdotally feel that taking coenzyme Q10 helps to avoid myalgias and fatigue while taking statin medications, although high-quality evidence from randomized placebo-controlled trials do not support this belief. The above supplements do not have the same mechanism of action as statin medications (inhibition of HMG-CoA reductase) and therefore would not be expected to cause similar adverse effects.

EDUCATIONAL OBJECTIVE

List supplements commonly used to lower cholesterol and their mechanisms of action.

REFERENCE(S)

Gerards MC, Terlou RJ, Yu H, Koks CH, Gerdes VE. Traditional Chinese lipid-lowering agent red yeast rice results in significant LDL reduction but safety is uncertain - systematic review and meta-analysis. *Atherosclerosis.* 2015;240(2):415-423. PMID: 25897793

Fogacci F, Banach M, Mikhailidis DP, et al; Lipid and Blood Pressure Meta-Analysis Collaboration (LBPMC) Group; International Lipid Expert Panel (ILEP). Safety of red yeast rice supplementation: a systematic review and meta-analysis of randomized controlled trials. *Pharmacologic Res.* 2019;143: 1-16. PMID: 30844537

Li Y, Jiang L, Jia Z, Xin W, Yang S, Yang Q, Wang L. A meta-analysis of red yeast rice: an effective and relatively safe alternative approach for dyslipidemia. *PLoS One.* 2014;9(6):e98611. PMID: 24897342

Lu Z, Kou W, Du B, et al. Effect of Xuezhikang, an extract from red yeast Chinese rice, on coronary events in a Chinese population with previous myocardial infarction. *Am J Cardiol.* 2008;101(12): 1689-1693. PMID: 18549841

Barrios V, Escobar C, Cicero AF, et al. A nutraceutical approach (Armolipid Plus) to reduce total and LDL cholesterol in individuals with mild to moderate dyslipidemia: review of the clinical evidence. *Atheroscler Suppl.* 2017;24:1-15. PMID: 27998714

5 ANSWER: B) Lipoprotein (a) measurement

This patient has a first-degree relative with premature heart disease who sustained a myocardial infarction at age 45 years before being on lipid-lowering therapy. This history puts the patient at risk of early cardiovascular disease, possibly due to familial hyperlipidemia. Familial hyperlipidemia is a relatively common genetic disorder affecting 1 in 250 to 500 persons depending on the population. The American Heart Association recommends high-intensity statin treatment for individuals with an LDL-cholesterol concentration greater than 190 mg/dL (>4.92 mmol/L) due to the very high likelihood that they have familial hyperlipidemia and are at very high cardiovascular risk. However, some patients with familial hyperlipidemia may have LDL-cholesterol levels less than 190 mg/dL (<4.92 mmol/L) as well, particularly depending on their lifestyle habits in relation to diet and exercise. Even patients with familial hyperlipidemia can lower their LDL cholesterol through lifestyle changes, as this patient did by adopting a vegan diet. Although she lowered her LDL cholesterol by approximately 27%, her LDL-cholesterol concentration remains above 100 mg/dL (>2.59 mmol/L), and her triglycerides are also above target according to the 2018 American Heart Association/American College of Cardiology cholesterol management guidelines.

Other conditions can put patients at high risk of premature cardiovascular disease. Elevated lipoprotein (a) (Answer B), a highly atherogenic lipoprotein, is also associated with very high cardiovascular disease risk, as well as aortic stenosis. Lipoprotein (a) is produced by the liver and levels are predominantly genetically inherited. Lipoprotein (a) is a large lipoprotein in which apolipoprotein (a) is attached covalently to apolipoprotein B. Lipoprotein (a) may be modestly elevated in familial hyperlipidemia, but it is an independent risk factor for atherosclerotic disease. Persons with a lipoprotein (a) level in the upper tertile have an increased risk of cardiovascular disease (odds ratio, 1.7; 95% CI, 1.4-1.9) compared with persons whose level is in the lower tertile. Elevated lipoprotein (a) is a strong indication for aggressive lipid lowering through available pharmacologic options in addition to lifestyle medication and a low-cholesterol diet to target a non–HDL-cholesterol concentration less than 100 mg/dL (<2.59 mmol/L) (LDL cholesterol <70 mg/dL [<1.81 mmol/L]). New therapeutic agents are in development that target lipoprotein (a) and effectively lower it in a dose-dependent manner. However, longer trials are needed that demonstrate a reduction in cardiovascular events with these compounds.

Current guidelines recommend screening for lipoprotein (a) in individuals at very high cardiovascular risk and those with a history of premature cardiovascular disease, a first-degree relative with premature cardiovascular disease or known lipoprotein (a) elevation, progressive cardiovascular disease despite maximal LDL-cholesterol lowering, or borderline 10-year cardiovascular risk with need for additional information to inform treatment decisions.

The 2018 American Heart Association guidelines recommend intensified lifestyle modification if triglycerides are greater than 150 mg/dL (>1.70 mmol/L) and consideration of additional lipid-lowering therapy if triglycerides are persistently greater than 175 mg/dL (>1.98 mmol/L) in patients at high cardiovascular risk, particularly in the setting of diabetes which this patient does not have. For triglycerides in this range, therapy would start with a statin, which she does not want to initiate.

Non-HDL cholesterol is considered a marker of cardiovascular risk that includes all atherogenic particles, including triglyceride-rich particles, but it would not add any additional information. Thus, measuring non-HDL cholesterol (Answer A) is incorrect. Similarly, measurement of apolipoprotein B (Answer C) would also provide a measure of additional atherogenic triglyceride-rich lipoproteins, as apolipoprotein B is a structural component of all of them. Its measurement would not add additional information to what is already available in her lipid profile since her LDL-cholesterol and triglyceride concentrations are listed. Her triglycerides could be a secondary target clinically as they are above target for optimal cholesterol profiles. Circulating chylomicrons (Answer D) relate to dietary fat ingestion, and severe elevations increase risk for pancreatitis. This patient's triglyceride concentration is less than 400 mg/dL (<4.52 mmol/L), which makes chylomicronemia syndrome unlikely.

Nuclear magnetic resonance spectroscopy (Answer E) gives information about particle size and concentration. Nuclear magnetic resonance spectroscopy typically provides information on lipoprotein profiles notable for high concentrations of small, dense LDL particles that are typical of an insulin-resistant phenotype associated with type 2 diabetes. This patient does not have diabetes. Nuclear magnetic resonance spectroscopy is not likely to provide additional insight into her risk of cardiovascular disease beyond her cholesterol profile with elevated LDL cholesterol.

EDUCATIONAL OBJECTIVE

Determine when measurement of lipoprotein (a) is indicated in the assessment of cardiovascular risk.

REFERENCE(S)

Danesh J, Collins R, Peto R. Lipoprotein(a) and coronary heart disease. Meta-analysis of prospective studies. *Circulation.* 2000;102(10):1082-1085. PMID: 10973834

Ma L, Chan DC, Ooi EMM, Marcovina SM, Barrett PHR, Watts GF. Apolipoprotein(a) kinetics in statin-treated patients with elevated plama lipoprotein(a) concentration. *J Clin Endocrinol Metab.* 2019;104(12):6247-6255. PMID: 31393573

Tsimikas S, Karwatowska-Prokopczuk E, Gouni-Berthold I, et al; AKCEA-APO(a)-LRx Study Investigators. Lipoprotein(a) reduction in persons with cardiovascular disease. *N Engl J Metab.* 2020;382(3):244-255. PMID: 31893580

Grundy SM, Stone NJ, Bailey AL, et al. 2018 AHA/ACC/AACVPR/AAPA/ABC/ACPM/ADA/AGS/APhA/ASPC/NLA/PCNA guideline on the management of blood cholesterol. *Circulation.* 2019;139(25):e1082-e1143. PMID: 30586774

6 ANSWER: B) Microsomal triglyceride transfer protein (*MTTP*)

Hypolipidemia can be generic or acquired. Acquired disorders include malignancy (colorectal and prostate cancer, leukemias, myeloma), malabsorption (pancreatic exocrine insufficiency, celiac disease, post bowel surgery), infection (giardiasis, tuberculosis, schistosomiasis), and severe or critical illness. This patient was diagnosed as an infant, which is most consistent with a genetic disorder. Her very low total cholesterol (<50 mg/dL [<1.30 mmol/L]) with undetectable LDL cholesterol and apolipoprotein B suggests severe hypolipidemia from alterations in genes regulating lipid metabolism. This patient has abetalipoproteinemia, a rare autosomal recessive disorder (1 in 1 million persons) caused by microsomal triglyceride transfer protein (MTTP) deficiency. Multiple variants in the *MTTP* gene (Answer B) cause MTTP deficiency. MTTP is produced in the liver and intestines where it is crucial for the formation of apolipoprotein B–containing lipoproteins in the endoplasmic reticulum through transfer of triglyceride or phospholipids. The absence of MTTP results in no synthesis or secretion of apolipoprotein B into the circulation where it is undetectable. Lack of MTTP in intestinal cells impairs chylomicron formation and severe malabsorption of fat and fat-soluble vitamins (A, D, E, and K). If not diagnosed early and treated aggressively, the severe vitamin deficiencies can lead to a range of complications, including retinal degeneration and blindness, degenerative neurologic disorders, anemias, and osteoporosis. Affected patients are treated with high-dosage oral supplements, as well as intravenous infusion of lipids and vitamins.

Two other rare genetic disorders in the differential diagnosis of severe hypolipidemias are the homozygous form familial hypobetalipoproteinemia and chylomicron retention syndrome (Anderson disease). Familial hypobetalipoproteinemia is a disorder of low cholesterol due to defective apolipoprotein B. The heterozygous form of familial hypobetalipoproteinemia occurs in 1 in 500 persons and is characterized by a cholesterol concentration less than 100 mg/dL (<2.59 mmol/L), or half of typical values but not severely low levels less than 50 mg/dL (<1.30 mmol/L). Affected patients are generally asymptomatic and identified with screening lipid profiles. The homozygous form is rare and presents with very low cholesterol levels and a clinical presentation similar to that of abetalipoproteinemia, although the defect is in the *APOB* gene and not in the *MTTP* gene.

Chylomicron retention syndrome (Anderson disease) is a rare autosomal recessive disorder due to pathogenic variants in the *SAR1B* gene. In this disorder, chylomicrons cannot be secreted from the intestines, which results in very low circulating cholesterol and triglycerides with a clinical presentation similar to that of abetalipoproteinemia. Neither of these severe forms of hypolipidemias were presented as an option in this vignette.

Lipoprotein lipase deficiency (Answer A) is a primary hypertriglyceridemia disorder with severely elevated triglycerides (>1000 mg/dL [>11.30 mmol/L]), not low cholesterol. Lipoprotein lipase is located on endothelial cells where it hydrolyzes triglycerides from chylomicrons and VLDL particles, effectively clearing triglyceride. The absence of lipoprotein lipase activity results in very high triglycerides.

Apolipoprotein CII (Answer C) is a cofactor of lipoprotein lipase and its deficiency leads to very high triglycerides (>1000 mg/dL [>11.30 mmol/L]).

Apolipoprotein A1 (Answer D) is an important protein for HDL cholesterol, and its absence leads to very low HDL cholesterol but not low LDL cholesterol or low triglycerides.

Cholesterol ester transfer protein (Answer E) transfers cholesterol esters from HDL to VLDL, IDL, and remnant particles in exchange for triglyceride, essentially clearing HDL cholesterol. The absence of cholesterol ester transfer protein results in high circulating levels of HDL cholesterol with concentrations usually greater than 100 mg/dL (>2.59 mmol/L).

EDUCATIONAL OBJECTIVE

Describe the causes of hypolipidemias and key management considerations.

REFERENCE(S)

Welty FK. Hypobetalipoproteinemia and abetalipoproteinemia. *Curr Opin Lipidol.* 2014;31(2): 49-55. PMID: 32039990

Olsson AG, Angelin B, Assmann G, et al. Can LDL cholesterol be too low? Possible risks of extremely low levels. *J Intern Med.* 2017;281(6):281-534. PMID: 28295777

Sharp D, Blinderman L, Combs KA, et al. Cloning and gene defects in microsomal triglyceride transfer protein associated with abetalipoproteinaemia. *Nature.* 1993;365(6441):65-69. PMID: 8361539

Wetterau JR, Aggerbeck LP, Bouma ME, et al. Absence of microsomal triglyceride transfer protein in individuals with abetalipoproteinemia. *Science.* 1992;258(5084):999-1001. PMID: 1439810

Peretti N, Sassolas A, Roy CC, et al. Guidelines for the diagnosis and management of chylomicron retention disease based on a review of the literature and experience of the two centers. *Orphanet J Rare Dis.* 2010;5:24. PMID: 20920215

7 ANSWER: E) Colesevelam

This patient most likely has heterozygous familial hyperlipidemia (FH) with an LDL-cholesterol concentration of 300 mg/dL (7.77 mmol/L) before pregnancy. This diagnosis puts her at very high risk for cardiovascular disease. All adults with familial hyperlipidemia and LDL-cholesterol concentrations greater than 190 mg/dL (>4.92 mmol/L) should be started on lipid-lowering therapy with a high-intensity statin followed by additional medications as needed to target at least a 50% reduction in LDL cholesterol and ideally an LDL-cholesterol concentration less than 100 mg/dL (<2.59 mmol/L). A long-term study of children with genetically confirmed FH treated with statins for an average of 20 years showed less subclinical atherosclerosis as indicated by carotid intima-media thickness measurement and reduced cardiovascular disease compared with their affected parents and unaffected siblings. Women of reproductive age who have FH should be counseled regarding treatment during pregnancy and lactation. In a 40-year observation cohort study of the Medical Birth Registry of Norway (1967-2006), there was no increased risk of preterm delivery (<37 weeks), low birth weight (<2500 g), or congenital malformations in 1869 women with FH compared with other women. Women of reproductive age who have FH should be treated with lipid-lowering treatment with cessation of statins and/or other lipid-lowering medications 3 months before planned conception. All lipid-lowering therapy is recommended to be stopped during pregnancy due to risk to the fetus. Cholesterol levels increase by approximately one-third during pregnancy, including LDL cholesterol, which means it will be higher during gestation.

Breastfeeding presents another challenge, although cholesterol levels generally return to prepregnancy levels over time while lactating. Lipid-lowering medication is generally not recommended while breastfeeding, including any intensity statin and PCSK9 inhibitors (Answers A, B, C, and D). However, the time without lipid-lowering therapy in the context of term pregnancy and lactation can extend to 2 years with high circulating LDL-cholesterol levels in patients with FH. If lipid-lowering therapy is going to be started, bile-acid resins such as colesevelam (Answer E) can be initiated while breastfeeding. For patients with severely elevated levels or homozygous FH, apheresis has been used in some cases to remove LDL cholesterol during pregnancy and lactation, but it was not a choice in this vignette.

EDUCATIONAL OBJECTIVE

Manage heterozygous familial hyperlipidemia in women of reproductive age.

REFERENCE(S)

Arnett DK, Blumenthal RS, Albert MA, et al. 2019 ACC/AHA guideline on the primary prevention of cardiovascular disease: a report of the American College of Cardiology/American Heart Association Task Force on Clinical Practice Guidelines. *J Am Coll Cardiol.* 2019;74(10): 1376-1414. PMID: 30894319

Luirink IK, Wiegman A, Kusters DM, et al. 20-year follow-up of statins in children with familial hyperlipidemia. *N Engl J Metab.* 2019;381(16): 1547-1556. PMID: 31618540

Toleikyte I, Retterstol K, Leren TP, Iversen PO. Pregnancy outcomes in familial hypercholesterolemia: a registry-based study. *Circulation.* 2011;124(15):1606-1614. PMID: 21911783

deGoma EM, Ahmad ZS, O'Brien EC, et al. Treatment gaps in adults with heterozygous familial hypercholesterolemia in the United States: data from the CASCADE-FH Registry. *Circ Cardiovasc Genet.* 2016;9(3):240-249. PMID: 27013694

8 ANSWER: D) Biliopancreatic diversion

Because of the increasing prevalence of severe obesity, patients regularly ask their endocrinologists for advice on the risks and benefits of bariatric surgery. It is important, therefore, for clinical endocrinologists to have a sense of both the amount of weight loss that a patient might expect from the commonly performed bariatric surgical procedures, as well as the potential problems associated with each.

Biliopancreatic diversion (Answer D) is a more extensive operation that is not often performed. It is important for endocrinologists to be aware of this procedure, however, as they may see patients who are thinking of having it or who have had it. It is associated with the greatest degree of weight loss (32%-35%) and has the largest effects on glucose levels, but it is not widely used because of more frequent complications and adverse effects, including severe and potentially difficult-to-treat vitamin deficiencies.

Roux-en-Y gastric bypass (Answer B) remains the criterion standard operation. Of the first 3 operations listed, it provides the most weight loss (25%-28%) and often dramatically improves glucose levels in patients with type 2 diabetes. However, it results in a lifelong need for vitamin supplementation and most likely puts patients at risk for metabolic bone disease.

The laparoscopic banding procedure (Answer C) was popular for a number of years because it was relatively easy for the surgeon to perform and had low perioperative risk. Because it was potentially reversible, it satisfied many patients' desire to not have their "plumbing changed." However, as time has passed, it has become clear that the weight loss provided by this option is less (18%-22% of baseline weight) than that of other procedures and that mechanical problems are more common with this procedure in the long run.

Sleeve gastrectomy (Answer A) is gaining in popularity because it does not require ongoing adjustment (as does the band), results in better weight loss (22%-25%), and is relatively easy for the surgeon to perform. Despite these advantages, recent studies have shown that the sleeve gastrectomy is not as effective as gastric bypass in either producing weight loss or improving glucose control in patients with type 2 diabetes.

The endoscopically placed dual balloon device (Answer E) is a newly approved device that creates a sense of fullness and is used for temporary weight loss. The limited data available in humans suggest that it produces roughly a 7% weight loss 6 months after placement.

EDUCATIONAL OBJECTIVE

Describe the expected weight loss associated with different bariatric surgical procedures.

REFERENCE(S)

Dumon KR, Murayama KM. Bariatric surgery outcomes. *Surg Clin North Am.* 2011;91(6): 1313-1338. PMID: 22054156

Chang SH, Stoll CR, Song J, Varela JE, Eagon CJ, Colditz GA. The effectiveness and risks of bariatric surgery: an updated systematic review and meta-analysis, 2003-2012. *JAMA Surg.* 2014;149(3): 275-287. PMID: 24352617

Padwal R, Klarenbach S, Wiebe N, et al. Bariatric surgery: a systematic review and network meta-analysis of randomized trials. *Obes Rev.* 2011;12(8):602-621. PMID: 21438991

9 ANSWER: Answer: A) Melanocortin 4 receptor *(MC4R)*

Although knowledge of the monogenic forms of severe childhood obesity is most relevant for pediatric endocrinologists, adult endocrinologists will on occasion encounter a patient with one of these syndromes, and genetic forms of obesity provide insights into important pathways that regulate body weight.

The most common monogenic form of early-onset obesity is caused by pathogenic variants in the gene than encodes the melanocortin 4 receptor (*MC4R*) (Answer A). The melanocortin 4 receptor is involved in hypothalamic signaling along the neural pathway that responds to leptin. The hypothalamus has a central role in the regulation of food intake. Leptin and insulin act on proopiomelanocortin (POMC) neurons in the arcuate nucleus to increase the expression and release of a-melanocyte–stimulating hormone, which then binds to melanocortin 4 receptors on postsynaptic cells to reduce food intake. A pathogenic variant that impairs receptor function would lead to the loss of satiety and unblocked hunger leading to hyperphagia. These patients present with childhood obesity.

Individuals who have pathogenic variants in the genes encoding leptin (Answer B) or the leptin receptor (Answer C) have hypothalamic hypogonadism and subtle impairments in GH and immune function.

A pathogenic variant in the gene encoding proopiomelanocortin (POMC) (Answer D) causes a rare form of early-onset, childhood obesity due to hyperphagia. POMC has an important role in regulating satiety and energy expenditure. POMC is cleaved into melanocyte-stimulating hormone and ACTH, which is necessary for normal adrenal function. Affected patients present with childhood obesity, as well as adrenal insufficiency, which may present with hypoglycemia in the neonatal period. The adrenal insufficiency is treated with glucocorticoid replacement, but the obesity is difficult to treatment. Two affected individuals were treated with setmelanotide, a melanocortin 4 receptor agonist that reduced hunger and induced weight loss of 44 to 110 lb (20-50 kg) over 12 to 42 weeks.

Pathogenic variants in the fat mass and obesity-associated protein gene (*FTO*) (Answer E) are most commonly associated with generalized obesity, not early childhood-onset obesity. The *FTO* gene, in addition to variants in more than 90 other genes, collectively explains less than 5% of the variation in BMI.

EDUCATIONAL OBJECTIVE

Identify monogenic forms of early-onset childhood obesity.

REFERENCE(S)

Kuhnen P, Clement K, Wiegand S, et al. Proopiomelanocortin deficiency treated with a melanocortin-4 receptor agonist. *N Engl J Med.* 2016;375(3):240-246. PMID: 27468060

Farooqi S, O'Rahilly S. Genetics of obesity in humans. *Endocr Rev.* 2006;27(7):710-718. PMID: 17122358

Ranadive SA, Vaisse C. Lessons from extreme human obesity: monogenic disorders. *Endocrinol Metab Clin North Am.* 2008;37(3):733-751. PMID: 18775361

Schwartz MW, Woods SC, Porte D Jr, Seeley RJ, Baskin DG. Central nervous system control of food intake. *Nature.* 2000;404(6778): 661-671. PMID: 10766253

10 ANSWER: Answer: D) Atorvastatin

Many commonly prescribed medications are associated with weight gain. Of the available antihypertensive medications, β-adrenergic blockers (Answer A) are associated with weight gain, while ACE inhibitors, angiotensin receptor blockers, calcium-channel blockers, and diuretics are not. Many diabetes medications are associated with weight gain, up to 10 to 20 lb (4.5-9.1 kg) in the first 6 to 12 months, including the anabolic hormone insulin, insulin secretagogues (eg, sulfonylureas, meglitinides), and thiazolidinediones (Answer B). Metformin is weight neutral in general, although it is associated with mild weight loss in some patients. DPP-4 inhibitors and α-glucosidase inhibitors are weight neutral, and GLP-1 receptor agonists promote weight loss in addition to blood glucose control. SGLT-2 inhibitors are associated with mild weight loss in the context of glucosuria and water loss. More recently, antihistamines (Answer C) have been recognized as weight promoting. The more potent the antihistamine, the more likely the patient is to gain weight with long-term use. The H1-antihistamines such as cetirizine are the most likely to be associated with weight gain. Inhaled glucocorticoids (Answer E) are associated with weight gain. Other medication classes that can lead to weight gain include glucocorticoids, antidepressants, antipsychotic agents, and hormonal contraceptives. The statin class of medications (Answer D) is not associated with significant weight gain.

EDUCATIONAL OBJECTIVE

Identify weight-promoting and weight-neutral medications among commonly prescribed medications for adults.

REFERENCE(S)

Apovian CM, Aronne LJ, Bessesen DH, et al; Endocrine Society. Pharmacological management of obesity: an Endocrine Society clinical practice guideline. *J Clin Endocrinol Metab.* 2015;100(2): 342-362. PMID: 25590212

11 ANSWER: C) Phentermine/topiramate

Selection of weight-loss medications should be based on a patient's individual characteristics and clinical profile. Polycystic ovary syndrome is associated with overweight and obesity and significant metabolic dysfunction, including insulin resistance, type 2 diabetes, metabolic syndrome, and fatty liver disease. Weight loss will improve this patient's metabolic and reproductive dysfunction. There are no data to suggest one medication works better than another for weight loss in patients with polycystic ovary syndrome specifically. However, her clinical picture should guide selection of a weight-loss medication, particularly her history of migraines and gallbladder disease.

Phentermine/topiramate (Answer C) is a combination medication containing phentermine (increasing doses up to 15 mg daily) and topiramate (increasing doses up to 92 mg daily). Topiramate is approved by the US FDA for use in patients with chronic migraines to reduce the frequency of migraines and for patients with seizure disorders to reduce the frequency of seizures. Although topiramate itself is not approved for weight loss, topiramate in combination with phentermine is in the combination medication phentermine/topiramate. Given this patient's chronic migraines, phentermine/topiramate is a good choice for her.

One of the most common adverse effects of naltrexone/bupropion (Answer A) is headache, which would make it a poor choice in a patient with chronic migraines. Liraglutide, 3.0 mg daily, (Answer B) is associated with gallbladder disease, including cholecystitis and gallstone pancreatitis. Over 3 years, treatment with liraglutide, 3.0 mg daily, for weight loss was associated with gallbladder disease in 4.9% of patients with consistent risk of gallbladder problems throughout the 3-year observation period. Given this patient's recurrent abdominal pain and known gallstones, liraglutide is not a good choice for her, although it would most likely improve her insulin resistance. Weight loss itself is associated with increased gallbladder dysfunction believed to be due to decreased gallbladder contractility, and GLP-1 receptor agonists are associated with added risk of gallbladder disease irrespective of the degree of weight loss.

Semaglutide (Answer D), a GLP-1 receptor agonist, is FDA approved for the treatment of diabetes but not for weight loss or prediabetes. Semaglutide, which comes in both subcutaneous and oral formulations, is, however, associated with weight loss when used to treat patients with type 2 diabetes. Semaglutide is currently being developed as a treatment for weight loss as an adjunct to changes in diet and increased physical activity.

EDUCATIONAL OBJECTIVE

Select appropriate medical therapy for weight loss based on a patient's individual characteristics and risk profile.

REFERENCE(S)

Apovian CM, Aronne LJ, Bessesen DH, et al; Endocrine Society. Pharmacological management of obesity: an Endocrine Society clinical practice guideline. *J Clin Endocrinol Metab.* 2015;100(2): 342-362. PMID: 25590212

Yanovski SZ, Yanovski JA. Long-term drug treatment for obesity: a systematic and clinical review. *JAMA.* 2014;311(1):74-86. PMID: 24231879

Garvey WT, Ryan DH, Look M, et al. Two-year sustained weight loss and metabolic benefits with controlled-release phentermine/topiramate in obese and overweight adults (SEQUEL): a randomized, placebo-controlled, phase 3 extension study. *Am J Clin Nutr.* 2012;95(2):297-308. PMID: 22158731

le Roux CW, Astrup A, Fujioka K, et al; SCALE Obesity Prediabetes NN8022-1839 Study Group. 3 years of liraglutide versus placebo for type 2 diabetes risk reduction and weight management in individuals with prediabetes: a randomised, double-blind trial. *Lancet.* 2017;389(10077): 1399-1409. PMID: 28237263

12 ANSWER: A) Liraglutide

Obesity is an independent risk factor for cardiovascular disease, and it can adversely affect other risk factors for cardiovascular disease, including hypertension, type 2 diabetes, and dyslipidemia. Weight loss can lower cardiovascular risk for both primary and secondary prevention. Care must be taken when selecting a weight-loss medication for use in patients with a recent coronary heart disease event or who are at risk for tachyarrhythmias, as most of the currently approved weight-loss medications can affect blood pressure and heart rate. Furthermore, resting tachycardia is commonly present in obese patients, even in the absence of known heart disease.

GLP-1 receptor agonists, including liraglutide (Answer A), are recognized as being "cardioprotective" with multiple formulations being associated with lower risk of cardiovascular events, which makes liraglutide a good choice in this patient. Of note, GLP-1 receptor agonists are known to increase resting heart rate, although they are not associated with increased blood pressure. Liraglutide, 3.0 mg daily, is associated with an average 2 to 3 beat/min increase in heart rate, but a proportion of patients may experience an increase in resting heart rate of greater than 10 beats/min (34% compared with 19% on placebo) or greater than 20 beats/min (5% compared with 2% on placebo), but only 0.9% develop a resting heart rate higher than 100 beats/min compared with 0.3% on placebo.

Phentermine (Answer B) and diethylpropion (Answer E) are sympathomimetic agents, or stimulants, that suppress appetite and are known to increase both blood pressure and heart rate and would thus be contraindicated in this patient. Phentermine/topiramate (Answer C) is a combination medication containing phentermine, which makes it a poor choice for weight loss in this patient.

Naltrexone/bupropion (Answer D) is contraindicated in patients with uncontrolled hypertension.

EDUCATIONAL OBJECTIVE

Select weight-loss medications for a patient with a history of cardiovascular disease and arrhythmic potential.

REFERENCE(S)

Apovian CM, Aronne LJ, Bessesen DH, et al; Endocrine Society. Pharmacological management of obesity: an Endocrine Society clinical practice guideline. *J Clin Endocrinol Metab.* 2015;100(2): 342-362. PMID: 25590212

Yanovski SZ, Yanovski JA. Long-term drug treatment for obesity: a systematic and clinical review. *JAMA.* 2014;311(1):74-86. PMID: 24231879

Pi-Sunyer X, Astrup A, Fujioka K, et al; SCALE Obesity and Prediabetes NN8022-1839 Study Group. A randomized, controlled trial of 3.0 mg of liraglutide in weight management. *N Engl J Med.* 2015;373(1):11-22. PMID: 26132939

13 ANSWER: C) Thiamine

The symptoms displayed by this patient are characteristic of Wernicke encephalopathy, which is caused by thiamine deficiency (Answer C). Thiamine deficiency causes neuronal death due to metabolic dysfunction of astrocytes within the central nervous system. The classic triad of this condition is confusion, ataxia, and nystagmus. A wide range of other abnormalities can be seen, including cranial nerve dysfunction, peripheral neuropathies, seizures, and psychosis. Because thiamine is a water-soluble vitamin, body stores can be depleted within days to weeks of inadequate intake. The condition typically presents 4 to 12 weeks after bariatric surgery but can occur as early as 2 weeks and as late as 18 months after surgery. Although most commonly reported following gastric bypass surgery, Wernicke encephalopathy can occur after any type of bariatric surgery. The most common antecedent is persistent vomiting, which then severely limits thiamine intake. Other less common precipitating factors are intravenous glucose or parenteral nutrition administration without thiamine supplementation. The condition is important to recognize, as treatment with parenteral thiamine (100 mg daily for 7 to 14 days, or 500 mg 3 times daily for 3 days) must be administered to prevent serious morbidity.

Although vitamin B_{12} deficiency (Answer A) can cause neurologic symptoms and signs, body stores of B_{12} are sizable, so deficiency does not usually occur until 6 to 24 months after bariatric surgery. Folate deficiency (Answer D) is uncommon and typically presents as anemia. Zinc deficiency (Answer E) is rare; it is associated with skin and hair findings and primarily occurs after biliary pancreatic diversion. Vitamin D deficiency (Answer B) can cause generalized weakness, but vitamin D is fat-soluble, so deficiency typically occurs months or years after bariatric surgery. In addition, vitamin D deficiency would not be expected to cause the focal neurologic signs that this patient exhibits.

EDUCATIONAL OBJECTIVE

Differentiate among the vitamin deficiencies that can occur after gastric bypass surgery.

REFERENCE(S)

Aasheim ET. Wernicke encephalopathy after bariatric surgery, a systematic review. *Ann Surg.* 2008;248(5):714-720. PMID: 18948797

Serra A, Sechi G, Singh S, Kumar A. Wernicke encephalopathy after obesity surgery: a systematic review. *Neurology.* 2007;69(6):615. PMID: 17679686

Mechanick JI, Apovian C, Brethauer S, et al. Clinical practice guidelines for the perioperative nutrition, metabolic, and nonsurgical support of patients undergoing bariatric procedures – 2019 update: cosponsored by American Association of Clinical Endocrinologists/American college of Endocrinology, The Obesity Society, American Society for Metabolic and Bariatric Surgey, Obesity Medicine Association, and American Society of Anesthesiologists. *Obesity (Silver Spring).* 2020;28(4):O1-O58. PMID: 32202076

14 ANSWER: Answer: A) Hypobetalipoproteinemia

This patient has hypobetalipoproteinemia (Answer A) with a reduction in production of both LDL (cholesterol) and VLDL (triglyceride). This condition is most often due to a defect in liver production of apolipoprotein B–containing lipoproteins because of defective production of apolipoprotein B. With apolipoprotein B, a defective protein is associated with lower than one-half normal LDL-cholesterol levels. In hypobetalipoproteinemia, inability to efficiently secrete lipoproteins from the liver can lead to nonalcoholic fatty liver disease.

Hypobetalipoproteinemia should be distinguished from abetalipoproteinemia (Answer B), a rare autosomal recessive disorder caused by a pathogenic variant in the gene encoding the microsomal transfer protein causing low levels of apolipoproteins used in the synthesis and export of chylomicrons and VLDL. LDL-cholesterol and triglyceride levels are much lower in this setting, and affected patients develop deficiencies of fat-soluble vitamins with neurologic symptoms, including weakness and balance problems as adults. This profile can also be the result of drugs that inhibit microsomal triglyceride transfer protein or antisense therapies to reduce apolipoprotein B secretion. Dysbetalipoproteinemia (Answer C) is an autosomal recessive disorder associated with an *APOE*E2/APOE*E2* genotype and clinically characterized by palmar xanthomas with roughly equal and significant elevations in both total cholesterol and triglycerides, not low levels. This is the same genetic locus that is associated with risk for Alzheimer disease (*APOE*E4/APOE*E4* genotype). Persons with hypoalphalipoproteinemia (Answer D), also known as apolipoproteinemia A1 deficiency, lack a structural protein associated with HDL and consequently have very low HDL-cholesterol levels but the other lipid fractions are not as low as in this vignette.

EDUCATIONAL OBJECTIVE

Identify conditions characterized by very low cholesterol levels and associated health risks.

REFERENCE(S)

Musunuru K, Pirruccello JP, Do R, et al. Exome sequencing, ANGPTL3 mutations, and familial combined hypolipidemia. *N Engl J Med.* 2010;363(23):2220-2227. PMID: 20942659

Cuchel M, Bloedon LT, Szapary PO, et al. Inhibition of microsomal triglyceride transfer protein in familial hypercholesterolemia. *N Engl J Med.* 2007;356(2):148-156. PMID: 17215532

Tanoli T, Yue P, Yablonskiy D, Schonfeld G. Fatty liver in familial hypobetalipoproteinemia: roles of the APOB defects, intra-abdominal adipose tissue, and insulin sensitivity. *J Lipid Res.* 2004;45(5):941-947. PMID: 14967820

Mahley RW, Huang Y, Rall SC Jr. Pathogenesis of type III hyperlipoproteinemia (dysbetalipoproteinemia). Questions, quandaries, and paradoxes. *J Lipid Res.* 1999;40(11):1933-1949. PMID: 10552997

15 ANSWER: B) Myositis

A number of medications increase the risk of myositis (Answer B) with statins. This is thought to be due to reduced statin clearance by the liver. In this situation, the concern is that interaction with the protease inhibitor will increase risk of myositis, which might lead to statin discontinuation. Reintroduction of the statin at a lower dosage or after a change in HIV therapy is, however, a possibility. The best-studied drug interaction is that with gemfibrozil, which leads to a marked increase in circulating statin levels. Cyclosporine, which is often used as a long-term treatment in transplant recipients, also increases myositis risk. Greater LDL-cholesterol reduction in patients such as this one may be achieved with the use of low statin dosages supplemented with other LDL-cholesterol reduction therapies such as ezetimibe. Resins are likely to increase the patient's triglyceride levels. Other drugs that increase myositis risk include ketoconazole and erythromycin (Answer D). Patients taking a short-term course of these drugs are advised to stop their statins.

Patients such as the one in this vignette often develop diabetes mellitus (Answer A). High-dosage statin therapy will probably increase this risk, but it would not be a reason to avoid lowering the LDL cholesterol in a patient with great cardiovascular disease risk. Statins do not inhibit antiviral agents (Answer C). Increased transaminases in patients taking statins are common (1% to 2% of patients). However, liver disease (Answer E) caused by statins is rare, and provided the increases in transaminase levels are less than 3 times the upper normal limit, it is acceptable to continue the lipid-lowering therapy. For this reason, the

US FDA has recently changed its guidelines on monitoring liver function in statin-treated patients—it now recommends checking liver enzymes "as clinically indicated."

EDUCATIONAL OBJECTIVE

Identify the potential interaction of statins with protease inhibitors, which may lead to an increased risk of myositis.

REFERENCE(S)

Venero CV, Thompson PD. Managing statin myopathy. *Endocrinol Metab Clin North Am.* 2009;38(1):121-136. PMID: 19217515

Thompson PD, Clarkson P, Karas RH. Statin-associated myopathy. *JAMA.* 2003;289(13):1681-1690. PMID: 12672737

Kirchner JT. Clinical management considerations for dyslipidemia in HIV-infected individuals. *Postgrad Med.* 2012;124(1):31-40. PMID: 22314112

16 ANSWER: D) Add evolocumab

Given that this patient had progressive coronary disease while on high-intensity statin therapy (atorvastatin, 80 mg daily), with an LDL-cholesterol concentration of 109 mg/dL (2.82 mmol/L), he would benefit from the addition of a PCSK9 inhibitor (Answer D) to target an LDL-cholesterol concentration less than 70 mg/dL (<1.81 mmol/L). Thus, advising no further treatment (Answer A) is incorrect. PCSK9 is a hepatic-produced protein that is secreted, binds to cell-surface LDL receptors, and mediates their intracellular degradation. Antibodies to PCSK9 prevent this and lead to increased LDL-receptor levels, which in turn reduce circulating LDL-cholesterol levels. Up-regulation of LDL receptors is also the mechanism for statin-mediating LDL-cholesterol reductions because inhibition of de novo cholesterol biosynthesis increases sterol-responsive element–binding protein (SREBP)–mediated transcription of the LDL receptor. Oligonucleotide inhibition of apolipoprotein B and inhibition of microsomal triglyceride transfer protein are therapies recently approved for treatment of the rare homozygous form of familial hypercholesterolemia.

Current indications for PCSK9 inhibitors include heterozygous familial hyperlipidemia and clinical atherosclerotic cardiovascular disease such as acute coronary syndromes, stable and unstable angina, myocardial infarction, peripheral vascular disease, history of coronary of other arterial revascularization, transient ischemic attack, and stroke for secondary prevention.

Icosapent ethyl (Answer B) is a purified n-3 fatty acid that lowers triglycerides and the risk of cardiovascular events in studies of individuals with coronary disease who have optimized their LDL-cholesterol levels to less than 100 mg/dL (<2.59 mmol/L) but have residually elevated triglycerides between 135 and 499 mg/dL (1.53-5.64 mmol/L), commonly with type 2 diabetes. This patient does have type 2 diabetes but his triglycerides are not persistently elevated. Also, given that his LDL cholesterol is not yet optimized, the addition of a PCSK9 inhibitor is the best next treatment, not icosapent ethyl. Niacin (Answer C) will not lower his risk of cardiovascular events. Lipopheresis (Answer E) could lower his LDL cholesterol further, but he has not yet tried all available medications, including ezetimibe, which could also be used as a second-line agent in addition to a statin but was not presented as an option, or a PCSK9 inhibitor. Lipopheresis should only be considered once all other medical therapies are exhausted.

EDUCATIONAL OBJECTIVE

List the indications for addition of PCSK9 inhibitors to statin therapy to reduce risk of cardiovascular disease events.

REFERENCE(S)

Sabatine MS, Giugliano RP, Keech AC, et al; FOURIER Steering Committee and Investigators. Evolocumab and clinical outcomes in patients with cardiovascular disease. *N Engl J Med.* 2017;376(18):1713-1722. PMID: 28304224

Sabatine MS, Giugliano RP, Wiviott SD, et al; Open-Label Study of Long-Term Evaluation against LDL Cholesterol (OSLER) Investigators. Efficacy and safety of evolocumab in reducing lipids and cardiovascular events. *N Engl J Med.* 2015;372(16):1500-1509. PMID: 25773607

Ajufo E, Rader DJ. Recent advances in the pharmacological management of hypercholesterolaemia. *Lancet Diabetes Endocrinol.* 2016;4(5): 436-446. PMID: 27012540

17 ANSWER: C) Apolipoprotein *E2/E2*

The apolipoprotein *E2/E2* phenotype (Answer C) is present in patients with dysbetalipoproteinemia, which is also referred to as type III hyperlipidemia. Classic skin manifestations include tuberoeruptive lesions at the elbows and palmar xanthomas as observed in this patient. The apolipoprotein *E2/E2* phenotype occurs in about 1 per 100 persons, but the development of characteristic dyslipidemia is infrequent and usually appears later in life due to acquired medical conditions such as hypothyroidism, obesity, diabetes mellitus, or estrogen replacement therapy. The lipoprotein that accumulates is a remnant of triglyceride metabolism (beta VLDL) and is associated with an increased risk of atherosclerotic vascular disease. Although the calculated LDL-cholesterol level is increased in this patient, it is spurious due to accumulation of the beta VLDL. This remnant is cholesterol ester–enriched and has "balanced" concentrations of cholesterol and triglyceride, which accounts for the "near-equal" serum cholesterol and triglyceride levels.

ABCA1 is a protein involved in moving cholesterol from peripheral tissues onto HDL particles. Deficiency of this protein results in the condition known as Tangier disease, characterized by very low HDL-cholesterol levels (<20 mg/dL [<0.52 mmol/L]), and the classic physical examination finding of orange tonsils, which this patient does not have. Thus, ABCA1 deficiency (Answer A) is incorrect. LDL-receptor deficiency (Answer B) results in the condition known as familial hyperlipidemia. Patients with familial hyperlipidemia have very high LDL-cholesterol levels but not triglycerides unless there is an additional defect. They present with tendinous xanthomas and premature coronary artery disease. Lipoprotein lipase is an enzyme that acts in the vascular bed to hydrolyze triglycerides. Lipoprotein lipase deficiency (Answer E) results in very high triglyceride levels (>1000 mg/dL [>11.30 mmol/L]), which this patient does not have. Apolipoprotein CII is a cofactor for lipoprotein lipase. Deficiency of apolipoprotein CII (Answer D) results in marked hypertriglyceridemia such as that seen in lipoprotein lipase deficiency, typically greater than 1000 mg/dL (>11.30 mmol/L).

EDUCATIONAL OBJECTIVE

Identify the clinical features of dysbetalipoproteinemia.

REFERENCE(S)

Garg A, Simha V. Update of dyslipidemia. *J Clin Endocrinol Metab.* 2007;92(5):1581-1589. PMID: 17483372

Walden CC, Hegele RA. Apolipoprotein E in hyperlipidemia. *Ann Intern Med.* 1994;120(12): 1026-1036. PMID: 8185134

Marais AD, Solomon GA, Blom DJ. Dysbetalipoproteinaemia: a mixed hyperlipidaemia of remnant lipoproteins due to mutations in apolipoprotein E. *Crit Rev Clin Lab Sci.* 2014;51(1):46-62. PMID: 24405372

18 ANSWER: E) Accumulation of lipoprotein X

Primary biliary cirrhosis is a progressive liver disease that most commonly presents in older women and can be associated with marked elevation of serum lipid levels. Elevated total cholesterol levels in these patients are most often due to the presence of an abnormal LDL-like particle named lipoprotein X (Answer E). Lipoprotein X is made up in part by biliary lipids that are not being excreted by the liver. A number of clinical series do not show an increased risk of coronary artery disease in these patients, despite high levels of what would be considered LDL cholesterol if the Friedewald formula were used to estimate LDL-cholesterol levels. Individuals with high levels of lipoprotein X can develop coronary artery disease, and they do have a reduction in cholesterol levels with statins, but they just do not appear to have a degree of risk for coronary artery disease that would be expected given the high level of "LDL-like" lipoprotein particles.

Lecithin-cholesterol acyltransferase (LCAT) is the enzyme that converts free cholesterol to cholesterol esters, thereby trapping the cholesterol in HDL to be taken to the liver. LCAT deficiency (Answer C) is a genetic disorder that is associated with very low levels of HDL cholesterol, hemolytic anemia, corneal opacities, renal insufficiency, and, uncommonly, atherosclerosis. While LCAT deficiency may be part of the pathogenesis of lipoprotein X production, it is not the only mechanism at work. Lipoprotein (a) (Answer A) is an LDL particle that has apolipoprotein (a) covalently attached to the apolipoprotein B, which is the structural backbone of LDL. It is not associated with primary biliary cirrhosis. Ursodeoxycholic acid treatment (Answer B) does not worsen serum lipids in patients with primary biliary cirrhosis; in fact, data suggest that cholesterol levels fall with the use of this medication. Liver disease is a secondary cause of hyperlipidemia that should routinely be screened for when caring for a patient with hyperlipidemia. Increased production of apolipoprotein B is the underlying cause of hyperlipidemia in familial combined hyperlipidemia. However, increased production of apolipoprotein B (Answer D) is not typical in primary biliary cirrhosis and would not be expected to increase total cholesterol levels to the degree seen in this patient.

EDUCATIONAL OBJECTIVE

Identify the lipid abnormalities associated with primary biliary cirrhosis.

REFERENCE(S)

Sorokin A, Brown JL, Thompson PD. Primary biliary cirrhosis, hyperlipidemia, and atherosclerotic risk: a systematic review. *Atherosclerosis.* 2007;194(2): 293-299. PMID: 17240380

Longo M, Crosignani A, Battezzati PM, et al. Hyperlipidaemic state and cardiovascular risk in primary biliary cirrhosis. *Gut.* 2002;51(2): 265-269. PMID: 12117892

19 ANSWER: B) Switch metoprolol to amlodipine

Patients with collagen-vascular disease can develop severe hyperlipidemias. On occasion, these are due to the production of antibodies that can inhibit lipoprotein lipase or heparin (and lipase binding to endothelium). Antibodies can also be directed to apolipoproteins: antibodies to apolipoprotein B lead to hypobetalipoproteinemia, and antibodies to apolipoprotein AI lead to low HDL-cholesterol levels. Several medications in this setting, as well as in patients without collagen-vascular disease, can exacerbate hypertriglyceridemia. One such class of medications is β-adrenergic blockers. Thus, substituting a calcium-channel blocker for metoprolol (Answer B) is correct.

Changing from one steroid to another (Answer A) should not affect the hypertriglyceridemia. Neither infliximab nor lisinopril affects triglyceride levels (thus, Answers C and E are incorrect). Apremilast (Answer C) is a treatment for plaque psoriasis, not lupus. Although thiazide diuretics increase triglycerides, so does chlorthalidone (Answer D).

EDUCATIONAL OBJECTIVE

Advise patients on medications, such as β-adrenergic blockers, that increase triglyceride levels.

REFERENCE(S)

Stone NJ. Secondary causes of hyperlipidemia. *Med Clin North Am.* 1994;78(1):117-141. PMID: 8283927

Dinu AR, Merrill JT, Shen C, Antonov IV, Myones BL, Lahita RG. Frequency of antibodies to the cholesterol transport protein apolipoprotein A1 in patients with SLE. *Lupus.* 1998;7(5): 355-360. PMID: 9696140

20 ANSWER: A) Cholesterol ester transfer protein (CETP) deficiency

HDL-cholesterol levels are highly genetically determined. Deficiencies of both cholesterol ester transfer protein (CETP) and hepatic lipase lead to increased plasma HDL cholesterol. CETP deficiency is most commonly seen in patients of Japanese ancestry (thus, Answer A is the most likely explanation). The protective value of this very high HDL cholesterol is unclear; however, these patients do not have premature disease. Pharmacologic inhibition of CETP is being studied as a method to raise HDL cholesterol, and these inhibitors also reduce plasma LDL cholesterol and lipoprotein (a). It should be noted that the first generation of these drugs increased blood pressure and, unexpectedly, cardiac events.

Hepatic lipase deficiency (Answer C) is very rare. Aside from increased HDL cholesterol (not usually to this degree), affected the patients also have increased cholesterol and triglycerides, suggestive of an accumulation of remnant lipoproteins. Moreover, they have premature coronary artery disease. The SR-B1 receptor is associated with delivery of HDL cholesterol to the liver, and its deficiency (Answer D) has been rarely reported (not in Asian patients) and is associated with increased HDL cholesterol, although not to this degree. Carriers of pathogenic variants in the gene encoding SR-B1 have higher HDL-cholesterol levels than noncarriers (70.4 mg/dL [1.82 mmol/L] vs 53.4 mg/dL [1.38 mmol/L]). The other options lead to reduced HDL-cholesterol levels. Lecithin cholesterol acyltransferase (LCAT) is needed to esterify cholesterol and create spherical HDL (thus, Answer B is incorrect). ABCA1 transports cholesterol from hepatocytes and enterocytes to mature, newly formed HDL (thus, Answer E is incorrect).

EDUCATIONAL OBJECTIVE

Describe the metabolic role of enzymes affecting HDL cholesterol.

REFERENCE(S)

Cannon CP, Shah S, Dansky HM, et al; Determining the Efficacy and Tolerability Investigators. Safety of anacetrapib in patients with or at high risk for coronary heart disease. *N Engl J Med.* 2010;363(25):2406-2415. PMID: 21082868

Nicholls SJ, Brewer HB, Kastelein JJ, et al. Effects of the CETP inhibitor evacetrapib administered as monotherapy or in combination with statins on HDL and LDL cholesterol: a randomized controlled trial. *JAMA.* 2011;306(19):2099-2109. PMID: 22089718

Barter PJ, Caulfield M, Eriksson M, et al; ILLUMINATE Investigators. Effects of torcetrapib in patients at high risk for coronary events. *N Engl J Med.* 2007;357(21):2109-2122. PMID: 17984165

Hegele RA, Tu L, Connelly PW. Human hepatic lipase mutations and polymorphisms. *Hum Mutat.* 1992;1(4):320-324. PMID: 1301939

Vergeer M, Korporaal SJ, Franssen R, et al. Genetic variant of the scavenger receptor BI in humans. *N Engl J Med.* 2011;364(2):136-145. PMID: 21226579

21 ANSWER: C) Avoid alcohol

The changes in circulating triglyceride levels due to alcohol intake are sometimes dramatic. This college student most likely has underlying hypertriglyceridemia that is exacerbated by alcohol. Some such patients will, however, normalize their triglyceride levels without drugs. In this situation, switching to nonalcoholic beer is often the single most impactful diet change. Alcohol has a number of effects on liver triglyceride metabolism, including reducing fatty acid oxidation and increasing de novo triglyceride production. Thus, avoiding alcohol (Answer C) is the most important immediate lifestyle change.

Several other dietary changes also reduce triglyceride levels, but the impact would probably be less dramatic than that due to elimination of alcohol. Reducing intake of foods with simple sugars (sugar, bread, rice, potatoes, and pasta) (Answer B) and high-fat foods should lead to some triglyceride reduction. Omega-3 fatty acids reduce triglycerides, and fruit juice is a source of free sugars (thus, Answers A and D are incorrect).

Although reducing consumption of high-fat foods, such as fried foods (Answer E), is an important dietary change, it is not the most likely culprit here. Losing weight and exercising more are important lifestyle changes, but their effects on this patient's hypertriglyceridemia are likely to be less acute than those of avoiding alcohol.

EDUCATIONAL OBJECTIVE

Recommend avoidance of alcohol as an important lifestyle modification in a patient with severe hypertriglyceridemia.

REFERENCE(S)

Pownall HJ. Alcohol: lipid metabolism and cardioprotection. *Curr Atheroscler Rep.* 2002;4(2):107-112. PMID: 11822973

Goldberg IJ, Mosca L, Piano MR, Fisher EA. AHA Science Advisory. Wine and your heart: a science advisory for healthcare professionals from the Nutrition Committee, Council on Epidemiology and Prevention, and Council on Cardiovascular Nursing of the American Heart Association. *Stroke.* 2001;32(2):591-594. PMID: 11157206

22 ANSWER: A) Start a statin

While there has been concern for some time about the potential risk of treating individuals who have abnormal liver function tests with lipid-lowering drugs, there is no evidence that these drugs cause severe or progressive hepatic damage or that they cannot be safely used in patients with chronic liver disease. The GREACE study (Greek Atorvastatin and Coronary Heart Disease Evaluation) demonstrated that in individuals with liver function test results less than 3 times the upper normal limit, there are no adverse effects of lipid-lowering drugs on liver function tests over time and there are significant benefits to lipid-lowering therapy in cardiovascular disease risk reduction.

Approximately 3 million persons in the United States have chronic hepatitis C viral infection and a larger but unquantified number of obese patients have nonalcoholic fatty liver disease or nonalcoholic steatohepatitis. Fibrates, metformin, and thiazolidinediones reverse nonalcoholic fatty liver disease/nonalcoholic steatohepatitis. Some patients with chronic liver disease have lipid or lipoprotein abnormalities that, in the big scheme of things, require therapy because they are potentially as important as or more important than the liver disease. This patient has familial combined hyperlipidemia and a family history of coronary heart disease; she fits the criteria for a statin benefit group (no diabetes, aged 40-75 years, LDL-cholesterol concentration 70-189 mg/dL [1.81-4.90 mmol/L], >7.5%-20% risk of cardiovascular disease event in the next 10 years).

In the absence of serious or progressive liver disease, she first requires therapy with a statin (Answer A). While diet alone (Answer B) might provide modest reduction in cardiovascular disease risk, the benefit would be substantially lower than that resulting from statin therapy. Likewise, neither a fibrate (Answer C), ezetimibe (Answer D), nor niacin (Answer E) would provide the cardiovascular disease risk reduction comparable to that of a statin. Since a statin is safe to use in this patient and it has the greatest benefits, it is the treatment of choice.

EDUCATIONAL OBJECTIVE

Assess the risk of liver toxicity from statin use.

REFERENCE(S)

Athyros VG, Tziomalos K, Gossios TD, et al; GREACE Study Collaborative Group. Safety and efficacy of long-term statin treatment for cardiovascular events in patients with coronary heart disease and abnormal liver tests in the Greek Atorvastatin and Coronary Heart Disease Evaluation (GREACE) Study: a post-hoc analysis. *Lancet.* 2010;376(9756):1916-1922. PMID: 21109302

Khorashadi S, Hasson NK, Cheung RC. Incidence of statin hepatotoxicity in patients with hepatitis C. *Clin Gastroenterol Hepatol.* 2006;4(7):902-907. PMID: 16697272

Demyen M, Alkhalloufi K, Pyrsopoulos NT. Lipid-lowering agents and hepatotoxicity. *Clin Liver Dis.* 2013;17(4):699-714. PMID: 24099026

23 ANSWER: B) Corneal arcus

Premature development of corneal arcus (Answer B) (under age 40 years per the Dutch Lipid Criteria for diagnosis of familial hyperlipidemia) is one of the signature signs of familial genetic hypercholesterolemia. The cardinal feature of the disorder on physical examination is tendon xanthoma affecting either the Achilles tendon or the tendons on the dorsum of the hands. The reason why lipid accumulates in the tendons is not completely understood, but it is thought to be secondary to recurrent inflammation and macrophage recruitment to where the tendon interacts with its overlying sheath. Tendon xanthomas are usually most prominent in the Achilles tendon. Some patients with familial hypercholesterolemia do not have tendon xanthomas but do have premature corneal arcus. In current practice, many patients with heterozygous familial hyperlipidemia do not exhibit these 2 signs, as they have been on lipid-lowering therapy for years before their specific genetic disorder is diagnosed.

Most often, patients with familial hypercholesterolemia have a heterozygous pathogenic variant in the gene encoding the LDL receptor. Defective apolipoprotein B, the ligand for the receptor, and a defect in an intracellular adaptor protein cause a similar phenotype. Persons who are heterozygous have total cholesterol concentrations of 350 to 600 mg/dL (9.06-15.54 mmol/L), LDL-cholesterol concentrations greater than 250 mg/dL (>6.48 mmol/L), premature coronary artery disease, and aortic stenosis.

This patient is being treated with atorvastatin, 80 mg daily; his off-therapy LDL-cholesterol concentration is most likely around 300 mg/dL (7.77 mmol/L). The homozygous form of this disease leads to atherosclerosis before age 20 years (sometimes before age 10 years). Liver transplant is often the treatment. Genetic testing does not alter therapy and is not usually performed.

Lipemia retinalis (Answer A) is the milky appearance of the retina and retinal vessels that accompanies severe hypertriglyceridemia. Eruptive xanthomas (Answer C) are acne-like papules that are found on extensor surfaces of the arms and on the back and buttocks. They are also a sign of severe hypertriglyceridemia. Palmar xanthomas (Answer D) are lipid depositions in the creases of the palms that occur with dysbetalipoproteinemia (formerly called type 3 hyperlipoproteinemia). Arthropathy (Answer E) is not a sign of a dyslipoproteinemia.

EDUCATIONAL OBJECTIVE
Identify physical findings of hyperlipidemias.

REFERENCE(S)

Semenkovich CF, Goldberg AC, Goldberg IJ. Disorders of lipid metabolism. In: Melmed S, Polonsky KS, Larsen PR, Kronenberg HM, eds. *Williams Textbook of Endocrinology*. 12th ed. Philadelphia, PA: Elsevier Saunders; 2011:1633-1674.

24 ANSWER: C) Oral contraceptive use

Hypertriglyceridemia has a number of causes including genetic pathogenic variants, medications, and other medical conditions. The described patient has both high triglycerides and high HDL-cholesterol levels. This can be observed in the setting of alcohol use or estrogen use. The history lists oral contraceptives (Answer C) as a medication, and this is the most likely culprit. The frank hypertriglyceridemia that this patient exhibits can occur in someone with an underlying predisposition to hypertriglyceridemia who then begins oral estrogens. This typically does not occur with transdermal estrogens, but it can occur with oral estrogens given for postmenopausal symptoms.

Lipoprotein lipase is the key enzyme in the catabolism of circulating triglyceride-rich lipoproteins VLDL and chylomicrons. Apolipoprotein C2 is a cofactor for lipoprotein lipase, so both lipoprotein lipase deficiency (Answer A) and apolipoprotein C2 deficiency (Answer B) can cause marked hypertriglyceridemia. Triglyceride levels in affected individuals are typically greater than 1000 mg/dL (>11.30 mmol/L) and can be 2000 to 3000 mg/dL (22.60-33.90 mmol/L). The enzyme cholesteryl ester transfer protein (CETP) exchanges cholesterol esters in HDL for triglyceride in VLDL and chylomicrons, resulting in increased clearance of HDL cholesterol. This process is increased when triglyceride levels are high. This explains the common association between increased triglyceride levels and decreased HDL-cholesterol levels. CETP deficiency (Answer D) is associated with very high HDL-cholesterol levels but not hypertriglyceridemia. Lipoprotein lipase deficiency and apolipoprotein C2 deficiency cause high triglyceride levels, but because of CETP, HDL-cholesterol levels are typically low. Soy isoflavones (Answer E) do not have a clinical impact on cholesterol, including HDL cholesterol.

EDUCATIONAL OBJECTIVE

Identify the most likely cause of high triglycerides in a patient with high HDL-cholesterol levels.

REFERENCE(S)

Baksu B, Davas I, Agar E, Akyol A, Uluocak A. Do different delivery systems of estrogen therapy influence serum lipids differently in surgically menopausal women? *J Obstet Gynaecol Res.* 2007;33(3):346-352. PMID: 17578365

Brien SE, Ronksley PE, Turner BJ, Mukamal KJ, Ghali WA. Effect of alcohol consumption on biological markers associated with risk of coronary heart disease: systematic review and meta-analysis of interventional studies. *BMJ.* 2011;342:d636. PMID: 21343206

25 ANSWER: E) Lecithin-cholesterol acyltransferase deficiency

The most striking feature of this patient's clinical presentation is his very low HDL-cholesterol level. His phenotype is typical for lecithin-cholesterol acyltransferase (LCAT) deficiency (Answer E). The enzyme LCAT is responsible for converting the relatively polar free cholesterol in the developing HDL particle into nonpolar cholesterol esters. Cholesterol esters are then "trapped" in the HDL particle to be taken back to the liver. When LCAT is deficient, free cholesterol does not stay associated with the HDL particle, resulting in low circulating HDL-cholesterol levels. This condition is associated with cholesterol accumulation in the eyes resulting in corneal clouding. Affected patients also have proteinuria that develops in childhood, progressive renal dysfunction leading eventually to end-stage renal disease, and anemia due to red cell fragility secondary to abnormal membrane lipids.

ATP-binding cassette A1 (ABCA1) deficiency (Answer A), or Tangier disease, is also a cause of very low HDL cholesterol, but it is not associated with abnormal renal function. Tangier disease is associated with accumulation of cholesterol in lymphoid tissue giving a classic physical finding: orange tonsils. Surreptitious testosterone abuse (Answer B) can lower HDL-cholesterol levels—even dramatically. However, individuals abusing testosterone would be expected to exhibit findings of excess androgens (increased muscle mass, acne) that are not described here, and such individuals would not have the eye or kidney problems described in this patient. Defective apolipoprotein B (Answer C) looks clinically like familial hypercholesterolemia with tendinous xanthomas and very high LDL-cholesterol levels. Lipoprotein lipase deficiency (Answer D) results in very high triglyceride levels (>1000 mg/dL [>11.3 mmol/L]) and a more modest decrease in HDL cholesterol.

EDUCATIONAL OBJECTIVE

Describe the clinical features of conditions that cause very low HDL-cholesterol levels.

REFERENCE(S)

Rader DJ, deGoma EM. Approach to the patient with extremely low HDL-cholesterol. *J Clin Endocrinol Metab.* 2012;97(10):3399-3407. PMID: 23043194

Schaefer EJ, Anthanont P, Asztalos BF. High-density lipoprotein metabolism, composition, function, and deficiency. *Curr Opin Lipidol.* 2014;25(3): 194-199. PMID: 24785961

Rader DJ, Hovingh GK. HDL and cardiovascular disease. *Lancet.* 2014;384(9943): 618-625. PMID: 25131981

26 ANSWER: D) Familial combined hyperlipidemia

This vignette is typical of a person from a family with familial combined hyperlipidemia (Answer D), the most common lipid abnormality among patients with coronary artery disease.

Familial combined hyperlipidemia was discovered from studies of families that had many individuals afflicted with coronary artery disease and high serum lipid levels. In a large percentage of patients, it is also associated with insulin resistance and the metabolic syndrome. Although familial, the phenotype is typically not expressed until the third or later decades of life. Affected family members can have 1 of 3 lipid abnormalities: hypercholesterolemia, hypertriglyceridemia, or both. The lipid abnormality may change and vary from time to time in a given patient, probably because of nutritional factors (weight gain/weight loss). Familial combined hyperlipidemia is caused by an overproduction of apolipoprotein B by the liver. The variable serum lipid phenotype reflects individual differences in the metabolism of VLDL depending on diet composition and other genes present in a particular individual.

Individuals with lipoprotein lipase deficiency (Answer B) have very high triglyceride levels, often greater than 1000 mg/dL (>11.30 mmol/L). Familial hypercholesterolemia (Answer A) and familial defective apolipoprotein B (Answer C) are characterized by very high LDL-cholesterol levels (200-300 mg/dL [5.18-7.77 mmol/L]) and specific physical features including tendinous xanthomas. Apolipoprotein A1 is the structural lipoprotein associated with HDL. Patients with apolipoprotein A1 deficiency (Answer E), also known as hypoalphalipoproteinemia, have very low HDL-cholesterol levels (<20 mg/dL [<0.52 mmol/L]).

EDUCATIONAL OBJECTIVE

List the features of familial combined hyperlipidemia.

REFERENCE(S)

Brunzell JD, Albers JJ, Chait A, Grundy SM, Groszek E, McDonald GB. Plasma lipoproteins in familial combined hyperlipidemia and monogenic familial hypertriglyceridemia. *J Lipid Res.* 1983;24(2):147-155. PMID: 6403642

Hopkins PN, Heiss G, Ellison RC, et al. Coronary artery disease risk in familial combined hyperlipidemia and familial hypertriglyceridemia: a case-control comparison from the National Heart, Lung, and Blood Institute Family Heart Study. *Circulation.* 2003;108(5):519-523. PMID: 12847072

27 ANSWER: D) Continue atorvastatin and add fenofibrate

This patient has known cardiovascular disease in the context of type 2 diabetes and mixed hyperlipidemia, with both elevated LDL cholesterol and triglycerides. She is at very high risk for another cardiovascular event and will benefit from continuing the statin for cardiovascular risk reduction (thus, Answers A and C are incorrect). The most common inherited lipid disorder in type 2 diabetes is familial combined hyperlipidemia, which has a very variable clinical phenotype regarding LDL-cholesterol and triglyceride elevations, which can shift over time within the same patient. This patient most likely had a triglyceride concentration greater than 1000 mg/dL (>11.3 mmol/L), as she had several episodes of pancreatitis. Her current fasting triglyceride concentration of 760 mg/dL (8.59 mmol/L) while on a statin (≥500 mg/dL [≥5.65 mmol/L]) does put her risk for pancreatitis. The 2013 American College of Cardiology/American Heart Association Guidelines on the Treatment of Blood Cholesterol to Reduce Atherosclerotic Cardiovascular Risk in Adults recommend treating triglycerides as a secondary target when levels remain above 500 mg/dL. She would benefit from lipid-lowering therapy targeted at lowering triglycerides.

Both fibrates gemfibrozil and fenofibrate effectively lower triglycerides, but gemfibrozil is contraindicated due to concurrent use of a statin because of the increased risk of muscle-related adverse effects, including myositis and rhabdomyolysis (thus, Answers A and B are incorrect). Adding fenofibrate to a statin (Answer D) is the safer choice for additional triglyceride lowering. Niacin (Answer E) may help to lower triglycerides, but it would also most likely worsen her diabetes and is therefore not the best choice.

EDUCATIONAL OBJECTIVE

Recommend when and how to treat hypertriglyceridemia in patients with cardiovascular disease.

REFERENCE(S)

Stone NJ, Robinson JG, Lichtenstein AH, et al; American College of Cardiology/American Heart Association Task Force on Practice Guidelines. 2013 ACC/AHA guideline on the treatment of blood cholesterol to reduce atherosclerotic cardiovascular risk in adults: a report of the American College of Cardiology/American Heart Association Task Force on Practice Guidelines [published correction appears in *Circulation.* 2014;129(25 Suppl 2):S46-S48]. *Circulation.* 2014;129(25 Suppl 2):S1-S45. PMID: 24222016

Stone NJ, Robinson JG, Lichtenstein AH, et al; 2013 ACC/AHA Cholesterol Guideline Panel. Treatment of blood cholesterol to reduce atherosclerotic cardiovascular disease risk in adults: synopsis of the 2013 American College of Cardiology/American Heart Association cholesterol guideline. *Ann Intern Med.* 2014;160(5):339-343. PMID: 24474185

Berglund L, Brunzell JD, Goldberg AC, et al; Endocrine Society. Evaluation and treatment of hypertriglyceridemia: an Endocrine Society clinical practice guideline. *J Clin Endocrinol Metab.* 2012;97(9):2969-2989. PMID: 22962670

Pituitary Board Review

Laurence Katznelson, MD

1 ANSWER: B) Pathogenic variant in the *POU1F1* gene

This patient has childhood-onset GH deficiency, recent-onset central hypothyroidism, and hypoprolactinemia. Her history and biochemical assessment are notable for the presence of menses, consistent with adequate gonadotropin function, as well as normal adrenal reserve. These findings suggest that she has a pathogenic variant in the gene encoding the transcription factor POU1F1 (*POU1F1* [formerly *PIT1*]) (Answer B). POU1F1 is important for the development of the somatotroph, lactotroph, and thyrotroph lineages, and *POU1F1* pathogenic variants lead to deficiencies of their respective hormones. The secretion of ACTH, FSH, and LH is preserved.

In patients with pathogenic variants in *PROP1* (Answer A), which is the most common cause of congenital combined pituitary hormone deficiency, gonadotropin deficiency is usually present as well. This is not the case in this patient. POU1F1 is the transcription factor that acts temporally just after PROP1. Patients with pathogenic variants in *TBX19 (TPIT)* (Answer C) present with isolated ACTH deficiency (not present in this case), as the *TBX19* gene product is necessary for differentiation of corticotroph cells. Histiocytosis (Answer D) is not the diagnosis in this patient, as she does not have diabetes insipidus and the imaging does not reveal an enhancing posterior sellar mass. Hypopituitarism occurs in up to 30% of individuals following moderate to severe brain injury (Answer E). However, her trauma occurred recently, far after the onset of her endocrine findings, and her injury was most likely too mild to result in hypopituitarism.

EDUCATIONAL OBJECTIVE

Determine the cause of childhood-onset combined hypopituitarism.

REFERENCE(S)

Prince KL, Walvoord EC, Rhodes SJ. The role of homeodomain transcription factors in heritable pituitary disease. *Nat Rev Endocrinol.* 2011;7(12): 727-737. PMID: 21788968

Bertko E, Klammt J, Dusatkova P, et al. Combined pituitary hormone deficiency due to gross deletions in the POU1F1 (PIT-1) and PROP1 genes. *J Hum Genet.* 2017;62(8):755-762. PMID: 28356564

Majdoub H, Amselem S, Legendre M, Rath S, Bercovich D, Tenenbaum-Rakover Y. Extreme short stature and severe neurological impairment in a 17-year-old male with untreated combined pituitary hormone deficiency due to POU1F1 mutation. *Front Endocrinol (Lausanne).* 2019;10: 381. PMID: 31316460

Mendonca BB, Osorio MG, Latronico AC, Estefan V, Lo LS, Arnhold IJ. Longitudinal hormonal and pituitary imaging changes in two females with combined pituitary hormone deficiency due to deletion of A301,G302 in the PROP1 gene. *J Clin Endocrinol Metab.* 1999;84(3):942-945. PMID: 10084575

2 ANSWER: D) Metastasis

The key features in this vignette are the rapid growth of the mass and the presence of diabetes insipidus, and they are most consistent with metastasis (Answer D). Diabetes insipidus occurs because the metastasis involves the posterior pituitary gland. Common cancers causing such metastases include breast cancer, renal cell cancer, and lung cancer. This patient's history of renal cell cancer makes this the most likely diagnosis.

Clinically nonfunctioning pituitary adenomas (Answer A) are usually slow growing and are rarely associated with diabetes insipidus. Prolactinoma (Answer B) is unlikely given the modestly elevated serum prolactin, the rapid increase in tumor size, and the presence of diabetes insipidus (rarely associated). Nivolumab (Answer C) is an anti-PD-1 antibody that is used as immunotherapy, and it has been associated with hypophysitis. However, because this patient has a discrete mass and diabetes insipidus, and because hypophysitis is uncommon with PD-1 inhibitors (more common with CTLA-4 checkpoint inhibitors), nivolumab is an unlikely culprit. In addition, immunotherapy-induced hypophysitis is usually associated with a hyperenhancing—not a hypoenhancing—mass on imaging, although this is a variable finding. Histiocytosis (Answer E) is a sellar lesion that can cause diabetes insipidus, but histiocytosis is contrast enhancing and is thus incorrect.

EDUCATIONAL OBJECTIVE

Differentiate metastases from other pituitary mass lesions.

REFERENCE(S)

Al-Aridi R, El Sibai K, Fu P, Khan M, Selman WR, Arafah BM. Clinical and biochemical characteristic features of metastatic cancer to the sella turcica: an analytical review. *Pituitary.* 2014;17(6):575-587. PMID: 24337713

Ariel D, Sung H, Coghlan N, Dodd R, Gibbs IC, Katznelson L. Clinical characteristics and pituitary dysfunction in patients with metastatic cancer to the sella. *Endocr Pract.* 2013;19(6):914-919. PMID: 23757610

Barroso-Sousa R, Barry WT, Garrido-Castro AC, et al. Incidence of endocrine dysfunction following the use of different immune checkpoint inhibitor regimens: a systematic review and meta-analysis. *JAMA Oncol.* 2018;4(2):173-182. PMID: 28973656

3 ANSWER: B) Glucagon-stimulation test with measurement of GH

Given this patient's history of pituitary adenoma and subsequent surgery, he is at risk for hypopituitarism. He has normal thyroid and adrenal function. His serum testosterone is slightly low, but this is unlikely to account for his more recent symptoms. He is at risk for GH deficiency, which can present with change in body composition with an increase in abdominal girth, change in well-being with fatigue and worsening cognitive function (including reduced short-term memory), lower bone density, and cardiovascular risk. He does have signs and symptoms of GH deficiency, so further testing is important. A glucagon-stimulation test (Answer B) is the best next step. This patient's erectile dysfunction is not likely related to GH deficiency.

Measurement of IGFBP-3 (Answer C), an IGF-binding protein stimulated by GH, is not useful for the diagnosis of GH deficiency. Morning GH measurement (Answer A) is incorrect, as a random level is not useful in the diagnosis of GH deficiency. Given the patient's adequate morning cortisol, a cosyntropin-stimulation test (Answer D) would not be useful to search further for adrenal insufficiency and would not add to the evaluation. A novel oral GH secretagogue, macimorelin, is an additional available option for GH-stimulation testing. IGF-1, a marker of GH levels, can be normal even if an acceptable stimulation test documents GH deficiency. In this case, the IGF-1 is low-normal. If 3 or more axes are deficient, then no stimulation test is needed if the IGF-1 level is low. This patient has 1 deficient axis, so a stimulation test is necessary to determine whether he is GH deficient. Thus, no testing (Answer E) is incorrect.

EDUCATIONAL OBJECTIVE

Determine the most appropriate test to diagnose GH deficiency.

REFERENCE(S)

Toogood AA, Stewart PM. Hypopituitarism: clinical features, diagnosis, and management. *Endocrinol Metab Clin North Am.* 2008;37(1):235-261. PMID: 18226739

Yuen KC, Tritos NA, Samson SL, Hoffman AR, Katznelson L. American Association of Clinical Endocrinologists and American College of Endocrinology Disease State Clinical Review: update on growth hormone stimulation testing and proposed revised cut-point for the glucagon stimulation test in the diagnosis of adult growth hormone deficiency. *Endocr Pract.* 2016;22(10): 1235-1244. PMID: 27409821

Molitch ME, Clemmons DR, Malozowski S, Merriam GR, Vance ML; Endocrine Society. Evaluation and treatment of adult growth hormone deficiency: an Endocrine Society clinical practice guideline. *J Clin Endocrinol Metab.* 2011;96(6):1587-1609. PMID: 21602453

Yuen KCJ, Biller BMK, Radovick S, et al. American Association of Clinical Endocrinologists and American College of Endocrinology guidelines for management of growth hormone deficiency in adults and patients transitioning from pediatric to adult care. *Endocr Pract.* 2019;25(11):1191-1232. PMID: 31760824

4 ANSWER: B) α-Subunit measurement

This patient has hyperthyroidism, a goiter with high iodine uptake, and the unexpected finding of a TSH value that is not suppressed—an indication that a TSH-secreting tumor is the cause of her hyperthyroidism. Pituitary MRI would be an appropriate next test to confirm an adenoma, but imaging was not listed as an answer choice. Elevation of α-subunit is present in up to 85% of patients with a TSH-secreting pituitary adenoma, and its measurement (Answer B) would be an appropriate next test in this patient's evaluation. The relative increase in serum α-subunit is greater than that of serum TSH, resulting in a high molar ratio of α-subunit to TSH.

In patients with TSH-secreting adenomas, the tumor and TSH secretion are relatively resistant to dopamine agonists, so a trial of cabergoline (Answer A) would not be effective. Assessment for a pathogenic variant in the thyroid hormone receptor gene (Answer C) may be diagnostic in a patient with presumed resistance to thyroid hormone, but this patient does not have evidence of thyroid hormone resistance despite the elevated free T_4 and inappropriately normal TSH. As such, administration of thyroid hormone (Answer D) to overcome a relative resistance may be necessary in the setting of thyroid hormone resistance but would not be appropriate in this patient with clinical and biochemical hyperthyroidism. Although she has hyperthyroidism with an increased and diffuse iodine uptake consistent with Graves disease, she does not have Graves disease given the inappropriately normal TSH. Thus, measurement of thyroid-stimulating immunoglobulin (Answer E) is not warranted. Surgery would be the best management option.

EDUCATIONAL OBJECTIVE

Confirm the diagnosis of a TSH-secreting tumor.

REFERENCE(S)

Teramoto A, Sanno N, Tahara S, Osamura YR. Pathological study of thyrotropin-secreting pituitary adenoma: plurihormonality and medical treatment. *Acta Neuropathol.* 2004;108(2):147-153. PMID: 15185102

Beck-Peccoz P, Persani L, Mannavola D, Campi I. TSH-secreting adenomas. *Best Pract Res Clin Endocrinol Metab.* 2009;23(5);597-606. PMID: 19945025

Dieu X, Sueur G, Moal V, et al. Apparent resistance to thyroid hormones: from biological interference to genetics. *Ann Endocrinol (Paris).* 2019;80(5-6): 280-285. PMID: 31590893

5 ANSWER: C) A need to increase the hydrocortisone dosage

A number of interactions can occur following initiation of GH replacement. Due to increased metabolism of cortisol by GH, relative adrenal insufficiency may result. Therefore, the hydrocortisone dosage may need to be increased (Answer C). Similarly, GH may metabolize free T_4, leading to an increased levothyroxine requirement, not a decreased requirement (Answer A). Oral estrogens can act on the liver to decrease the liver's responsiveness to GH with respect to IGF-1 production. Therefore, higher GH dosages may be necessary to maintain a steady IGF-1 level in such patients. A change in the oral contraceptive dosage (Answer B) is not indicated in this case, although one could consider switching to transdermal estrogen to potentially reduce the impact of estrogen on the GH dosage. GH replacement does not regulate prolactin secretion, thus increased serum prolactin (Answer D) is unlikely. GH therapy may lead to hyperglycemia, not a decrease in blood glucose (Answer E).

EDUCATIONAL OBJECTIVE

Describe interactions among hormonal replacement therapies.

REFERENCE(S)

Cook DM, Ludlam WH, Cook MB. Route of estrogen administration helps to determine growth hormone (GH) replacement dose in GH-deficient adults. *J Clin Endocrinol Metab.* 1999;84(11): 3956-3960. PMID: 10566634

Fleseriu M, Hashim IA, Karavitaki N, et al. Hormonal replacement in hypopituitarism in adults: an Endocrine Society clinical practice guideline. *J Clin Endocrinol Metab.* 2016;101(11):3888-3921. PMID: 27736313

Yuen KCJ, Biller BMK, Radovick S, et al. American Association of Clinical Endocrinologists and American College of Endocrinology guidelines for management of growth hormone deficiency in adults and patients transitioning from pediatric to adult care. *Endocr Pract.* 2019;25(11):1191-1232. PMID: 31760824

6 **ANSWER: C) Start tolvaptan**

This patient has severe hyponatremia following pituitary surgery, which is usually due to the syndrome of inappropriate antidiuretic hormone secretion (SIADH). Because the hyponatremia occurred rapidly, it is possible to increase the serum sodium rapidly. She has no evidence of cognitive dysfunction, but the serum sodium is very low, so it is critical to manage this appropriately. Tolvaptan (Answer C) is an oral vasopressin receptor antagonist that is administered daily for up to 4 days, and it is very effective in the treatment of moderate to severe hyponatremia following pituitary surgery.
A vasopressin receptor antagonist may facilitate recovery from syndrome of inappropriate antidiuretic hormone secretion in this setting. Tolvaptan administration (15 mg) will result in the most rapid normalization of sodium compared with the other listed options. Hypertonic saline can also be used in this setting, usually at a recommended dose and rate of 0.5 to 1.0 mL/kg body weight per hour, which, in a patient weighing 130 lb (59 kg), translates to 30 to 60 mL per hour. A rate of 5 mL/h (Answer D) is too low.

If fluid restriction is to be successful, it should be to less than 500 to 1000 mL/24 h. A 1500-mL limit (Answer A) is too high. In addition, the severity of this patient's hyponatremia dictates that fluid restriction alone would not be appropriate. Demeclocycline (Answer B) causes partial nephrogenic diabetes insipidus and can be useful for patients with chronic, symptomatic hyponatremia, such as that associated with malignancy; it is generally not used when hyponatremia develops acutely. Administration of normal saline (Answer E) is not appropriate for this patient, as she does not appear to be hypovolemic, and normal saline administration may further lower the serum sodium in a patient with SIADH.

EDUCATIONAL OBJECTIVE

Manage severe hyponatremia in the postoperative setting following transsphenoidal surgery.

REFERENCE(S)

Verbalis JG, Goldsmith SR, Greenberg A, et al. Diagnosis, evaluation, and treatment of hyponatremia: expert panel recommendations. *Am J Med.* 2013;126(10 Suppl 1):S1-S42. PMID: 24074529

Jahangiri A, Wagner J, Tran MT, et al. Factors predicting postoperative hyponatremia and efficacy of hyponatremia management strategies after more than 1000 pituitary operations. *J Neurosurg.* 2013;119(6):1478-1483. PMID: 23971964

Woodmansee WW, Carmichael J, Kelly D, Katznelson L; AACE Neuroendocrine and Pituitary Scientific Committee. American Association of Clinical Endocrinologists and American College of Endocrinology disease state clinical review: postoperative management following pituitary surgery. *Endocr Pract.* 2015;21(7):832-838. PMID: 26172128

Gross P. Clinical management of SIADH. *Ther Adv Endocrinol Metab.* 2012;3(2):61-73. PMID: 23148195

7 **ANSWER: B) Lanreotide depot monthly**

Somatostatin analogues are effective in managing acromegaly and are often used as first-line medical therapy. Therefore, lanreotide depot, a somatostatin analogue, given monthly (Answer B) would be the initial treatment choice in this patient. Pegvisomant (Answer D) is effective and, in the most recent Endocrine Society guidelines, was recommended to be considered as first-line medical therapy when administered as daily, not weekly, dosing. Repeated surgery (Answer C) is probably not indicated if the residual tumor is within the cavernous sinus and is hence not surgically accessible. Irradiation (Answer A) could certainly be done if cabergoline, somatostatin analogue, or daily pegvisomant is ineffective. However, radiation can take 5 to 10 years for effect, and she is currently symptomatic, so immediate therapy with medication is necessary. Cabergoline (Answer E) may be used to treat acromegaly, but this is usually most effective with more modest disease. She has persistent residual tumor, as well as a relatively high IGF-1 level, and cabergoline would not likely be effective in such a patient.

EDUCATIONAL OBJECTIVE

Manage persistent acromegaly after transsphenoidal surgery.

REFERENCE(S)

Katznelson L, Laws ER Jr, Melmed S, et al. Acromegaly: an endocrine society clinical practice guideline. *J Clin Endocrinol Metab.* 2014;99(11): 3933-3951. PMID: 25356808

Giustina A, Chanson P, Kleinberg D, et al; Acromegaly Consensus Group. Expert consensus document: a consensus on the medical treatment of acromegaly. *Nat Rev Endocrinol.* 2014;10(4): 243-248. PMID: 24566817

8 ANSWER: C) Discuss surgery

Of concern in this patient is the discrepancy between her prolactin level of only 152 ng/mL (6.8 nmol/L) and the size of the adenoma—24 mm. Although this discrepancy could be due to inefficient production of prolactin by a prolactinoma, it is more likely due to stalk dysfunction caused by a nonfunctioning adenoma or some other mass lesion such as a meningioma or Rathke cleft cyst. A dopamine agonist could indeed reduce if not normalize prolactin levels and correct amenorrhea and galactorrhea but have no effect on the growth of a mass lesion that is not a prolactinoma. Given the size of the lesion and its proximity to the optic chiasm, transsphenoidal surgery should be strongly considered and discussed (Answer C). Visual field testing would be indicated to ascertain impact on chiasmal function, but this was not an offered answer choice.

Given the fact that this lesion is most likely not a prolactinoma, increasing the bromocriptine dosage (Answer A) or switching from bromocriptine to cabergoline (Answer B) is not indicated, as this would be unlikely to shrink the tumor further. Performing a pituitary-directed MRI in 6 months (Answer D) to assess for an increase in tumor size could be considered, but, given the proximity of the tumor to the chiasm, surgery would be the best next step. The somatostatin analogues octreotide (Answer E) and lanreotide are not useful in the management of patients with prolactinoma.

EDUCATIONAL OBJECTIVE

Distinguish prolactinomas from clinically nonfunctioning adenomas and recommend appropriate management.

REFERENCE(S)

Melmed S, Casanueva FF, Hoffman AR, et al; Endocrine Society. Diagnosis and treatment of hyperprolactinemia: an Endocrine Society clinical practice guideline. *J Clin Endocrinol Metab.* 2011;96(2):273-288. PMID: 21296991

Karavitaki N, Thanabalasingham G, Shore HC, et al. Do the limits of serum prolactin in disconnection hyperprolactinaemia need re-definition? A study of 226 patients with histologically verified non-functioning pituitary macroadenoma. *Clin Endocrinol (Oxf).* 2006;65(4):524-529. PMID: 16984247

9 ANSWER: A) Temozolomide

This patient has a rapidly enlarging macroprolactinoma that is unresponsive to cabergoline, surgery, and stereotactic radiosurgery. The tumor is certainly acting in a malignant fashion. However, distant metastases would have to be demonstrated for this to qualify as a true malignancy. About 75% of these very aggressive tumors, and some true pituitary carcinomas, respond to temozolomide (Answer A), an alkylating agent used primarily for the treatment of glioblastomas. However, even patients who respond to this agent for a while may have, over time, a bad outcome. Additional radiotherapy (Answer C) within 2 years of prior radiation may lead to excessive radiation exposure to the local brain structures, so this would not be advised now. Surgery (Answer B) is unlikely to help given the location of the tumor mass. No data have been published regarding the use of pasireotide (Answer D) to treat prolactinomas, nor are there sufficient data on the use of octreotide long-acting release (Answer E) in this setting.

EDUCATIONAL OBJECTIVE

Recommend a treatment strategy for aggressive pituitary tumors and pituitary carcinomas.

REFERENCE(S)

Di Ieva A, Rotondo F, Syro LV, Cusimano MD, Kovacs K. Aggressive pituitary adenomas--diagnosis and emerging treatments. *Nat Rev Endocrinol.* 2014;10(7):423-435. PMID: 24821329

McCormack AI, Wass JA, Grossman AB. Aggressive pituitary tumours: the role of temozolomide and the assessment of MGMT status. *Eur J Clin Invest.* 2011;41(10):1133-1148. PMID: 21496012

Whitelaw BC, Dworakowska D, Thomas NW, et al. Temozolomide in the management of dopamine agonist-resistant prolactinomas. *Clin Endocrinol (Oxf).* 2012;76(6):877-886. PMID: 22372583

10 ANSWER: B) Ipilimumab

Ipilimumab (Answer B) is a monoclonal antibody used in the treatment of patients with metastatic melanoma. Hypophysitis has been reported in 10% to 15% of treated patients. Pituitary enlargement can occur within 2 months of treatment initiation, and corticotrophs and thyrotrophs are the most common cell types affected. This form of hypophysitis is different from lymphocytic hypophysitis that occurs peripartum in women. Ipilimumab is an immune checkpoint inhibitor that enhances immune response by working through the cytotoxic T-lymphocyte–associated antigen 4 (CTLA-4). Although prednisone (Answer A) can certainly suppress ACTH secretion, it does not cause pituitary enlargement. High-dosage steroids are not effective in treating this hypophysitis.

Temozolomide (Answer C) is an alkylating agent used in the treatment of gliomas and has been useful in the treatment of some patients with pituitary carcinomas and very aggressive macroadenomas. Sunitinib (Answer D) is a tyrosine kinase inhibitor that has been used to treat thyroid cancer, among other cancers, but it has not been implicated as a cause of hypophysitis. Hemochromatosis due to iron overload (Answer E) could cause a pituitary abnormality, but it would not cause homogeneous pituitary enlargement or severe hypopituitarism.

EDUCATIONAL OBJECTIVE

Identify medications that can cause hypophysitis.

REFERENCE(S)

Corsello SM, Barnabei A, Marchetti P, De Vecchis L, Salvatori R, Torino F. Endocrine side effects Induced by immune checkpoint inhibitors. *J Clin Endocrinol Metab.* 2013;98(4):1361-1375. PMID: 23471977

Faje AT, Sullivan R, Lawrence D, et al. Ipilimumab-induced hypophysitis: a detailed longitudinal analysis in a large cohort of patients with metastatic melanoma. *J Clin Endocrinol Metab.* 2014;99(11): 4078-4085. PMID: 25078147

Albarel F, Gaudy C, Castinetti F, et al. Long-term follow-up of ipilimumab-induced hypophysitis, a common adverse event of the anti-CTLA-4 antibody in melanoma. *Eur J Endocrinol.* 2015;172(2):195-204. PMID: 25416723

Barroso-Sousa R, Barry WT, Garrido-Castro AC, et al. Incidence of endocrine dysfunction following the use of different immune checkpoint inhibitor regimens: a systematic review and meta-analysis. *JAMA Oncol.* 2018;4(2):173-182. PMID: 28973656

11 ANSWER: A) Radiotherapy

Transsphenoidal surgery is the first-line treatment for clinically nonfunctioning pituitary adenomas, but tumor tissue that is left in the sellar area has the potential for subsequent regrowth. Although it is not recommended as routine for every case, radiotherapy (Answer A) may be used to reduce tumor mass or prevent remnant regrowth. There are no randomized controlled trials of radiotherapy vs other treatment options, but several retrospective series have shown that individuals who undergo postoperative radiotherapy for clinically nonfunctioning pituitary adenomas have a 50% lower rate of recurrence than those who are simply observed when there is residual tumor seen on MRI.

Although repeated surgery (Answer C) would be useful for management of residual disease, the current tumor is in the cavernous sinus and is unlikely to be accessible for resection. Pegvisomant (Answer B) is a treatment for acromegaly, and it has no role in the management of gonadotroph adenomas. Although GnRH antagonists (Answer D) make theoretical sense to try in patients with gonadotroph adenomas based on the assumption that GnRH may stimulate gonadotroph cells, in practice their use has not been shown to be beneficial. There are no data on use of pasireotide (Answer E) for patients with nonfunctioning adenomas.

Thus, of the choices presented in this vignette, radiotherapy is most likely to be effective in preventing further growth of the remnant nonfunctioning pituitary adenoma after surgery.

EDUCATIONAL OBJECTIVE

Guide the long-term management of clinically nonfunctioning pituitary adenomas.

REFERENCE(S)

Molitch ME. Nonfunctioning pituitary tumors and pituitary incidentalomas. *Endocrinol Metab Clin North Am.* 2008;37(1):151-171. PMID: 18226735

Freda PU, Beckers AM, Katznelson L, et al; Endocrine Society. Pituitary incidentaloma: an Endocrine Society clinical practice guideline. *J Clin Endocrinol Metab.* 2011;96(4):894-904. PMID: 21474686

Greenman Y, Tordjman K, Osher E, et al. Postoperative treatment of clinically nonfunctioning pituitary adenomas with dopamine agonists decreases tumour remnant growth. *Clin Endocrinol (Oxf).* 2005;63(1):39-44. PMID: 15963059

12 ANSWER: E) Pasireotide

Somatostatin analogues such as octreotide (Answer A), lanreotide (Answer B), and pasireotide (Answer E) decrease GH and IGF-1 and therefore improve insulin resistance. However, all 3 also inhibit insulin secretion to some extent, and when large groups of patients treated with octreotide and lanreotide have been analyzed, some were found to have improvement in diabetes status, some to have worsening, and some to have no change. The situation is worse with pasireotide (Answer E) because it decreases GLP-1 and glucose insulinotropic peptide (GIP) and worsens glucose tolerance in many patients. Pegvisomant (Answer C) works entirely by blocking the GH receptor, thereby decreasing insulin resistance, and it has no effect on insulin. Therefore, an improvement in glycemic status occurs in virtually everyone. Cabergoline (Answer D) is generally much less effective than pegvisomant, and the improvement that can be expected in glycemic status is therefore also less.

EDUCATIONAL OBJECTIVE

In the treatment of acromegaly, identify which medications may worsen diabetes mellitus.

REFERENCE(S)

Baldelli R, Battista C, Leonetti F, et al. Glucose homeostasis in acromegaly: effects of long-acting somatostatin analogues treatment. *Clin Endocrinol (Oxf).* 2003;59(4);492-499. PMID: 14510913

Barkan AL, Burman P, Clemmons DR, et al. Glucose homeostasis and safety in patients with acromegaly converted from long-acting octreotide to pegvisomant. *J Clin Endocrinol Metab.* 2005;90(10): 5684-5691. PMID: 16076947

Colao A, Bronstein M, Freda P, et al; Pasireotide C2305 Study Group. Pasireotide versus octreotide in acromegaly: a head-to-head superiority study. *J Clin Endocrinol Metab.* 2014;99(3): 791-799. PMID: 24423324

13 ANSWER: D) Oral contraceptives

Because this woman does not desire pregnancy in the near future, there is no critical need to restore ovulation. However, she has had amenorrhea for 4 years, implying hypoestrogenemia and an increased risk for osteoporosis. Oral contraceptives (Answer D) will supply needed estrogen and simultaneously provide contraception. Studies have shown that oral contraceptive use is safe in women with microadenomas and there is minimal risk of tumor enlargement. If the patient's course were followed with observation only (Answer E), her hypoestrogenemic state would persist, putting her at even higher risk of osteoporosis. The dopamine agonists bromocriptine (Answer B) and cabergoline (Answer C) can restore ovulatory cycles in more than 80% of women, but an additional mode of contraception would be needed. Furthermore, oral contraceptives are much cheaper than either bromocriptine or cabergoline, an important consideration in this woman with poor insurance coverage. A dopamine agonist would be indicated if pregnancy were desired. In this clinical setting, transsphenoidal surgery (Answer A) is less effective than dopamine agonists and carries with it considerably higher risk and cost.

EDUCATIONAL OBJECTIVE

Compare and contrast the treatment options for women with prolactin-secreting microadenomas.

REFERENCE(S)

Gillam MP, Molitch ME, Lombardi G, Colao A. Advances in the treatment of prolactinomas. *Endocr Rev.* 2006;27(5):485-534. PMID: 16705142

14 ANSWER: A) Another transsphenoidal surgery

In patients truly cured of Cushing disease, ACTH and cortisol levels are very low because they have been suppressed by the previously high cortisol levels. Therefore, it is expected that adrenal insufficiency will be detected following curative surgery. In the current patient, the cortisol concentration never fell to a level consistent with adrenal insufficiency. Therefore, she has residual disease. Consideration should be given to repeated surgery (Answer A).

This patient is not currently truly hypocortisolemic nor hypercortisolemic, so neither hydrocortisone replacement therapy (Answer B) nor medical therapy (Answer C), respectively, is indicated now. Furthermore, an attempt should be made to cure her surgically before committing to medical therapy. Stereotactic radiosurgery (Answer D) would be indicated only if repeated surgery, and perhaps medical therapy, has failed. Cortisol levels are usually less than 5 µg/dL (<137.9 nmol/L) when patients are surgically cured and hydrocortisone is generally needed for several months, initially for both maintenance therapy and stress management, and then later just for stress. Cosyntropin-stimulation testing (Answer E) is not useful in the immediate postoperative period because the adrenal glands themselves are not suppressed and should respond vigorously to exogenous ACTH, thereby giving a falsely reassuring result.

EDUCATIONAL OBJECTIVE

Assess patients with Cushing disease postoperatively.

REFERENCE(S)

Esposito F, Dusick JR, Cohan P, et al. Clinical review: early morning cortisol levels as a predictor of remission after transsphenoidal surgery for Cushing's disease. *J Clin Endocrinol Metab.* 2006;91(1):7- 13. PMID: 16234305

Hameed N, Yedinak CG, Brzana J, et al. Remission rate after transsphenoidal surgery in patients with pathologically confirmed Cushing's disease, the role of cortisol, ACTH assessment and immediate reoperation: a large single center experience. *Pituitary.* 2013;16(4):452-458. PMID: 23242860

Salmon PM, Loftus PD, Dodd RL, et al. Utility of adrenocorticotropic hormone in assessing the response to transsphenoidal surgery for Cushing's disease. *Endocr Pract.* 2014;20(11):1159-1164. PMID: 24936567

15 ANSWER: B) Continue the mifepristone dosage at 600 mg daily

Mifepristone is a glucocorticoid receptor blocker that is effective in the treatment of patients with all forms of Cushing syndrome. Because it blocks the glucocorticoid receptor, cortisol and ACTH levels may actually rise during treatment, but these higher levels are biologically unimportant because of the receptor blockade. Therefore, it is not recommended that cortisol and ACTH measurements be used for dosage adjustment during mifepristone treatment; the dosage should be adjusted solely based on clinical parameters of the activity of Cushing syndrome while avoiding symptoms of adrenal insufficiency. Thus, this patient is doing very well clinically and no dosage adjustment is needed (thus, Answer B is correct and Answers A and C are incorrect). There is no need to add pasireotide (Answer D) or to perform stereotactic radiosurgery (Answer E).

EDUCATIONAL OBJECTIVE

Guide the use of mifepristone in the treatment of Cushing syndrome.

REFERENCE(S)

Fleseriu M, Molitch ME, Gross C, Schteingart DE, Vaughan TB 3rd, Biller BM. A new therapeutic approach in the medical treatment of Cushing's syndrome: glucocorticoid receptor blockade with mifepristone. *Endocr Pract.* 2013;19(2):313-326. PMID: 23337135

Katznelson L, Loriaux DL, Feldman D, Braunstein GD, Schteingart DE, Gross C. Global clinical response in Cushing's syndrome patients treated with mifepristone. *Clin Endocrinol (Oxf).* 2014;80(4):562-569. PMID: 24102404

16 ANSWER: D) Obtain a semen analysis

The first thing to establish in this patient is whether he is truly infertile. Although one might expect that he would be, given his panhypopituitarism and being on testosterone replacement, he may have adequate sperm counts and morphology for fertility. Drincic et al found adequate spermatogenesis for fertility in about 50% of such men. Therefore, the first management step is to obtain a semen analysis (Answer D). If he has azoospermia or oligospermia, he might respond to hCG injections and may also need FSH injections. Trying these therapies before assessing his fertility status (Answers A and B) would be inappropriate. In the context of this vignette, a blockage in the patient's duct system is unlikely and testicular sperm extraction (Answer C) would not be a technique used. The chances for fertility in a patient such as this are well over 50%, and suggesting adoption at this point (Answer E) would be premature.

EDUCATIONAL OBJECTIVE

Evaluate for infertility in men with hypopituitarism.

REFERENCE(S)

Drincic A, Arseven OK, Sosa E, Mercado M, Kopp P, Molitch ME. Men with acquired hypogonadotropic hypogonadism treated with testosterone may be fertile. *Pituitary.* 2003;6(1):5-10. PMID: 14674718

Farhat R, Al-zidjali F, Alzahrani AS. Outcome of gonadotropin therapy for male infertility due to hypogonadotrophic hypogonadism. *Pituitary.* 2010;13(2):105-110. PMID: 19838805

17 ANSWER: A) Perform a GH-stimulation test one month after stopping GH

More than two-thirds of children with idiopathic isolated GH deficiency diagnosed by conventional criteria have normal GH secretion as adults. Consequently, retesting such patients as adults with a stimulation test is important before continuing GH treatment. Because one-third of these patients may have persistent GH deficiency, simply discontinuing GH therapy because he has reached peak growth (Answer C) is incorrect. Testing should be done one month after stopping GH. In this setting, IGF-1 measurement alone (Answer B) is not sufficient to document persistent GH deficiency, and a GH-stimulation test is needed (Answer A). GH treatment can be resumed at a lower dosage than that used in childhood because of its known benefits on body composition

(Answer D), but only if GH deficiency is documented to still be present. Measuring a morning GH level following discontinuation of GH therapy (Answer E) is not useful diagnostically to assess for ongoing GH deficiency.

EDUCATIONAL OBJECTIVE

Perform GH-stimulation testing in a young adult with a childhood diagnosis of GH deficiency to determine whether therapy is still needed.

REFERENCE(S)

Tauber M, Moulin P, Pienkowski C, Jouret B, Rochiccioli P. Growth hormone (GH) retesting and auxological data in 131 GH-deficient patients after completion of treatment. *J Clin Endocrinol Metab.* 1997;82(2):352-356. PMID: 9024217

Molitch ME, Clemmons DR, Malozowski S, Merriam GR, Vance ML; Endocrine Society. Evaluation and treatment of adult growth hormone deficiency: an Endocrine Society clinical practice guideline. *J Clin Endocrinol Metab.* 2011;96(6):1587-1609. PMID: 21602453

18 ANSWER: B) Transsphenoidal surgery now

All of these treatment modalities can improve Cushing disease, and treatment during pregnancy is advocated because it results in better fetal outcomes. Transsphenoidal surgery has a cure rate of 80% to 90% in expert neurosurgical hands, with very low complication and fetal loss rates when done in the second trimester. Surgery now (Answer B) should be strongly considered in this patient. Because of the presence of active Cushing disease, it is not safe for either the fetus or the mother to have uncontrolled hypercortisolism through the rest of her pregnancy. Thus, delaying surgery until after delivery (Answer A) is not acceptable.

Mifepristone (Answer C) was originally developed as a progesterone receptor blocker and is a potent abortifacient (RU486); therefore, its use in pregnancy is absolutely contraindicated. There is experience with only about 50 cases in which somatostatin analogues have been used to treat acromegaly during pregnancy, with relatively minor adverse effects. However, somatostatin analogues cross the placenta and have unknown effects on the fetus. There is no documented experience with pasireotide (Answer D) during pregnancy, and it would be expected to worsen glucose tolerance in this population susceptible to gestational diabetes. Although cabergoline (Answer E) is safe when stopped after conception, there is little experience when used throughout pregnancy, and its ability to normalize cortisol levels in Cushing disease is only modest.

EDUCATIONAL OBJECTIVE

Guide treatment of Cushing disease during pregnancy.

REFERENCE(S)

Marions L. Mifepristone dose in the regimen with misoprostol for medical abortion. *Contraception.* 2006;74(1):21-25. PMID: 16781255

Lindsay JR, Jonklaas J, Oldfield EH, Nieman LK. Cushing's syndrome during pregnancy: personal experience and review of the literature. *J Clin Endocrinol Metab.* 2005;90(5):3077-3083. PMID: 15705919

Cohen-Kerem R, Railton C, Oren D, Lishner M, Koren G. Pregnancy outcome following non- obstetric surgical intervention. *Am J Surgery.* 2005;190(3):467-473. PMID: 16105538

19 ANSWER: A) DDAVP, 0.1 mg orally as needed for polyuria and hypernatremia

This patient has acute onset of diabetes insipidus. In this setting, the cause of the diabetes insipidus is central, due to deficiency of vasopressin. The goal of therapy is to control the free water depletion from polyuria, as well as maintain comfort. DDAVP should be administered in a short-acting regimen with avoidance of prescheduled dosing given the risk of hyponatremia from syndrome of inappropriate antidiuretic hormone secretion (SIADH) in the subsequent days as part of the triphasic response following surgery. Therefore, DDAVP should be administered as needed (0.1 mg orally, and higher doses of 0.2 to 0.3 mg may be necessary) (Answer A) or as subcutaneous aqueous DDAVP, 0.5 to 1.0 mcg (not offered as an option in this vignette). Scheduled dosing (Answer D) should be avoided. Administration of DDAVP immediately following endonasal surgery should be given through oral or parenteral routes. Intranasal administration (Answer E) would not be absorbed sufficiently given trauma to the mucosal membranes from surgery, but may be considered in the future if the diabetes insipidus persists and the mucosal membranes have healed. Fluid restriction (Answer C) is contraindicated in these patients who are prone to dehydration and is used to treat hyponatremia. Tolvaptan (Answer B) is an oral vasopressin receptor antagonist used for the treatment of severe hyponatremia, not present in this patient.

EDUCATIONAL OBJECTIVE

Manage diabetes insipidus following pituitary surgery.

REFERENCE(S)

Woodmansee WW, Carmichael J, Kelly D, Katznelson L; AACE Neuroendocrine and Pituitary Scientific Committee. American Association of Clinical Endocrinologists and American College of Endocrinology disease state clinical review: postoperative management following pituitary surgery. *Endocr Pract.* 2015;21(7):832-838. PMID: 26172128

Fleseriu M, Hashim IA, Karavitaki N, et al. Hormonal replacement in hypopituitarism in adults: an Endocrine Society clinical practice guideline. *J Clin Endocrinol Metab.* 2016;101(11):3888-3921. PMID: 27736313

20 ANSWER: B) GH deficiency

Hypopituitarism occurs following both penetrating and blunt head trauma in approximately 25% of individuals (range 15%-68%). The pathophysiology of hypopituitarism in patients with traumatic brain injury includes direct injury to the gland, vasospasm of the hypothalamo-hypophyseal blood supply, and compression of the hypothalamus and pituitary gland by edema, hemorrhage, or elevated intracranial pressure. Genetic factors, including certain apolipoprotein E haplotypes, may influence this risk. Also, there are studies showing that antipituitary and antihypothalamic antibodies are found in patients with traumatic brain injury, although the pathogenic role is unclear. Autopsy series have shown necrotic glands in up to 80% of fatal cases. GH deficiency (Answer B) is the most common deficiency found, and this has critical implications, as GH deficiency may impact full convalescence.

All patients with moderate to severe traumatic brain injury should be evaluated for hypopituitarism during the acute and chronic course of their recovery. Immediately following the traumatic brain injury, emphasis on care during the first 2 weeks after traumatic brain injury should be on the adrenal axis and posterior pituitary function. In the subsequent months after injury, the entire anterior and posterior pituitary hormonal axes should be assessed. In addition, symptomatic patients with mild traumatic brain injury (including those with repetitive mild traumatic brain injury) and impaired quality of life are also at risk for hypopituitarism and neuroendocrine testing should be considered. Testing for chronic hypopituitarism following traumatic brain injury is usually performed at least 6 to 12 months following the event. Hormone replacement should be administered accordingly.

This patient does not have evidence of significant testosterone deficiency (Answer A), adrenal insufficiency (Answer C), or hypothyroidism (Answer D) to explain his symptoms. There are no clear clinical findings of hypoprolactinemia (Answer E).

EDUCATIONAL OBJECTIVE

Diagnose hypopituitarism after head trauma and review its manifestations.

REFERENCE(S)

Tritos NA, Yuen KC, Kelly DF; AACE Neuroendocrine and Pituitary Scientific Committee. American Association of Clinical Endocrinologists and American College of Endocrinology Disease State Clinical Review: A Neuroendocrine Approach to Patients with Traumatic Brain Injury. Endocrine practice: official journal of the American College of Endocrinology and the American Association of Clinical Endocrinologists. *Endocr Pract.* 2015;21(7): 823-831. PMID: 26172127

Klose M, Feldt-Rasmussen U. Chronic endocrine consequences of traumatic brain injury - what is the evidence? *Nat Rev Endocrinol.* 2018;14(1):57-62. PMID: 28885623

Giuliano S, Talarico S, Bruno L, Nicoletti FB, Ceccotti C, Belfiore A. Growth hormone deficiency and hypopituitarism in adults after complicated mild traumatic brain injury. *Endocrine.* 2017;58(1): 115-123. PMID: 27878771

21 ANSWER: C) Refer for transsphenoidal surgery

Most patients with prolactinomas respond very well to cabergoline, and the overall success rate in normalizing prolactin levels with cabergoline is higher than it is for bromocriptine. A few studies have shown that more than 50% of patients whose prolactin levels do not normalize on bromocriptine therapy will experience normalization when switched to cabergoline. For this patient, neither bromocriptine nor cabergoline at routine dosages was able to normalize her prolactin level. It is possible that increasing the cabergoline dosage further may have some effect, but this was not an answer choice in this vignette. Switching cabergoline back to bromocriptine (Answer A) is unlikely to be more effective.

Transsphenoidal surgery (Answer C) can provide a long-term cure in patients with microprolactinomas and should be strongly considered in this patient who has not had a clear and successful response to a dopamine agonist and has a tumor that abuts the chiasm.

Clomiphene (Answer D) would be an option for a patient interested in fertility but attempt at prolactinoma control in this patient is the priority. Radiation therapy (Answer B) is indicated for management of prolactinomas that are growing despite dopamine agonist therapy, are treatment resistant, and cannot be managed surgically. The risk of hypopituitarism following radiation therapy is substantial, making fertility management more complex. In addition, the tumor abuts the chiasm, so radiation would have risk of chiasmal damage. Therefore, radiation therapy is not recommended. Temozolomide (Answer E) is an alkylating agent that may have a role in treating aggressive or malignant pituitary tumors. As this tumor does not show such characteristics, temozolomide would not be appropriate.

EDUCATIONAL OBJECTIVE

Manage a patient with a prolactinoma unresponsive to dopamine agonist therapy.

REFERENCE(S)

Gillam MP, Molitch ME, Lombardi G, Colao A. Advances in the treatment of prolactinomas. *Endocr Rev.* 2006;27(5):485-534. PMID: 16705142

Melmed S, Casanueva FF, Hoffman AR, et al; Endocrine Society. Diagnosis and treatment of hyperprolactinemia: an Endocrine Society clinical practice guideline. *J Clin Endocrinol Metab.* 2011;96(2):273-288. PMID: 21296991

22 ANSWER: C) Lymphocytic hypophysitis

This pregnant woman has pituitary enlargement presenting near term, and it is most likely to be lymphocytic hypophysitis (Answer C). MRI shows diffuse pituitary enlargement, which is more compatible with hypophysitis than pituitary adenoma (Answer A). Had gadolinium been given, there would have been diffuse enhancement rather than focal enhancement. No data show adverse effects of performing MRI or giving gadolinium during pregnancy, although it is recommended to withhold gadolinium during pregnancy. One of the striking features of hypophysitis occurring during pregnancy is the high risk of ACTH deficiency, and this should be evaluated.

Histiocytosis (Answer B) is not more common in pregnancy, and it usually presents with diabetes insipidus and a posterior sellar mass. The radiographic characteristics of the lesion are not consistent with a Rathke cyst (Answer D). Malignant metastasis (Answer E) to the sella is usually seen in the presence of known primary neoplastic disease, and it often presents with diabetes insipidus.

EDUCATIONAL OBJECTIVE

Diagnose lymphocytic hypophysitis in a pregnant woman.

REFERENCE(S)

Rivera JA. Lymphocytic hypophysitis: disease spectrum and approach to diagnosis and therapy. *Pituitary.* 2006;9(1):35-45. PMID: 16703407

Molitch ME. Pituitary disorders during pregnancy. *Endocrinol Metab Clin North Am.* 2006;35(1):99-116. PMID: 16310644

Khare S, Jagtap VS, Budyal SR, et al. Primary (autoimmune) hypophysitis: a single centre experience. *Pituitary.* 2015;18(1):16-22. PMID: 24375060

Thyroid Board Review

Jacqueline Jonklaas, MD, PhD, MPH

1 **ANSWER: E) Hold enteral feeding from 5:30 AM to 7:30 AM daily**

Each of the listed options would most likely lower this patient's serum TSH. However, increasing the levothyroxine dosage to 125 mcg daily (Answer B) is incorrect, as the relatively small increase in levothyroxine dosage would be insufficient to lower TSH into the normal range. Discontinuing enteral feeding (Answer A) is incorrect; although it might normalize the patient's TSH, caloric restriction would not the in the best interests of a patient requiring a prolonged hospital stay.

Switching to a liquid levothyroxine formulation (Answer C), switching to intravenous levothyroxine (Answer D), or holding enteral feeding from 5:30 AM to 7:30 AM (Answer E) would all be reasonable approaches to correcting the patient's elevated TSH. Liquid levothyroxine, either given directly in liquid form (recently available in the United States) or delivered within a gelatin capsule (available in the United States), has the advantage of improved absorption in several levothyroxine-malabsorptive states, including those associated with proton-pump inhibitors, celiac disease, and coexistent food consumption or coexistent enteral feeding administration. Although this option is reasonable, it is probably not the most cost-effective, as levothyroxine tablets are generally cheaper than levothyroxine in gel capsules or as a liquid and are also covered by most insurance plans. Many hospital formularies do not yet carry the gel capsule or liquid formulations.

Certainly switching to intravenous levothyroxine (Answer D) is simple and would be guaranteed to reverse the problem of elevated TSH. The dose of intravenous levothyroxine should be 70% to 80% of the oral dose (78-89 mcg). Single-use vials containing either 100 mcg, 200 mcg, or 500 mcg of levothyroxine as a lyophilized powder are available. Reconstitution using 5 mL of isotonic saline is recommended. Although this option is effective and the dosage of levothyroxine can be readily adjusted based on trough levels of free T_4 and based on TSH values over a longer period, many hospitals discourage its use because of the increased cost of intravenous levothyroxine preparations compared with that of tablet preparations. Some hospitals may also require an endocrinology consultation before intravenous levothyroxine can be used.

In the outpatient setting, a separation of 30 to 60 minutes between levothyroxine administration and food intake is recommended. An even longer separation of up to 4 hours is recommended for calcium and iron. In a 2014 study by Pirola et al, normal serum TSH values were maintained in hospitalized patients being given enteral tube feeds if the feeds were held for 1 hour in order to administer crushed levothyroxine tablets. Temporarily suspending the patient's tube feeding for 1 to 2 hours (Answer E) would allow for better levothyroxine absorption and would be the most cost-effective approach. Although this option avoids the cost of intravenous levothyroxine preparations, it is probably not the most convenient choice from the standpoint of the nursing staff. Interestingly, in general, administration of levothyroxine in the hospital setting is associated with errors that result in out-of-range TSH values. Elevated TSH values seem to be associated with increased length of hospital stay.

EDUCATIONAL OBJECTIVE

Differentiate among the options available to reverse elevated TSH due to reduced levothyroxine absorption in a hospitalized patient.

REFERENCE(S)

Pirola I, Daffini L, Gandossi E, et al. Comparison between liquid and tablet levothyroxine formulations in patients treated through enteral feeding tube. *J Endocrinol Invest.* 2014;37(6):583-587. PMID: 24789541

Dickerson RN, Maish GO 3rd, Minard G, Brown RO. Clinical relevancy of the levothyroxine-continuous enteral nutrition interaction. *Nutr Clin Pract.* 2010;25(6):646-652. PMID: 21139130

2 ANSWER: C) TSH, 0.01 mIU/L; free T_4, 2.5 ng/dL; total T_3, 210 ng/dL; thyroglobulin, 100 ng/mL

Both the position of the thyroid gland on the anterior surface of the neck and its vascularity contribute to it being a gland that is susceptible to trauma, both blunt and penetrating. Injury can result in destructive thyroiditis associated with release of preformed thyroid hormones from the injured thyroid gland and manifestation of thyrotoxicosis, as occurred in this patient. Causes of blunt trauma that have been documented to be associated with thyrotoxicosis include palpation, vigorous use of an ultrasonography probe, massage, strangulation, manipulation of the thyroid during nonthyroid surgery, and motor vehicle or bicycle accidents. Examples of penetrating trauma include civilian or military injuries related to weapons, assault, flying objects, or sharp objects. An extreme example is a case of thyroid storm associated with a spear-fishing gun trident.

This particular patient sustained a blunt injury to his thyroid gland due to the pressure from the noose used for strangulation. This subsequently resulted in thyrotoxicosis, as illustrated in Answer C. As the thyrotoxicosis is due to release of preformed thyroid hormones from the stores within the thyroid gland, a relatively modest elevation of T_3 is often observed, as is the case here. This is in contrast to the thyroid hormone profile associated with hyperthyroidism due to Graves disease or toxic nodular disease in which the T_3 elevation is more substantial. In some cases, the T_3 may, in fact, be the only elevated thyroid hormone, as seen in the pattern of thyroid hormones in Answer D. Answer B, with elevated TSH, represents central or TSH-driven hyperthyroidism. This is incorrect as it is inconsistent with the history provided in the vignette. Answers A and E are incorrect as they illustrate a hypothyroid and euthyroid thyroid function profile, respectively, and are not consistent with the signs and symptoms of thyrotoxicosis displayed by the patient.

The course of trauma-induced thyroiditis is similar, for example, to that of the more common subacute thyroiditis. The thyrotoxic phase is self-limited and gradually resolves. There may be a period of hypothyroidism as the thyroid gland recovers from the injury, and eventual return to euthyroidism is anticipated, as long as the injury to the thyroid gland can be repaired. The degree of thyrotoxicosis from trauma can even result in thyroid storm. Destructive thyroiditis can be distinguished from Graves disease by a low uptake of radiotracer on a thyroid uptake and scan and by reduced blood flow on color-flow Doppler, compared with the prominent vascularity seen in Graves disease. Serum thyroglobulin levels are elevated with both destructive thyroiditis and Graves disease but would be low in iatrogenic thyrotoxicosis associated with administration of thyroid hormone.

EDUCATIONAL OBJECTIVE

Recognize the presentation of trauma-induced thyroiditis.

REFERENCE(S)

Kasagi K, Hattori H. A case of destructive thyrotoxicosis induced by neck trauma. *Thyroid.* 2008;18(12):1333-1335. PMID: 19067641

Hari Kumar KV, Pasupuleti V, Jayaraman M, Abhyuday V, Rayudu B R, Modi KD. Role of thyroid Doppler in differential diagnosis of thyrotoxicosis. *Endocr Pract.* 2009;15(1):6-9. PMID: 19211390

3 ANSWER: D) An hCG value of greater than 6,000,000 mIU/mL

This patient presented with combined symptoms of thyrotoxicosis and advanced malignancy. Assuming that the patient's hyperthyroidism is directly related to his choriocarcinoma and that he does not have 2 separate etiologies for his hyperthyroidism, positive TSH-receptor antibodies (Answer B) is incorrect. Positive TSH-receptor antibodies would indicate Graves disease and a nonmalignancy-associated cause of his hyperthyroidism.

Germ-cell tumors, including choriocarcinoma, produce hCG, often in large amounts. hCG has enough structural similarity to TSH that high levels of this hormone can act upon the thyroid gland to cause hyperthyroidism. This is a well-documented, albeit rare, cause of hyperthyroidism. It is believed that hCG has a much lower potency for the TSH receptor than TSH itself, such that hCG concentrations greater than 400,000 to 500,000 mIU/mL are required to cause sufficient thyroid stimulation of thyroid hormone production to result in suppressed TSH. This patient's TSH was indeed suppressed at less than 0.001 mIU/mL, and an hCG value of 6000 mIU/mL (Answer C), if accurately measured, is insufficient to cause the thyrotoxicosis exhibited by this patient. In one study of patients with germ-cell tumors, mean hCG values of 346,686 mIU/mL were associated with subclinical hyperthyroidism, whereas mean hCG levels of 1,325,147 mIU/mL were associated with overt hyperthyroidism. Thus, an hCG value greater than 6,000,000 mIU/mL (Answer D) is correct. The initial hCG concentration is this patient was 6,760,713 mIU/mL.

Studies have shown that there is a consistent relationship between hCG and free T_4, such that free T_4 levels rise as hCG levels rise. In addition, TSH suppression is directly proportional to the hCG elevation. This patient's hyperthyroidism was initially treated with methimazole. However, following initiation of chemotherapy, his hCG levels decreased to 213,467 mIU/mL and his thyroid function normalized without the need for thionamides.

If ultrasonography of the thyroid is performed in an individual with hCG-induced thyrotoxicosis, it shows increased vascularity consistent with endogenous hyperthyroidism, as indeed was the case with this patient. Reduced vascularity (Answer A) would be more consistent with thyroiditis and is an incorrect answer. Metastasis of nonthyroid malignancies to the thyroid gland are rare but have been reported. Affected patients are mostly euthyroid or hypothyroid, but they can become hyperthyroid, usually in the setting of a destructive thyroiditis caused by malignant infiltration of the thyroid gland. Prominent features of a progressive malignancy causing destructive thyroiditis are a rapidly enlarging thyroid gland with tenderness and possibly compressive symptoms. These features are not described in this vignette, and a biopsy showing choriocarcinoma metastatic to the thyroid gland (Answer E) is not the best choice.

EDUCATIONAL OBJECTIVE

Describe the cause and mechanism of hCG-induced thyrotoxicosis associated with germ-cell tumors.

REFERENCE(S)

Lockwood CM, Grenache DG, Gronowski M. Serum human chorionic gonadotropin concentrations greater than 400,000 IU/L are invariably associated with suppressed serum thyrotropin concentrations. *Thyroid.* 2009;19(8):863-868. PMID: 19505185

Pallais JC, McInnis M, Saylor PJ, Wu RI. Case records of the Massachusetts General Hospital. Case 38-2015. A 21-year-old man with fatigue and weight loss. *N Engl J Med.* 2015;373(24):2358-2569. PMID: 26650156

Oosting SF, de Haas EC, Links TP, et al. Prevalence of paraneoplastic hyperthyroidism in patients with metastatic non-seminomatous germ-cell tumors. *Ann Oncol.* 2010;21(1):104-108. PMID: 19605510

4 ANSWER: D) Take levothyroxine at bedtime

The package insert on most levothyroxine products states that levothyroxine should be taken 30 to 60 minutes before food and 4 hours apart from calcium and iron supplements in order to avoid interference with levothyroxine absorption. Absorption of levothyroxine is approximately 75% to 80% in the fasting state and may drop to as little as 50% when taken with food. This patient clearly wishes to optimize her therapy for hypothyroidism and has consistently maintained euthyroidism. Another consideration when managing a chronic condition, in addition to treating to the desired goal, is to make the therapeutic regimen easy and convenient for the patient. This is not being achieved in this vignette. Her regimen is unnecessarily causing her to lose sleep, which could be detrimental over the long term. Therefore, continuing the current schedule (Answer C) is incorrect. Refraining from eating breakfast (Answer E) is not the best advice for someone who prefers to eat breakfast and has an active job. Weekly administration of levothyroxine (Answer A) is associated with accentuated peaks and troughs in free T_4 concentrations and should only be considered as a means of improving adherence in nonadherent patients.

With all other factors being stable, a higher TSH level would reflect less absorption of levothyroxine and a lower TSH level would reflect better absorption. Another consideration, in addition to the actual TSH value achieved, is the variability of TSH values over time. Many studies have examined the effect of different timings of levothyroxine on serum TSH with some variable results. However, not all these trials have been randomized or controlled. Three randomized crossover trials have been conducted. A 2-period crossover study examining administration 30 minutes before breakfast and bedtime showed the best absorption (lowest TSH) at bedtime. A 3-period crossover study examining administration 1 hour before breakfast, with breakfast, and at bedtime showed the lowest, least variable TSH values with 1 hour before breakfast. TSH values with administration at bedtime were slightly higher with more variability, while administration with breakfast had both the highest TSH values and the greatest variability. A 3-period crossover study examining administration 30 minutes before breakfast, 1 hour before the main meal of the day, and at bedtime showed no TSH differences between regimens.

Taking levothyroxine with breakfast (Answer B) and taking levothyroxine at bedtime (Answer D) are both regimens that could be considered for this patient. Reduced absorption associated with a "breakfast" regimen can be overcome by increasing the levothyroxine dosage. However, variable absorption could still be an issue, particularly in someone who eats different breakfast foods each morning. Overall, taking levothyroxine at bedtime may work best for this patient with her current schedule.

EDUCATIONAL OBJECTIVE

Explain how the timing of levothyroxine administration affects its absorption and thereby affects TSH values and the variability of TSH values.

REFERENCE(S)

Bolk N, Visser TJ, Nijam J, Jongste IJ, Tijssen JG, Berghout A. Effects of evening vs morning levothyroxine intake: a randomized double-blind crossover trial. *Arch Intern Med.* 2010;170(22):1996-2003. PMID: 21149757

Bach-Huynh TG, Nayak B, Loh J, Soldin S, Jonklaas J. Timing of levothyroxine administration affects serum thyrotropin concentration. *J Clin Endocrinol Metab.* 2009;94(10):3905-3912. PMID: 19584184

5 ANSWER: C) Normal thyroid function

This patient has had a stable TSH value that is slightly below the lower end of the standard laboratory reference range. However, he has normal thyroid hormone levels and a normal radioactive iodine uptake and scan. Although he has subcentimeter thyroid nodules, these would not be expected to be associated with any thyroid dysfunction.

The patient was hospitalized 2 months ago, but this should not be influencing his thyroid function now, as sufficient time has elapsed for his thyroid function to return to baseline. Recovery from euthyroid sick syndrome (Answer A) is most commonly manifest as transiently elevated serum TSH as the patient recovers from an illness and is not associated with low TSH.

Some drugs or supplements such as metformin or vitamin C can lower TSH, but fluoxetine (Answer D) is not known to do so.

There is no particular reason to consider central hypothyroidism (Answer E) due to TSH deficiency in a patient with no symptoms of hypothyroidism and no known reason for pituitary dysfunction. However, thyroid hormone values in the low end of the normal range and a low TSH value could be consistent with central hypothyroidism in the appropriate clinical setting.

Subclinical hyperthyroidism (Answer B) could be considered in this patient, but this diagnosis is made less likely by his thyroid hormone levels being in the lower half of the reference range, the absence of significant nodular thyroid disease, and normal findings on his radioactive iodine uptake and scan study.

This individual is of African American ancestry and he smokes cigarettes. Both of these factors could provide an explanation for his TSH value being in the range of 0.25 to 0.29 mIU/L. TSH values are generally lower in persons who smoke cigarettes, with the mean difference in TSH between smokers and nonsmokers being 0.26 mIU/L in one study. Data from United States population surveys also illustrate that a small proportion of persons of African American ancestry have TSH values below the 2.5th percentile of 0.45 mIU/L. When examining a disease-free population without known thyroid disease, goiter, or use of antithyroidal medications, 8% of black individuals have TSH values below 0.45 mIU/L. Thus, the most likely assessment is that this individual is euthyroid (Answer C). He can be safely followed, and future monitoring can be performed to ensure that he does not develop hyperthyroidism over time. Population data illustrate the fact that race, ethnicity, and age all affect TSH reference ranges. These factors should be considered when deciding whether thyroid disease is present.

EDUCATIONAL OBJECTIVE

Recognize that patients can be erroneously classified as having thyroid dysfunction if age- and race-specific limits for TSH values are not used.

REFERENCE(S)

Hollowell JG, Staehling NW, Flanders WD, et al. Serum TSH, T(4), and thyroid antibodies in the United States population (1988 to 1994): National Health and Nutrition Examination Survey (NHANES III). *J Clin Endocrinol Metab.* 2002;87(2):489-499. PMID: 11836274

Surks MI, Boucai L. Age- and race-based serum thyrotropin reference limits. *J Clin Endocrinol Metab.* 2010;95(2):496-502. PMID: 19965925

6 ANSWER: A) The risk of this patient having distant metastases was approximately 1%

At initial presentation, the patient described in this vignette would have been classified as falling into the American Thyroid Association low-risk category (thus, Answers C and D are incorrect). Her largest tumor focus was 1.5 cm, and there was no documented extrathyroidal extension or cervical lymph node involvement. If she had been treated with radioactive iodine and if she had been detected as having iodine uptake within her lungs, she would have been classified as having American Thyroid Association high-risk disease based on the distant metastases, but such information was not available at the time of diagnosis.

The scenario described in this patient is extremely uncommon and probably accounts for 1% to 2% of patients initially classified as having low-risk disease (thus, Answer A is correct and Answer E is incorrect). For example, in recent series in which patients at low risk were in fact treated with radioactive iodine, 2 of 345 patients, 3 of 272 patients, and 3 of 202 patients were identified as having distant metastases (6 in the lungs and 2 in the bones) based on posttherapy iodine scan. These unexpected distant metastases generally reveal themselves on posttherapy radioiodine scans, highlighting the importance of performing such a scan if radioactive iodine therapy is used.

There is no reason to suspect that cervical lymph node metastases were present but not detected (Answer B) at the time of this patient's initial diagnosis. Ultrasonography of the neck is a sensitive means of detecting cervical metastases. An upward trend in serum thyroglobulin may also be suggestive of the presence of lymph node metastases. The patient in this vignette did not have evidence of cervical disease on serial ultrasonography and thus most likely did not have metastases involving the cervical lymph nodes, either at presentation or subsequently.

The balance of benefits vs risks does not favor treatment of patients at apparently low risk with radioactive iodine. The risks include salivary gland damage, secondary malignancies, potential reproductive impact, and delay of conception, if desired. Many individuals would need to be treated with radioactive iodine without benefit in order to detect a case of distant metastases such as this at an earlier point in time.

EDUCATIONAL OBJECTIVE

Describe how, very rarely, patients with apparently low-risk differentiated thyroid cancer may in fact have distant metastases.

REFERENCE(S)

Agate L, Bianchi F, Brozzi F, et al. Less than 2% of the low- and intermediate-risk differentiated thyroid cancers show distant metastases at post-ablation whole-body scan. *Eur Thyroid J.* 2019;8(2):90-95. PMID: 31192148

Matrone A, Gambale C, Piaggi, et al. Postoperative thyroglobulin and neck ultrasound in the risk restratification and decision to perform 131I ablation. *J Clin Endocrinol Metab.* 2017;102(3): 893-902. PMID: 27929713

7 ANSWER: D

The uncertainty regarding whether radioactive iodine therapy is beneficial for patients with Hurthle-cell carcinoma is clearly reflected in the conflicting advice that this patient has received. In general, Hurthle-cell carcinoma has variable ability to accumulate and respond to radioactive iodine. However, some studies have shown that following radioactive iodine administration, iodine accumulation has been seen in metastatic lesions, thus raising the possibility of potential benefit of such therapy. Hurthle-cell carcinoma also has variable ability to synthesize thyroglobulin and may not respond well to TSH suppression therapy. In one study, patients with recurrent or persistent disease had thyroglobulin levels between 0.1 and 234,000 ng/mL (0.1-234,000 µg/L) while taking levothyroxine therapy. However, in the same study, 5 patients with metastatic disease had thyroglobulin levels that remained undetectable throughout their follow-up.

The National Comprehensive Cancer Network recommends that radioactive iodine be considered for tumors larger than 2 cm and that it be routinely administered for tumors larger than 4 cm. For tumor sizes less than 2 cm, radioactive iodine is not typically recommended. Additional considerations in this patient that may favor use of radioactive iodine are his elevated thyroglobulin and liver lesions. The National Comprehensive Cancer Network recommends that radioactive iodine be given if postoperative unstimulated thyroglobulin concentrations are greater than 5 to 10 ng/mL (>5-10 µg/L). This patient certainly falls within this category. The American Thyroid Association recommends the same treatment considerations for Hurthle-cell carcinomas as for other follicular thyroid carcinomas.

A recent analysis of the National Cancer Database was performed to examine the treatment administered to patients with Hurthle-cell carcinoma and their subsequent overall survival. Approximately 40% of patients with Hurthle-cell carcinoma did not receive radioactive iodine treatment. Patients were more likely to be treated with radioactive iodine if they were younger, had private medical insurance, and were seen at an academic medical center. Receipt of radioactive iodine was associated with improved 5- and 10-year survival rates. The studies that have examined the effect of radioactive iodine therapy on the outcomes of Hurthle-cell carcinoma have not demonstrated a decrease in recurrence rates. The answer that correctly combines these various recommendations and findings is Answer D.

EDUCATIONAL OBJECTIVE

Explain the challenge of treating Hurthle-cell carcinoma due to its diminished ability to accumulate and respond to radioactive iodine therapy.

REFERENCE(S)

Tuttle RM, Haddad RI, Ball DW, et al. Thyroid carcinoma, version 2.2014. *J Natl Compr Canc Netw.* 2014;12(12):1671-1680. PMID: 25505208

Jillard CL, Youngwirth L, Scheri RP, Roman S, Sosa JA. Radioactive iodine treatment is associated with improved survival for patients with Hürthle cell carcinoma. *Thyroid.* 2016;26(7):959-964. PMID: 27150319

8 ANSWER: E) Intravenous hydrocortisone followed by intravenous levothyroxine

This scenario describes an uncommon etiology of panhypopituitarism in which the coagulopathy caused by snake venom can cause bleeding and tissue necrosis in many different organs or glands, including the pituitary gland. The Russell viper responsible is distributed throughout Southeast Asia. The associated hypopituitarism is usually delayed and gradual in onset as described in this case, although acute-onset hypopituitarism has also been reported. In one case series of 8 such patients, duration of symptoms was 1 to 8 years, all anterior pituitary hormones were affected, and imaging showed an empty sella. This patient had become amenorrheic, but her current symptoms and presentation are due to a combination of central (secondary) adrenal insufficiency and central (secondary) hypothyroidism.

Another situation in which adrenal insufficiency and hypothyroidism may co-present is in the case of autoimmune polyglandular syndrome type 2 in which both of these conditions are primary. The manifestations of primary adrenal insufficiency can be more severe than those of secondary adrenal insufficiency due to the additional mineralocorticoid deficiency. Initiation of thyroid hormone therapy without simultaneously treating the adrenal insufficiency can precipitate an adrenal crisis. The crisis is due to both increased need for cortisol and enhanced disposal of cortisol in the euthyroid state, compared with the hypothyroid state. The same mechanism applies to central adrenal insufficiency and central hypothyroidism, although the crisis might be of somewhat lesser magnitude.

The delayed laboratory evaluation in this patient showed low free T_4, low cortisol, and low ACTH. With these results, the diagnosis is clear. However, even without these results, the clinical presentation of the patient with signs and symptoms of both adrenal insufficiency and hypothyroidism suggests the need for administration of hydrocortisone followed by administration of levothyroxine (Answer E). The intravenous route is preferred given the unstable condition of the patient. Thus, oral levothyroxine (Answer B) is incorrect. This answer is also incorrect because the adrenal insufficiency would not be treated. Intravenous levothyroxine only (Answer A) or intravenous hydrocortisone only (Answer D) is incorrect, as only 1 of 2 hormonal deficiencies would be treated. Levothyroxine alone could potentially precipitate an adrenal crisis. Methimazole (Answer C) is not indicated; although the patient does have a low TSH level, she does not have hyperthyroidism.

EDUCATIONAL OBJECTIVE

Recognize the presentation of central hypothyroidism as part of the overall presentation of hypopituitarism and explain why central adrenal insufficiency and central hypothyroidism must be treated concurrently.

REFERENCE(S)

Shivaprasad C, Aiswarya Y, Sridevi A, et al. Delayed hypopituitarism following Russell's viper envenomation: a case series and literature review. *Pituitary.* 2019;22(1):4-12. PMID: 30317419

Murray JS, Jayarajasingh R, Perros P. Lesson of the week: deterioration of symptoms after start of thyroid hormone replacement. *BMJ.* 2001; 323(7308):332-333. PMID: 11498494

9 ANSWER: A) Recommend radioactive iodine treatment at least 6 months before pregnancy with normalization of TSH on levothyroxine before conception

Preconception counseling is very important for women with Graves hyperthyroidism and should include a discussion of the risks and benefits of all treatment options and the patient's desired timeline to conception. All of the listed approaches could be appropriate in individual patients, depending on circumstances and the severity of hyperthyroidism. The safety and effectiveness of these approaches have not been directly compared in studies to date.

Methimazole use in pregnancy is associated with a syndrome of fetal anomalies, including dysmorphic facies, choanal or esophageal atresia, abdominal wall defects such as umbilical abnormalities, eye defects, urinary system defects, ventricular septal defects, and aplasia cutis. Recent studies have shown that these complications are more common than previously thought, affecting 2% to 4% of children exposed to methimazole in early pregnancy, especially during gestational weeks 6 through 10. Propylthiouracil was not previously considered teratogenic.

However, a recent Danish study demonstrated that 2% to 3% of children exposed to propylthiouracil in utero developed defects, including face cysts, neck cysts, and urinary tract abnormalities (in boys). Although propylthiouracil-associated birth defects appear to be less severe than methimazole-associated birth defects, they are not negligible. If antithyroid drugs are continued until pregnancy is diagnosed, there is still some first-trimester exposure. Infants of women who are switched from methimazole to propylthiouracil during the first trimester (Answer C) are at risk for both types of birth defects. Therefore, Answer A, which is the only approach that would not involve any antithyroid drug exposure in pregnancy, is associated with a lower risk of fetal malformations than Answers B, C, or D. Women who undergo thyroidectomy or radioactive iodine ablation before conception still may have detectable thyroid receptor–stimulating antibodies, which could pose a risk for fetal and neonatal hyperthyroidism.

A "block-and-replace" strategy (Answer E) involves using a higher dosage of an antithyroid drug to render the patient hypothyroid and then treating with levothyroxine to restore euthyroidism. This has been suggested to be a management strategy that may increase the rates of remission of Graves disease or make the Graves disease easier to control. However, this approach is generally not favored as it exposes the patient to a higher dose of the antithyroid drug and probably does not increase the likelihood of remission. In the case of an individual planning pregnancy, it does not reduce the exposure to antithyroidal drugs, so it would not reduce the risk of fetal malformations.

Another option, not mentioned here, might be offered if the patient's hyperthyroidism can ultimately be controlled on a low dosage of methimazole before pregnancy. Such patients may potentially be able to discontinue methimazole before conception and not require methimazole during pregnancy.

EDUCATIONAL OBJECTIVE

Counsel women about the teratogenic risks of antithyroid drugs in the first trimester.

REFERENCE(S)

Andersen SL, Olsen J, Wu CS, Laurberg P. Birth defects after early pregnancy use of antithyroid drugs: a Danish nationwide study. *J Clin Endocrinol Metab.* 2013;98(11):4373-4381. PMID: 24151287

Andersen SL, Olsen J, Laurberg P. Antithyroid drug side effects in the population and in pregnancy. *J Clin Endocrinol Metab.* 2016;101(4):1606-1614. PMID: 26815881

Alexander EK, Pearce EN, et al. 2017 guidelines of the American Thyroid Association for the diagnosis and management of thyroid disease during pregnancy and the postpartum. *Thyroid.* 2017;27(3): 315-389. PMID: 28056690

10 ANSWER: B) Lenvatinib

This patient has rapidly progressive metastatic differentiated thyroid cancer that is becoming increasingly symptomatic. He is not a good candidate for additional radioactive iodine treatment because the absence of uptake on his posttreatment scans indicates that his disease is ^{131}I refractory. Although doxorubicin is approved by the US FDA to be used for treatment of metastatic thyroid cancer, such cytotoxic chemotherapy (Answer A) is generally of limited utility in differentiated thyroid cancer. Given that his disease is refractory to radioactive iodine, diffuse, progressive, and symptomatic (which would be expected to produce morbidity or mortality within 6 months), he is a candidate for tyrosine kinase inhibitor therapy. This treatment has been shown in several trials to improve progression-free survival. Although several other tyrosine kinase inhibitors are currently being studied in differentiated thyroid cancer (*see table*), only 2—lenvatinib (Answer B) and sorafenib—are currently FDA approved for the treatment of differentiated thyroid cancer in patients with extensive local disease or distant metastases. Palbociclib (Answer D) is a cyclin-dependent kinase inhibitor used for metastatic breast cancer; it has not been studied in thyroid cancers. Ipilimumab (Answer C) is a monoclonal antibody that blocks the cytotoxic T-cell receptor 4 (CTLA-4) on activated T cells. It is used for the treatment of metastatic melanoma, but it has not been studied in differentiated thyroid cancer. Vandetinib (Answer E) is approved for the treatment of metastatic medullary thyroid cancer and thus would not be the best agent to use in this patient.

Table. Tyrosine Kinase Inhibitors Currently Approved for Use in Advanced Thyroid Cancer

Tyrosine kinase inhibitor	Type of thyroid cancer	Effectiveness: progression-free survival compared with placebo*
Vandetanib	Medullary	30.5 vs 19.3 months
Cabozantinib	Medullary	11.2 vs 4 months
Sorafenib	Differentiated	10.8 vs 5.8 months
Lenvatinib	Differentiated	18.3 vs 3.6 months
Dabrafenib and trametinib	Anaplastic	Open-label trial with 69% overall response rate**

*Enrolled populations were different; efficacy cannot be compared directly across studies.

**Phase II open label trial.

Many other multikinase inhibitors are currently being investigated for use in advanced thyroid cancer.

EDUCATIONAL OBJECTIVE

Recommend treatment options in radioactive iodine–refractory metastatic differentiated thyroid cancer.

REFERENCE(S)

Haugen BR, Alexander EK, Bible KC, et al. 2015 American Thyroid Association management guidelines for adult patients with thyroid nodules and differentiated thyroid cancer: the American Thyroid Association guidelines task force on thyroid nodules and differentiated thyroid cancer. *Thyroid.* 2016;26(1):1-133. PMID: 26462967

Berdelou A, Lamartina L, Klain M, Leboulleux S, Schlumberger M; TUTHTYREF Network. Treatment of refractory thyroid cancer. *Endocr Relat Cancer.* 2018;25(4):R209-R223. PMID: 29371330

11 ANSWER: E) Start dexamethasone, start SSKI, and optimize β-adrenergic blockade before surgery

This patient has experienced hepatotoxicity while taking methimazole. Although hepatic dysfunction on methimazole is frequently described as cholestatic in nature, a hepatocellular destructive pattern manifested by transaminitis may also occur. In 1 series of methimazole-induced hepatic dysfunction, 11 of 30 cases involved noncholestatic hepatocellular injury. In this particular case, the patient's regimen cannot be switched to the alternative antithyroid drug, propylthiouracil, because of her marked hepatic transaminase elevation. Her refusal to consider radioiodine leaves only thyroidectomy. Because she has moderate thyrotoxicosis, she will require preoperative preparation for thyroidectomy to reduce the risk of perioperative morbidity. Dexamethasone is a potent inhibitor of T_4-to-T_3 conversion. Supersaturated potassium iodide (SSKI) acutely inhibits thyroid hormone synthesis and release. Thus, Answer E summarizes the best approach now. At some centers, cholestyramine, which interferes with the enterohepatic circulation of thyroid hormone, is added in this setting as well.

The remaining options are not as attractive. Resuming methimazole at a lower dosage (Answer A) or starting propylthiouracil (Answer B) would expose the patient to continued hepatotoxicity. Patients treated with SSKI experience an escape from the acute inhibition of thyroid hormone synthesis (ie, they escape from the Wolff-Chaikoff effect), frequently after 10 to 14 days of therapy, so a prolonged course (Answer C) is not acceptable. Therapy with a β-adrenergic blocker (Answer D) as a single agent will not sufficiently contribute to attempts to lower the thyroid hormone level and is insufficient to prevent perioperative morbidity.

EDUCATIONAL OBJECTIVE

Devise a preoperative approach to a patient with thyrotoxicosis who cannot take antithyroid drugs because of hepatotoxicity.

REFERENCE(S)

Langley RW, Burch HB. Perioperative management of the thyrotoxic patient. *Endocrinol Metab Clin North Am.* 2003;32(2):519-534. PMID: 12800544

Ross DS, Burch HB, Cooper DS, et al. 2016 American Thyroid Association guidelines for diagnosis and management of hyperthyroidism and other causes of thyrotoxicosis. *Thyroid.* 2016;26(10):1343-1421. PMID: 27521067

12 ANSWER: E) Nephrotic syndrome

Nephrotic syndrome (Answer E) is the cause of this patient's progressive increase in levothyroxine dosage requirement, due largely to loss of thyroid-binding proteins (with thyroid hormone still bound to them) in the urine. Clues to this etiology include her lower-extremity edema, low albumin, and high lipid levels. This case and similar cases have been reported in the literature. In the setting of reversible nephrotic syndrome, levothyroxine dosage requirements return to baseline as the proteinuria resolves. Other sources of unexpected changes in levothyroxine dosage requirements include starting new medications that interfere either with absorption (iron, calcium, and binding resins) or with clearance (phenytoin, phenobarbital, and possibly sertraline) of thyroid hormone, significant weight gain or weight loss, and, of course, nonadherence to therapy.

Metformin therapy (Answer A) is associated with a slight decrease in serum TSH concentrations in levothyroxine-treated patients. It does not increase the levothyroxine dosage requirement. Although medication nonadherence (Answer B) and celiac disease (Answer C) could both increase the levothyroxine dosage requirement, they would not explain the clinical stigmata of nephrotic syndrome in the vignette. The patient is not acutely ill, so euthyroid sick syndrome (Answer D) is not pertinent, and even if it were, this syndrome does not result in an increased thyroid hormone dosage requirement.

EDUCATIONAL OBJECTIVE

Explain the effect of thyroid-binding protein loss in urine on the thyroid hormone dosage requirement.

REFERENCE(S)

Karethimmaiah H, Sarathi V. Nephrotic syndrome increases the need for levothyroxine replacement in patients with hypothyroidism. *J Clin Diagn Res.* 2016;10(12):OC10-OC12. PMID: 28208903

Halma C. Thyroid function in patients with proteinuria. *Neth J Med.* 2009;67(4):153. PMID: 19581660

Lupoli R, Di Minno A, Tortora A, Ambrosino P, Lupoli GA, Di Minno MN. Effects of treatment with metformin on TSH levels: a meta-analysis of literature studies. *J Clin Endocrinol Metab.* 2014;99(1):E143-E148. PMID: 24203069

13 ANSWER: C) Increase levothyroxine by 30%

Most thyroid hormone–treated women need to increase their levothyroxine dosage during pregnancy to maintain normal serum TSH values. The absolute increase required depends in part on the underlying etiology of the hypothyroidism, as well as on the preconception serum TSH level. A randomized controlled trial has demonstrated that euthyroid women receiving once-daily dosing of levothyroxine (regardless of the dose) who took 9 tablets per week instead of 7 tablets per week (a 29% increase) starting early in gestation were able to maintain euthyroidism in the first trimester. Current recommendations are to increase thyroid hormone doses empirically by 25% to 30% as soon as pregnancy is confirmed, with close follow-up of serum TSH levels through midgestation.

The remaining answer options either fail to recognize the rapid increase in thyroid hormone requirements in most women during early pregnancy (Answers A and B) or overreact by recommending a potentially excessive increase in the levothyroxine dosage (Answers D and E).

Another approach not mentioned here is an "ongoing adjustment approach" in which TSH is measured every 2 weeks during the first and second trimesters and the levothyroxine dosage is adjusted accordingly. This approach results in fewer low TSH values than the "empiric approach."

EDUCATIONAL OBJECTIVE

Recommend that hypothyroid women who become pregnant promptly increase their levothyroxine dosage by approximately 30%.

REFERENCE(S)

Yassa L, Marqusee E, Fawcett R, Alexander EK. Thyroid hormone early adjustment in pregnancy (the THERAPY) trial. *J Clin Endocrinol Metab.* 2010;95(7):3234-3241.

Alexander EK, Marqusee E, Lawrence J, Jarolim P, Fischer GA, Larsen PR. Timing and magnitude of increases in levothyroxine requirements during pregnancy in women with hypothyroidism. *N Engl J Med.* 2004;351(3):241-249. PMID: 15254282

Sullivan SD, Downs E, Popoveniuc G, Zeymo A, Jonklaas J, Burman KD. Randomized trial comparing two algorithms for levothyroxine dose adjustment in pregnant women with primary hypothyroidism. *J Clin Endocrinol Metab.* 2017;102(9): 3499-3507. PMID: 28911144

Alexander EK, Pearce EN, Brent GA, et al. 2017 guidelines of the American Thyroid Association for the diagnosis and management of thyroid disease during pregnancy and the postpartum. *Thyroid.* 2017;27(3):315-389. PMID: 28056690

14 ANSWER: D) Repeat complete blood cell count with differential

This patient has most likely developed agranulocytosis due to antithyroid drug therapy, which would be confirmed by repeating the complete blood cell count with differential (Answer D). His normal complete blood cell count 2 weeks earlier should not be considered reassuring because this disorder can develop rapidly and unpredictably. A recent large review of agranulocytosis cases in Japan showed that more than half of agranulocytosis cases occur within 2 weeks of a previously normal granulocyte count. Therefore, patients receiving antithyroid drugs should be reminded at each clinical interaction of the need to seek medical attention immediately for fever or sore throat, for the explicit purpose of excluding this rare complication, which affects approximately 1 in 200 patients treated.

After a diagnosis of antithyroid drug–related agranulocytosis, patients should not receive any form of thionamide therapy again (thus, Answers A and B are incorrect). A throat culture (Answer C), even if positive, does not prove agranulocytosis. There is no clinical evidence of thyroid storm (Answer E) in this patient.

Thionamide antithyroid drugs are associated with other important minor and major adverse effects. The most common minor adverse effect is a pruritic rash that affects 3% to 5% of treated patients. This may require antihistamines or switching to the alternative antithyroid drug. Major adverse effects include hepatotoxicity, antineutrophil cytoplasmic antibodies (ANCA)–positive vasculitis (more common with propylthiouracil), and agranulocytosis, as illustrated in this vignette.

EDUCATIONAL OBJECTIVE

Diagnose agranulocytosis and review appropriate management.

REFERENCE(S)

Nakamura H, Miyauchi A, Miyawaki N, Imagawa J. Analysis of 754 cases of antithyroid drug-induced agranulocytosis over 30 years in Japan. *J Clin Endocrinol Metab.* 2013;98(12):4776-4783. PMID: 24057289

Ross DS, Burch HB, Cooper DS, et al. 2016 American Thyroid Association guidelines for diagnosis and management of hyperthyroidism and other causes of thyrotoxicosis. *Thyroid.* 2016;26(10):1343-1421. PMID: 27521067

15 ANSWER: E) Heterophilic antibody interference with the TSH assay

This pattern of laboratory test results is typical of heterophilic antibody interference with the TSH assay (Answer E). The interference occurs in patients possessing antibodies that recognize the mouse monoclonal antibody used in the sandwich assay for TSH, creating a link between the capture and signal antibodies in the absence of antigen (in this case, TSH). The human antimouse monoclonal antibodies (HAMA) may occur naturally in up to 10% of the general population (not just laboratory workers with mouse exposure, as was first described), and they result in a false elevation of serum TSH. Preincubation of the patient's serum with nonimmune mouse antibodies is an added step in the assay intended to eliminate the effect of HAMA. A clue to the presence of HAMA in this case is the unchanged serum TSH despite progressively increasing free T_4 values as the levothyroxine dosage was increased. If the patient were absorbing levothyroxine poorly (Answer A) or were poorly adherent to therapy (Answer D), free T_4 values would not increase with an increasing levothyroxine dosage. If this patient had resistance to thyroid hormone (Answer B), the free T_4 level would have been elevated, rather than normal, at baseline. In the setting of a TSH-secreting pituitary adenoma (Answer C), the patient would be expected to be clinically hyperthyroid.

EDUCATIONAL OBJECTIVE

Identify heterophilic antibody interference with the thyrotropin assay.

REFERENCE(S)

SanthanaKrishnan SG, Pathalapati R, Kaplan L, Cobbs RK. Falsely raised TSH levels due to human anti-mouse antibody interfering with thyrotropin assay [published correction appears in *Postgrad Med J.* 2007;83(977):186]. *Postgrad Med J.* 2006;82(973):e27. PMID: 17099084

Ross HA, Menheere PP; Endocrinology Section of SKML (Dutch Foundation for Quality Assessment in Clinical Laboratories), Thomas CM, Mudde AH, Kouwenberg M, Wolffenbuttel BH. Interference from heterophilic antibodies in seven current TSH assays. *Ann Clin Biochem.* 2008;45(Pt 6):616. PMID: 18782812

16 ANSWER: A) Type 3 deiodinase

Type 3 deiodinase (DIO3) (Answer A) is an inactivating enzyme located in the placenta, brain, skin, and fetal liver. This enzyme inactivates T_4 to reverse T_3 and to 3,3'-T_2 and most likely has a major role in modulating the thyroid hormone status of the early fetus. The considerably elevated reverse T_3 levels in this patient point to high levels of type 3 deiodinase. In contrast to the type 3 deiodinase, both type 1 and type 2 deiodinases (DIO1 and DIO2) are activating enzymes, converting T_4 to T_3. Ectopic or paraneoplastic expression of DIO3 has been described in hepatocellular carcinoma and recently in patients with hepatic hemangioblastomas. Patients with paraneoplastic synthesis of this enzyme require very large amounts of exogenous T_4 and T_3 to keep up with the enhanced deactivation occurring through tumor expression of DIO3. This process has been referred to as "consumptive hypothyroidism."

Ectopic production of the sodium-iodine transporter (Answer C), the protein responsible for iodine transport, would not be expected to result in consumptive hypothyroidism. Tumor production of monocarboxylase transporter 8 (Answer B), the transmembrane protein responsible for intracellular transport of thyroid hormone, could in theory decrease circulating thyroid hormone levels, but this has not been described. Thyroid peroxidase (Answer D) in thyroid follicular cells catalyzes the oxidation of iodide and is required for thyroid hormone organification. Defects in the gene encoding thyroid peroxidase are a common cause of congenital hypothyroidism, but they would not explain this patient's presentation and thyroid peroxidase production from tumor cells has not been reported. Pendrin (Answer E) is a multifunctional anion exchanger that is believed to mediate iodine efflux from the apical membrane of thyroid follicular cells. Tumor production of pendrin has not been described.

EDUCATIONAL OBJECTIVE

Explain the consequences of overexpression of the type 3 deiodinase.

REFERENCE(S)

Huang SA, Tu HM, Harney JW, et al. Severe hypothyroidism caused by type 3 iodothyronine deiodinase in infantile hemangiomas. *N Engl J Med.* 2000;343(3):185-189. PMID: 10900278

Huang SA, Dorfman DM, Genest DR, Salvatore D, Larsen PR. Type 3 iodothyronine deiodinase is highly expressed in the human uteroplacental unit and in fetal epithelium. *J Clin Endocrinol Metab.* 2003;88(3):1384-1388. PMID: 1269133

Huang SA, Fish SA, Dorfman DM, et al. 21-year-old woman with consumptive hypothyroidism due to a vascular tumor expressing type 3 iodothyronine deiodinase. *J Clin Endocrinol Metab.* 2002;87(10): 4457-4461. PMID: 12364418

17 ANSWER: D) Repeat laboratory tests in 3 months

This patient has subclinical hyperthyroidism, most likely due to TSH receptor–stimulating antibodies. Her family history of autoimmune thyroid disease, her diffuse goiter, and the mildly positive thyroid-stimulating immunoglobulin are all consistent with this etiology. Patients with mild degrees of subclinical hyperthyroidism, particularly when it is due to thyroiditis or mild Graves disease, very often experience spontaneous resolution. Thus, the best course of action for this patient would be to repeat laboratory tests in 3 months (Answer D). Predictors of reversibility include having detectable (albeit subnormal) TSH values and having etiologies other than nodular hyperthyroidism (toxic adenoma or toxic multinodular goiter), such as thyroiditis or mild Graves disease, as is illustrated by the current case. Among patients with subclinical hyperthyroidism, the rate of progression to overt hyperthyroidism is 0.5% to 7% annually. Up to half of patients may spontaneously revert to normal TSH levels over time.

It is premature to start methimazole (Answer A) in this young patient who has a high likelihood of remission, but this could be considered in an elderly patient with similar findings because of the increased risk of arrhythmia or the concern about adverse effects on bone density, although the dosage of 20 mg daily would be excessive for this situation. This patient does not require atenolol (Answer B) because she is asymptomatic and has a resting pulse rate less than 90 beats/min. Although treatment with radioiodine therapy (Answer C) could be considered, it would most likely result in permanent hypothyroidism, and she may not require therapy at all with further observation. Most individuals in the United States do not necessarily require vitamin or iodine supplementation (Answer E) to achieve iodine sufficiency, although many may choose to take a multivitamin. However, this would not be a specific part of the management of her subclinical hyperthyroidism.

EDUCATIONAL OBJECTIVE

Describe the natural history of nonnodular causes of subclinical hyperthyroidism.

REFERENCE(S)

Mai VQ, Burch HB. A stepwise approach to the evaluation and treatment of subclinical hyperthyroidism. *Endocr Pract.* 2012;18(5):772-780. PMID: 22784850

Ross DS, Burch HB, Cooper DS, et al. 2016 American Thyroid Association guidelines for diagnosis and management of hyperthyroidism and other causes of thyrotoxicosis. *Thyroid.* 2016;26(10):1343-1421. PMID: 27521067

18 ANSWER: A) 70%-90%

The American Thyroid Association guidelines for the treatment of thyroid cancer have defined several risk categories for the likelihood of thyroid cancer associated with patterns observed on thyroid ultrasonography. Several other organizations have proposed risk stratification systems for classifying thyroid nodules on the basis of their sonographic appearance. These systems have good predictive value (thus, Answer E is incorrect). The image shows a nodule with a high risk of malignancy (70%-90% [Answer A]). It has classic features associated with papillary thyroid cancer, including hypoechogenicity, irregular margins, and scattered microcalcifications (*arrow*). Nodules with a very low risk for malignancy (Answer D) include spongiform nodules with clearly defined margins. Intermediate suspicion patterns associated with a 10% to 20% risk of malignancy (Answer C) include hypoechoic nodules with smooth margins but without microcalcifications, extrathyroidal extension, or a taller-than-wide shape. There is currently no American Thyroid Association–defined ultrasonography pattern associated with a 20% to 40% malignancy risk (Answer B).

EDUCATIONAL OBJECTIVE

Identify ultrasonographic features consistent with high risk for papillary thyroid carcinoma.

REFERENCE(S)

Haugen BR, Alexander EK, Bible KC, et al. 2015 American Thyroid Association management guidelines for adult patients with thyroid nodules and differentiated thyroid cancer: the American Thyroid Association Guidelines Task Force on Thyroid Nodules and Differentiated Thyroid Cancer. *Thyroid.* 2016;26(1):1-133. PMID: 26462967

Brito JP, Gionfriddo MR, Al Nofal A, et al. The accuracy of thyroid nodule ultrasound to predict thyroid cancer: systematic review and meta-analysis. *J Clin Endocrinol Metab.* 2014;99(4):1253-1263. PMID: 24276450

19 ANSWER: D) FNA biopsy again and measurement of thyroglobulin in aspirate

Measuring thyroglobulin in the fluid obtained from FNA biopsy aspirates of lymph nodes (Answer D) is referred to as thyroglobulin "washout" because the specimen is obtained by rinsing the hub of the needle used for lymph node FNA biopsy with 1 cc of normal saline. FNA biopsy alone, without thyroglobulin washout, may fail to diagnose thyroid cancer in up to 20% of cases. The utility of this technique in cases such as the one described is now well established. The higher the aspirate thyroglobulin level, the more accurate the result. Washout thyroglobulin concentrations greater than 10 ng/mL (>10 μg/L) are both sensitive and 90% specific for tumor metastatic to the sampled lymph node. Because of the risk of nonspecific PET uptake in reactive lymph nodes, "positive" PET images must generally be confirmed with tissue sampling before referring the patient for reoperation (Answer A). PET-CT uptake within the suspicious lymph node has already been demonstrated in this patient, so repeating PET-CT with recombinant human TSH stimulation (Answer B) is not required. MRI of the neck (Answer C) would not add to this case. Not treating this patient with strongly suspected persistent disease (Answer E) is inappropriate. After identifying metastatic disease to lymph nodes, the next step is generally to refer for surgical removal to include compartmental dissection in previously nonoperated compartments, as cervical lymph nodes are often relatively radioiodine resistant.

EDUCATIONAL OBJECTIVE

Appreciate that thyroglobulin "washout" may detect thyroid cancer, even if results on FNA biopsy are negative.

REFERENCE(S)

Urken ML, Milas M, Randolph GW, et al. Management of recurrent and persistent metastatic lymph nodes in well-differentiated thyroid cancer: a multifactorial decision-making guide for the thyroid cancer care collaborative. *Head Neck.* 2015;37(4):605-614. PMID: 24436291

Haugen BR, Alexander EK, Bible KC, et al. 2015 American Thyroid Association management guidelines for adult patients with thyroid nodules and differentiated thyroid cancer: the American Thyroid Association Guidelines Task Force on Thyroid Nodules and Differentiated Thyroid Cancer. *Thyroid.* 2016;26(1):1-133. PMID: 26462967

20 ANSWER: A) External beam radiation therapy to the thyroid bed

The tall cell variant of papillary thyroid cancer is associated with an aggressive presentation and may often not be iodine avid. This patient has persistent, nonresectable thyroid cancer involving the trachea and recurrent laryngeal nerve, and the tumor does indeed appear not to be radioiodine avid. These findings are an indication for external beam radiation therapy (Answer A). Tyrosine kinase inhibitor therapy (Answer B) may be used in these patients. However, the benefit of tyrosine kinase inhibitor therapy appears to be transient, whereas external beam radiation therapy is potentially tumoricidal. Repeated radioiodine therapy (Answer C) will not be helpful in this patient with non–radioiodine-avid disease. Conventional chemotherapy (Answer D) is of limited, if any, benefit in the treatment of thyroid cancer. Not treating this patient (Answer E) is inappropriate because he has known persistent, locally invasive disease.

EDUCATIONAL OBJECTIVE

Recommend external beam radiation therapy in a patient with persistent, nonresectable, non–radioiodine-avid thyroid cancer.

REFERENCE(S)

Haugen BR, Alexander EK, Bible KC, et al. 2015 American Thyroid Association management guidelines for adult patients with thyroid nodules and differentiated thyroid cancer: the American Thyroid Association Guidelines Task Force on Thyroid Nodules and Differentiated Thyroid Cancer. *Thyroid.* 2016;26(1):1-133. PMID: 26462967

Powell C, Newbold K, Harrington KJ, Bhide SA, Nutting CM. External beam radiotherapy for differentiated thyroid cancer. *Clin Oncol (R Coll Radiol).* 2010;22(6):456-463. PMID: 20427166

21 ANSWER: C) Plasmapheresis

This patient has developed thyroid storm after discontinuing methimazole. The diagnosis of thyroid storm can be made empirically with additional guidance from the use of diagnostic scoring systems. Both the Burch-Wartofsky point score (75 points) and the Japan Thyroid Association system ("Thyroid storm-1, Combination-2") would categorize this patient as having thyroid storm. Emergent thyroidectomy has been used in similar patients when other conventional medical therapies fail.

Because antithyroid drugs cannot be started in this patient, other means must be used to prepare him for thyroidectomy. Plasmapheresis (Answer C), as well as plasma exchange and charcoal perfusion, has been used successfully in this setting in the immediate preoperative period since it removes plasma-containing proteins such as immunoglobulins and thyroxine-binding globulin, along with its bound thyroid hormones. Hemodialysis (Answer A) does not remove the majority of thyroid hormone because it is bound to binding proteins. Changing from intravenous propranolol to intravenous esmolol would make sense because of the ability to rapidly titrate the latter. However, changing to atenolol (Answer B), which is even less titratable than propranolol and does not provide propranolol's beneficial effect on blocking conversion of T_4 to T_3, would be incorrect. Intravenous immunoglobulin therapy (Answer D) has not been used effectively in the treatment of thyroid storm. Cholestyramine (Answer E) can be used to treat hyperthyroidism and it acts by blocking the recirculation of thyroid hormones. However, its action is not likely to be of sufficient magnitude or speed to be helpful in this urgent situation.

EDUCATIONAL OBJECTIVE

Manage life-threatening thyrotoxicosis and use plasmapheresis in patients unable to take antithyroid drugs.

REFERENCE(S)

Warnock AL, Cooper DS, Burch HB. Life-threatening thyrotoxicosis: thyroid storm and adverse effects of antithyroid drugs. In: Mattfin G, ed. *Endocrine Medical Emergencies.* Endocrine Press: 2014.

Ross DS, Burch HB, Cooper DS, et al. 2016 American Thyroid Association guidelines for diagnosis and management of hyperthyroidism and other causes of thyrotoxicosis. *Thyroid.* 2016;26(10):1343-1421. PMID: 27521067

Akamizu T, Satch T, Isozaki O, et al; Japan Thyroid Association. Diagnostic criteria, clinical features, and incidence of thyroid storm based on nation-wide surveys. *Thyroid.* 2012;22(7):661-679. PMID: 22690898

Vyas AA, Vyas P, Fillipon NL, Vijayakrishnan R, Trivedi N. Successful treatment of thyroid storm with plasmapheresis in a patient with methimazole-induced agranulocytosis. *Endocr Pract.* 2010;16(4):673-676. PMID: 20439250

Carhill A, Gutierrez A, Lakhia R, Nalini R. Surviving the storm: two cases of thyroid storm successfully treated with plasmapheresis. *BMJ Case Rep.* 2012:bcr2012006696. PMID: 23087271

22 ANSWER: D) Surgical resection of the cystic mass

This patient has a thyroglossal duct cyst present in the midline superior to the thyroid gland (denoted by arrows on the CT images). The thyroglossal duct is the tract that the developing thyroid follows in its embryologic descent from the base of the tongue to its final anatomic position in the neck. When the tract persists, it is prone to cyst formation along its length. This patient's thyroglossal duct cyst is unlikely to completely resolve spontaneously at this stage. According to the literature, these lesions are prone to bacterial infection at a lifetime rate of approximately 50% if left untreated. Therefore, recommending no treatment now (Answer A) is not the ideal approach. The best means of definitively managing thyroglossal duct cysts is generally surgical resection together with removal of the central portion of the hyoid bone (this surgery is known as the Sistrunk procedure) (Answer D).

The incidence of thyroid cancer within a thyroglossal duct cyst is only 1%. There would be no indication to perform a total thyroidectomy as well as a Sistrunk procedure (Answer B) unless independent evidence suggested a malignancy within the thyroid gland itself. Thyroglossal duct cysts do not respond to thyroid hormone suppressive therapy (Answer E) or radioiodine therapy (Answer C).

EDUCATIONAL OBJECTIVE

Choose a management approach for a thyroglossal duct cyst based on the risk for cancer and infection.

REFERENCE(S)

Rayess HM, Monk I, Svider PF, Gupta A, Raza SN, Lin HS. Thyroglossal duct cyst carcinoma: a systematic review of clinical features and outcomes. *Otolaryngol Head Neck Surg.* 2017;156(5): 794-802. PMID: 28322121

Gioacchini FM, Alicandri-Ciufelli M, Kaleci S, Magliulo G, Presutti L, Re M. Clinical presentation and treatment outcomes of thyroglossal duct cysts: a systematic review. *Int J Oral Maxillofac Surg.* 2015;44(1):119-126. PMID: 25132570

23 ANSWER: D) Elevation of the head of the bed

Several scales are available to assess both the severity and activity of Graves eye disease. The Clinical Activity Score can be calculated with 1 point for the presence of each of the following features at initial evaluation: pain in primary gaze, pain with eye movement, chemosis, eyelid swelling, eyelid erythema, conjunctival redness, and caruncula swelling. A score greater than 3 is indicative of active disease; this patient has a Clinical Activity Score of 5. However, his disease severity is currently mild; symptoms consist only of mild soft-tissue involvement, tearing, and discomfort, without vision changes, corneal damage, or proptosis. He does not have signs or symptoms suggestive of sight-threatening disease. Therefore, orbital decompression surgery (Answer A) is incorrect. Corticosteroids (Answer E) are the mainstay of management of moderate to severe eye disease, but he does not have symptoms sufficient to warrant the institution of methylprednisolone therapy. There are conflicting recent clinical trial data regarding the efficacy of rituximab (Answer C) in patients with moderate to severe disease, but it is certainly not appropriate in this patient with only mild symptoms. Botulinum toxin injections of the extraocular muscles (Answer B) have been used to correct diplopia, but this patient does not currently have extraocular muscle dysfunction. Elevation of the head of the bed (Answer D) is the only option provided that could reasonably be considered for his mild, active eye disease. Other appropriate interventions for patients with active but mild disease include smoking cessation, use of artificial tears and sunglasses, and use of prisms to correct double vision. In addition, a single randomized clinical trial in patients with mild Graves orbitopathy suggested that treatment with 100 mcg of selenium twice daily may improve symptoms. Recently, a new drug, teprotumumab, has been approved for the treatment of active thyroid eye disease. However, it would be premature to consider such therapy without first assessing this patient's response to conservative measures.

EDUCATIONAL OBJECTIVE

Gauge activity and severity of Graves eye disease and recommend appropriate treatment for mild disease.

REFERENCE(S)

Bartalena L, Baldeschi L, Dickinson AJ, et al. Consensus statement of the European group on Graves' orbitopathy (EUGOGO) on management of Graves' orbitopathy. *Thyroid.* 2008;18(3): 333-346. PMID: 18341379

Marcocci C, Kahaly GJ, Krassas GE, et al; European Group on Graves' Orbitopathy. Selenium and the course of mild Graves' orbitopathy. *N Engl J Med.* 2011;364(20):1920-1931. PMID: 21591944

Fatourechi V. Medical management of extrathyroidal manifestations of Graves disease. *Endocr Pract.* 2014;20(12):1333-1344. PMID: 25370325

Douglass RS, Kahaly GJ, Patel A, et al. Teprotumumab for the treatment of active thyroid eye disease. *N Engl J Med.* 2020;382(4): 341-352. PMID: 31971679

24 ANSWER: A) Medullary thyroid cancer

The photograph shows cutaneous lichen amyloidosis, an autosomal dominant condition that has been strongly associated with multiple endocrine neoplasia type 2A, particularly in families harboring a pathogenic variant in codon 634 of the *RET* proto-oncogene, with a prevalence in some families as high as 36%. Cutaneous lichen amyloidosis typically occurs in the location shown (between the spine and the scapula) and is pruritic. It may occur in either or both interscapular areas. This lesion may precede the diagnosis of multiple endocrine neoplasia type 2A by many years. For example, in one study cutaneous lichen amyloidosis was diagnosed at an average age of 14 years, compared with an average age at diagnosis of medullary thyroid cancer of 31 years. The current theory regarding the pathogenesis of this lesion is that it is due to patient scratching to relieve a neurally mediated pruritus. Of the listed choices, only medullary thyroid cancer (Answer A) is associated with cutaneous lichen amyloidosis.

EDUCATIONAL OBJECTIVE

Identify cutaneous lichen amyloidosis and its association with multiple endocrine neoplasia type 2.

REFERENCE(S)

Verga U, Fugazzola L, Cambiaghi S, et al. Frequent association between MEN 2A and cutaneous lichen amyloidosis. *Clin Endocrinol (Oxf).* 2003;59(2):156-161. PMID: 12864791

Scapineli JO, Ceolin L, Punales MK, Dora JM, Maia AL. MEN 2A-related cutaneous lichen amyloidosis: report of three kindred and systematic literature review of clinical, biochemical and molecular characteristics. *Fam Cancer.* 2016;15(4):625-633. PMID: 26920351

25 ANSWER: D) Stop breastfeeding 3 months before the radioactive iodine treatment

The lactating breast expresses the sodium-iodide transporter, and iodine is actively concentrated in breast milk. Breastfeeding should ideally be stopped at least 3 months before radioactive iodine treatment (thus, Answer D is correct and Answer C is incorrect), both to avoid transmission of radioactive iodine to the breastfed infant and to avoid excessive radiation exposure to breast tissue. The half-life of ^{123}I is about 13 hours, so it is acceptable to pump and discard breast milk and then resume breastfeeding after diagnostic ^{123}I scanning. However, breastfeeding is contraindicated after any scanning or treatment with ^{131}I (thus, Answer B is incorrect). Deferring radioactive iodine treatment for a year in a patient with an aggressive tumor (Answer A) is not advisable. Dopamine agonist therapy with cabergoline has been used to lower prolactin levels, hasten the return of breast tissue to the nonlactating state, and reduce iodine uptake in breast tissue. This should shorten the time between cessation of lactation and the ability to treat with radioiodine without substantial breast exposure. Once this patient has been treated with ^{131}I, it is recommended by the Society of Nuclear Medicine and Molecular Imaging that she should not breastfeed her current infant, but that she can safely breastfeed future infants.

Amifostine (Answer E) is a potent scavenger of reactive oxygen species. It has been investigated as an agent that might protect the salivary glands from damage during therapy with radioactive iodine. It has also been investigated as a means of protecting normal breast tissue from external beam radiotherapy for breast cancer. However, it would not be expected to prevent iodine accumulation in breast tissue and, furthermore, would not be safe for a breastfeeding infant.

EDUCATIONAL OBJECTIVE

Assess safety issues related to radioactive iodine administration in lactating women.

REFERENCE(S)

Azizi F, Smyth P. Breastfeeding and maternal and infant iodine nutrition. *Clin Endocrinol (Oxf).* 2009;70(5):803-809. PMID: 19178515

Stagnaro-Green A, Abalovich M, Alexander E, et al; American Thyroid Association Taskforce on Thyroid Disease During Pregnancy and Postpartum. Guidelines of the American Thyroid Association for the diagnosis and management of thyroid disease during pregnancy and postpartum. *Thyroid.* 2011;21(10):1081-1125. PMID: 21787128

Brzozowska M, Roach PJ. Timing and potential role of diagnostic I-123 scintigraphy in assessing radioiodine breast uptake before ablation in postpartum women with thyroid cancer: a case series. *Clin Nucl Med.* 2006;31(11):683-687. PMID: 17053384

26 ANSWER: C) Repeated FNA biopsy with flow cytometry

The image shows multiple uniform-appearing lymphocytes. Features of anaplastic carcinoma, another potential cause of very rapid thyroid growth, are not seen. Thyroid lymphoma is rare, comprising 2% or less of all thyroid malignancies. The mean age at presentation is 65 to 75 years, and this occurs more frequently in women. The risk for thyroid lymphoma is 40 to 80 times higher in individuals with Hashimoto thyroiditis than in the general population. The most common presentation of thyroid lymphoma is a rapidly enlarging, painless goiter, often with compressive symptoms. The enlargement may be nodular or diffuse. Cytopathology showing uniform-appearing lymphocytes may be consistent with either Hashimoto thyroiditis or thyroid lymphoma. FNA biopsy with flow cytometry (Answer C) is typically needed to confirm a diagnosis of lymphoma. Treatment of thyroid lymphoma usually consists of chemotherapy with or without radiation. The role of thyroidectomy (Answer B) is controversial, but it has not been demonstrated to improve survival. Radioactive iodine scan (Answer A) may demonstrate a cold nodule, but it would not be helpful in diagnosing thyroid lymphoma. Gene classifier testing (Answer D) can be useful to predict the risk of differentiated thyroid cancer when an FNA biopsy result is indeterminate, but it is not useful in distinguishing between Hashimoto thyroiditis and thyroid lymphoma. Similarly, testing for pathogenic variants associated with differentiated thyroid cancer (Answer E) may aid decision-making when the FNA biopsy result is indeterminate, but it would not be helpful here where the clinical scenario is suggestive of thyroid lymphoma.

EDUCATIONAL OBJECTIVE

Identify the association between Hashimoto hypothyroidism and thyroid lymphoma and recommend initial workup.

REFERENCE(S)

Walsh S, Lowery AJ, Evoy D, McDermott EW, Prichard RS. Thyroid lymphoma: recent advances in diagnosis and optimal management strategies. *Oncologist.* 2013;18(9):994-1003. PMID: 23881987

Mancuso S, Carlisi M, Napolitano M, Siragusa S. Lymphomas and thyroid: bridging the gap. *Hematol Oncol.* 2018 [online ahead of print] PMID: 29484690

27 ANSWER: A) Refer for total thyroidectomy

In the Bethesda classification system for reporting thyroid cytopathology, nodules with indeterminate results, which include Bethesda class III (atypia of unknown significance/follicular lesion of unknown significance [AUS/FLUS]), and class IV (follicular neoplasm/suspicious for follicular neoplasm [FN/SFN]), and class V (suspicious for malignancy [SMC]), are sometimes selected for molecular testing. Testing using a small panel of pathogenic variants known to be associated with thyroid cancer is most helpful when a pathogenic variant or rearrangement is present (high positive predictive value) and is generally not helpful when a variant is absent (a low negative predictive value) because many cancers do not contain the limited set of abnormalities sought in the test. In this patient with a follicular neoplasm on FNA biopsy and a positive finding of a *PAX8/PPARG* rearrangement, there is a high enough risk of thyroid cancer (80%-90%) that total thyroidectomy (Answer A) is recommended (*see figure*).

Figure. FNA Prospective Genetic Analysis

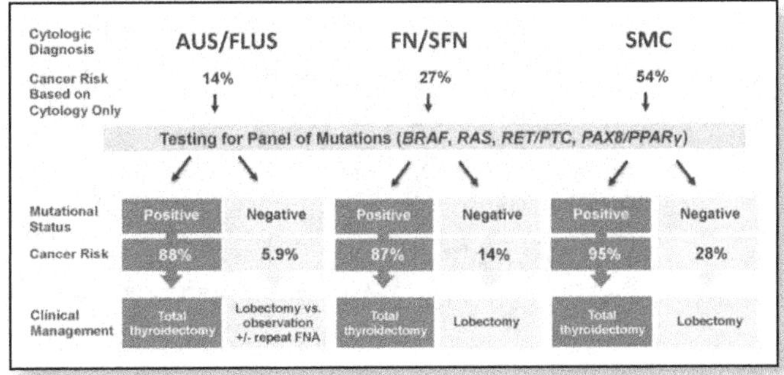

A total of 479 patients; 513 indeterminate FNAs. (247 AUS/FLUS, 214 FN/FSN, 52 suspicious). Pathogenic variants identified in 16% overall.

Reprinted from Nikiforov YE, Ohori NP, Hodak SP, et al. Impact of mutational testing on the diagnosis and management of patients with cytologically indeterminate thyroid nodules: a prospective analysis of 1056 FNA samples. *J Clin Endocrinol Metab.* 2011;96(11):3390-3397.

Another form of molecular testing—a gene expression classifier (uses a microarray of a large panel of genes associated with either benign or malignant thyroid nodules)—is currently only available from a single source. Limited data for this molecular classifier suggest that it is associated with a high negative predictive value, such that in general, if negative, no surgery would be required. No study to date has examined the tandem use of both methodologies, although the current cost of this approach could be prohibitive. A lobectomy (Answer E) is inappropriate because of the high risk of malignancy, as a completion thyroidectomy would then be required assuming pathologic examination confirms a malignant nodule. Performing thyroid ultrasonography, FNA biopsy, or molecular testing again in 6 months (Answers B, C, and D) would incorrectly avoid thyroid surgery. In addition, Answer D is also incorrect because the molecular profile is unlikely to change in 6 months.

EDUCATIONAL OBJECTIVE

Explain the role of molecular genetic testing in patients with thyroid nodules.

REFERENCE(S)

Nikiforov YE, Ohori NP, Hodak SP, et al. Impact of mutational testing on the diagnosis and management of patients with cytologically indeterminate thyroid nodules: a prospective analysis of 1056 FNA samples. *J Clin Endocrinol Metab.* 2011;96(11): 3390-3397. PMID: 21880806

Alexander EK, Kennedy GC, Baloch ZW, et al. Preoperative diagnosis of benign thyroid nodules with indeterminate cytology. *N Engl J Med.* 2012;367(8):705-715. PMID: 22731672

28 ANSWER: B) Ethanol injection of the cyst

Simple cysts are, by definition, benign, and do not require FNA biopsy to exclude malignancy. Fluid reaccumulation after aspiration occurs in 60% to 90% patients with cystic nodules. In controlled studies, percutaneous ethanol injection of a cyst (Answer B) is less likely to result in fluid reaccumulation than simple cyst aspiration (Answer A) and is now considered the first-line therapy. Up to 3 treatments may be required. Adverse effects are relatively minor but may include local pain and dysphonia. Thyroid function is not affected.

Radiofrequency ablation (Answer C) is a newer approach that is being used to manage benign thyroid nodules. Studies to date suggest that this is a promising nonsurgical option for reduction of the size of cold or hyperfunctioning solid, mixed solid-cystic nodules, or cystic nodules. Currently, ethanol ablation is generally used for volume reduction in cystic nodules as it is a less expensive option. Radiofrequency ablation is more costly and may be technically more difficult. However, in a recent study, an average of 1.7 sessions of radiofrequency ablation achieved a volume reduction of approximately 80% in cystic nodules, although none of the nodules were 100% cystic. This approach may be more commonly used in the future. Laser ablation (Answer D) can decrease the size of solid nodules by about 50%, but it does not effectively reduce cyst size. Radioactive iodine therapy (Answer E) would not be expected to affect cyst size and would most likely cause hypothyroidism. Thyroid lobectomy would be a reasonable option, but this patient prefers to avoid surgery.

EDUCATIONAL OBJECTIVE

Explain nonsurgical treatment options for benign nodules with compressive symptoms.

REFERENCE(S)

Gharib H, Hegedüs L, Pacella CM, Baek JH, Papini E. Clinical review: nonsurgical, image-guided, minimally invasive therapy for thyroid nodules. *J Clin Endocrinol Metab.* 2013;98(10):3949-3957. PMID: 23956350

Bennedbaek FN, Hegedüs L. Treatment of recurrent thyroid cysts with ethanol: a randomized double-blind controlled trial. *J Clin Endocrinol Metab.* 2003;88(12):5773-5777. PMID: 14671167

Cesareo R, Palermo A, Pasqualini V, et al. Radiofrequency ablation for the management of thyroid nodules: a critical appraisal of the literature. *Clin Endocrinol (Oxf).* 2017;87(6):639-648. PMID: 28718950

Lee GM, You JY, Kim HY, et al. Successful radiofrequency ablation strategies for benign thyroid nodules. *Endocrine.* 2019;64(2):316-321. PMID: 30569260

www.ingramcontent.com/pod-product-compliance
Lightning Source LLC
Chambersburg PA
CBHW080409190526
45161CB00003B/184

* 9 7 8 1 8 7 9 2 2 5 6 9 5 *